"Esther Gokhale's vision of what makes a healthy back will be startling to most Americans, because it is so different from what we have always learned…With the adoption of even a few of Esther's precepts, a life of bad habits can change to a life of healthy sitting and moving, and therefore a life of less pain and more freedom."

– Jessica Davidson, M.D., Internal Medicine, Palo Alto Medical Foundation, CA

"The fresh and thoughtful approach to preventing and treating back pain presented by Esther Gokhale in this book deserves the attention of the medical profession. We have not served our patients with back pain well, and the techniques so well-described in this book hold the promise of significant relief to a very common and distressing problem."

– Harvey J. Cohen, M.D., Ph.D., Professor Emeritus of Pediatrics, Stanford University School of Medicine, CA

"Esther Gokhale's unique expertise and the keen clinical acumen that fuel her work, displayed in her amazing, comprehensive and user-friendly book, will eventually be recognized by the medical community as the greatest-ever contribution to nonsurgical back treatment in this country."

– Helen Barkan, M.D., Ph.D., Neurology, Mayo Clinic, MN

"[Esther Gokhale] advocates exercises that are easily practiced during one's normal daily activities (e.g. stretches that can be done while walking, sitting in a chair, driving or while lying in bed). All of the exercises are gentle and are appropriate for patients of all ages and strengths."

– Teresa Nauenberg, M.D., Palo Alto Medical Foundation, CA

"The most lucid account I have read of how the human spine works."

– J.M. Coetzee, Nobel Prize Winner in Literature

"The patients I have referred to Esther have, without exception, found her work to be life changing."

– Salwan AbiEzzi, M.D., Palo Alto Medical Foundation

"Esther Gokhale's technique is totally unique and her research really backs it up. This is a great tool for all of us."

– Billie Jean King, Winner of 20 Wimbledon titles

"The Gokhale Method opens up a new level of health even to those of us who spend most of our week at a desk."

— **Susan Wojcicki**, Former CEO of YouTube

"The Gokhale Method turns much of conventional wisdom about pain and posture on its head. I now look forward to many years of a healthy neck and back."

— **Joan Baez**, Singer and Activist

"Esther Gokhale helped me resolve a five-year injury after nothing else had worked.

— **Patti Sue Plumer**, Olympian

"Gokhale's theory…seems almost too simple, but there is logic (and science) behind the fact that if the musculature is at rest, instead of being in a constant state of tension, discomfort can be avoided. Her book serves as a self-help manual that provides us a means to reclaim an active lifestyle without pain. Its step-by-step procedures, with excellent photos, can teach us how, once again, to stand, sit, and lie properly. It demonstrates how to allow the spine, rather than the muscles, to hold us upright. The Gokhale Method does not call for any special devices; all the reader needs is time and commitment."

— **Mary Martin**, Fitness Coordinator, NC

"Every year tens of thousands of patients undergo major back surgery without any benefits. By using the Gokhale Method's novel techniques, many of these patients can avoid such needless and expensive medical procedures, and quickly return to a pain-free life."

— **John R. Adler, M.D.**, Professor Emeritus of Neurosurgery, Stanford University Medical Clinic, CA

"I see tons of 'slouching and tucking' in my pediatric office and a surprising number of children and teens with back pain. I have been referring many of my patients to Esther and will be recommending this book routinely."

— **Tina McAdoo, M.D.**, Pediatrics, Sutter Health, CA

"The Gokhale Method is an extraordinary application of ancient wisdom to solve modern back problems. It explores intelligently the ancient wisdom accumulated in earlier times and forgotten in the modern world that can help us to improve on our number one way to happiness: health."

— **Luca Cavalli-Sforza, M.D.**, Professor Emeritus, Department of Genetics, Stanford University School of Medicine, CA

"*8 Steps to a Pain-Free Back* is a pleasure to read and a godsend to use. The lessons are easily accessible to anyone with an hour to spare. The account of why people in modern industrial society experience chronic back pain is fascinating in its own right. The photographs of people sitting, standing, and lifting in a preindustrial world are marvelously instructive and a joy to behold. While the principles of good posture are disarmingly simple, Esther Gokhale includes a wealth of pertinent detail to guide users through the eight lessons. As the pain goes away, you will not only experience relief; you will also come to understand why you feel so much better!"

— **David Riggs, Ph.D.**, Mark Pigott OBE Professor Emeritus in the School of Humanities and Sciences, Stanford University, CA

"As a scientist, I find Esther's approach to be very well thought out, based in extensive experience, integrated with the rest of one's life, and extremely effective."

— **Gretchen Daily, Ph.D.**, Professor of Biology, Stanford University, CA

"You are never too old to benefit from Esther Gokhale's artful, sound guide to better posture and freedom from pain."

— **Victor R. Fuchs, Ph.D.**, Henry J. Kaiser Jr. Professor Emeritus of Economics and of Health Research and Policy, Stanford University, CA

"Esther Gokhale's *8 Steps to a Pain-Free Back* is that rare instructional work that conveys information in a way the reader can readily understand. Among the many manuscripts I have read in the last two decades, this book stands out for its clarity of writing and selection of illustrations."

— **DeWitt Durham**, Former VP of Product Development, Klutz Press, Palo Alto, CA

"In 2005, taking up a visiting professorship at Stanford University and suffering from a bad back and extreme tension in my neck and shoulders, I was lucky enough to be recommended to Esther Gokhale's care. In a few weeks she taught me how to sit, lie, stand and walk in ways that would prevent the recurrence of that tension and pain. Now, far from Stanford, I can continue to put her method to work for me—not just through recalling that wise and clear voice but through this magnificent book and its compellingly beautiful photographs."

— **Dorothy Driver, Ph.D.**, Professor of English, Adelaide University, South Australia

"The power of pills is not absolute. You can go much further using the power of knowledge. This clearly written and richly illustrated book introduces a number of unique ideas that can help you regain your freedom of motion."

— **Andrei Linde, Ph.D.**, Professor Emeritus of Physics, Stanford University, CA

8 Steps to a Pain-Free Back.
Natural posture solutions for pain in the back, neck, shoulder, hip,
knee, and foot.

Printed and bound in China using plant-based inks on
Forest Stewardship Council™ (FSC™)-certified paper and other
controlled material in a BSCI and SEDEX-certified workplace.

MIX
Paper | Supporting
responsible forestry
FSC™ C007683

Published by Pendo Press, Fresno, California.

Publisher's Cataloging-in-Publication
(Provided by Quality Books, Inc.)

Gokhale, Esther.
        8 steps to a pain-free back : natural posture
    solutions for pain in the back, neck, shoulder, hip,
    knee, and foot / Esther Gokhale ; with Susan Adams.
        p. cm. -- (Move like you are meant to)
        Includes bibliographical references and index.
        Library of Congress Control Number: 2025900796
        ISBN: 978-0-9793036-3-0

        1. Back--Care and hygiene. 2. Backache--Treatment.
    3. Posture.   I. Adams, Susan, 1944- II. Title.
    III. Title: Eight steps to a pain-free back. IV. Series.

    RD771.B217G65 2008   617.5'64
                        QBI07-600232

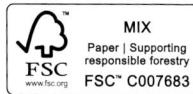

Attention: Quantity discounts are available for corporations, medical groups,
retirement homes, educational institutions, and sports organizations for
resale, teaching, subscription incentives, gifts, or fund raising. Organizations
interested in specialized books or excerpts: please contact Special Sales,
Pendo Press, 3790 El Camino Real #1033, Palo Alto, CA 94306.
Phone 1-844-777-0440.
Email: info@gokhalemethod.com.

Move Like You Are Meant To

8 STEPS to a PAIN-FREE BACK

Natural posture solutions for pain in the back, neck, shoulder, hip, knee, and foot

ESTHER GOKHALE, L.Ac.

WITH SUSAN ADAMS

PP Pendo Press

To the millions of people who suffer needlessly from back pain

ACKNOWLEDGMENTS

Many, many people helped make this book happen—friends, colleagues, teachers, subjects, patients, students, and family. In particular, I would like to thank:

My parents, Manohar Krishna Gokhale and Wilma Meijer, who gave me my first lessons in navigating multiple cultures and identifying what is positive and uplifting in them.

Noëlle Perez-Christiaens, for pioneering the field of anthropologically informed posture and movement work and for channeling the wisdom of B.K.S. Iyengar, André Delmas, and many other trailblazers in our understanding of the human body. What I learned from Noëlle and her teachers is the foundation of much of what I present in this book.

B.K.S. Iyengar (yoga), Elly Vunderink-de Vries (yoga), Kutti Krishnan (Bharata Natyam), Georgia Leconte (Aplomb®), Alain Girard (Aplomb), Angelika Thusius (Kentro), Karen Mattison (Pilates), Regine N'Dounda (Congolese dance), Wilfred Mark (Caribbean dance), Benny Duarte (Brazilian dance), Marsea Marquis (Brazilian dance), Beiçola (Capoeira, Brazilian dance), Dandha da Hora (Brazilian dance), and Massengo (Congolese drumming), for contributing to my work with techniques, understanding, or inspiration.

Susan Adams, for volunteering 18 months of invaluable help clarifying and polishing the text. Her remarkable stamina, perseverance, and linguistic skill kept the project in motion till the finish.

Gaith Kawar, for his patient instruction in InDesign at the Palo Alto Apple Store, followed by his expertise as the layout designer of the first edition. Nina Laurel, for her attention to detail in preparing the layout for the second edition.

Brett Miller, for drawing and redrawing almost all the illustrations in the book. Brett patiently and effectively rendered my unusual specifications on good and bad posture.

The late Tom Tworek, for shooting and editing all of the original instructional photographs. His good humor and reassuring manner made the photoshoots a pleasure.

Christophe Testi, who used his skill and patience to render the instructional photographs that appear in this edition.

Bryan Panesa and Erick Mangilit, for postproduction of the new instructional images.

Prudence Breitrose, for helping reedit the entire first edition and much improving it.

Tegan Kahn and Clare Chapman, who provided months of patient expertise as Gokhale Method® teachers to improve the text and images, making sure the many teaching enhancements over the last 15+ years are presented in this edition.

Cara Rosaen, for challenging me to refine my arguments in the Foundations chapter and then helping search the medical literature to enable me to do so.

George Foster, for delivering two excellent cover designs.

Janetti Marotta, for being my writing buddy during the year in which I wrote the first draft of the first edition.

Grant Barnes, Gertrude Bock, William Carter, Bridget Conrad, Laila Craveiro, Benjamin Davidson, Sheila dela Rosa, Julie Dorsey, DeWitt Durham, Elaine Gradman, Kevin Johnson, Leah McGarrigle, Susan Mellen, Michele Raffin, David Riggs, Beth Siegelman, Camille Spar, Julie Stanford, and Anne White, for valuable feedback on the content of the book.

Margo Davis, Angela Fischer/photokunst, Donald Greig, Ian Mackenzie, Randy Mont-Reynaud, Sandra Starkey-Simon, the family of Gerard Mackworth-Young, Dreamstime, iStockphoto, Unsplash, Pexels, AdobeStock, Shutterstock, and the Library of Congress for images that appear in the book.

Susan Adams, Deborah Addicott, Teresa Arnold, Suruchi Bhutani, Brian Danitz, Tushar Dave, Sheila dela Rosa, Vinod Dham, DeWitt Durham, Trish Hayes-Danitz, Miri Hutcherson, Kevin Johnson, Chloe Kamprath, Dan Leemon, Alon Maor, Michele Raffin, T.M. Ravi, Evan Roberts, Cara Rosaen, Beth Siegelman, Richard Williams, Julie Stanford, and Susan Wojcicki, for valuable advice on business matters related to the book.

Our team of Gokhale Method teachers, for contributing metaphors, additional techniques, refinements, and images to this endeavor, and for bringing the benefits of the method to people all around the world.

My team at Gokhale Method® Enterprise, including Julie Johnson, Susan van Niekerk, and Jonas Müller. Together, we are bringing the method to an increasing number of people who are happy to receive it.

The hundreds of subjects who gave me permission to interview them, photograph them, and use their pictures and stories for my work.

The hundreds of thousands of readers who purchased the first edition or borrowed it from a friend or library; your journey with back pain fuels my commitment to helping others live pain free. Your dedication to healing and improving your wellbeing is truly motivating. I hope the techniques presented in this book will guide you toward relief, help you feel better, and spread joy.

Brian White, my wonderful ex-husband, for championing my work for 40 years. Maya, Nathan, and Monisha White, who I am deeply grateful for having been able to bring into the world, and from whom I have learnt as much as I have taught.

CONTENTS

FOREWORD

Seventeen years ago, Esther Gokhale asked me if I would write a foreword to her soon-to-be-published book, *8 Steps to a Pain-Free Back*. I was introduced to Esther and her method at a lunchtime educational seminar at the Palo Alto Medical Clinic in the 1990s. I was riveted by the images on the screen and the words of the speaker. Esther's personal experience of debilitating lower back pain as a young woman—requiring spinal surgery that only provided temporary relief—started her on a journey to try and understand the root cause of why we see so much spinal pain in the present time.

As a primary care physician, I had puzzled over this, too. So many of my patients who worked in tech jobs were having wrist pain, neck pain and back pain, presumably from hunching over keyboards. My mother, who was born in 1915, and who had supported her family of nine as a secretary using the old-fashioned Remington typewriter, had none of these issues and worked until she was 70. Esther recognized that a significant change in posture from the Roaring Twenties onwards had something to do with it.

I was determined to learn more and quickly signed up for her program. In six sessions over the course of six weeks, I learned her simple steps of how to restore my spine to its natural alignment. My posture improved immediately. I could lengthen my spine as I slept, drove to work, or sat at my desk or on the stool in my exam room while I talked to my patients. Within weeks, I slept better, and my neck (which had given me trouble since childhood injuries) stopped hurting. I had more energy and a new sense of well-being! I was sold! Esther offered a dance class to interested students to extend their posture lessons, which proved popular. We danced Samba and traditional Indian steps to great music. We all missed it when it ended.

I began referring my patients, friends, and family, and their positive feedback led to a ground swell of support for Esther to write her book, which was published in 2008 to great acclaim. My 84-year-old mother-in-law, who had polio as a child, and had a hunch back and osteoporosis and couldn't get up off the floor,

took the class. Her posture changed, she walked better, and she lived the remaining nine years of her life with better function.

The world changed in 2020. We stopped gathering at home and work. Group classes came to a halt. Video medical visits became the norm. My personal life changed too. I had been working as a primary care Internist in Palo Alto for almost 40 years, but moved from San Mateo County to Alameda County in 2017 and the long hours and commute had taken a toll on my health and relationships. I even lost track of Esther! But not her teachings. I credit her program—which I had taken in about 1996—for the preservation of my height, my mood, and my sense of well-being.

In May 2023 I retired. This was a difficult transition as I really missed my patients and my colleagues. But the timing was right, as I became a grandmother that October and I had a lot more time to hike in the hills nearby! I resumed the glidewalking I learned from Esther, and I did not hurt my neck or back carrying my hefty grandson.

I was delighted when I heard from Esther in December 2024. She was updating *8 Steps* and invited me to bring the foreword up to date. We met and I quickly got up to speed about how, in the past 10 years, the Gokhale Method had transformed into a "Worldwide Experience." Esther now has a team of teachers all over the world helping people to address their posture and alleviate their pain. She shared a list of all the different classes available online, which are remarkable! She calls these "Gokhale Active," including Gokhale Fitness, Gokhale Yoga, Moving Meditation, and a dance-based program called 123-Move. One can take them in real time or on replay, and 123-Move even includes a "freestyle dance party!" I was psyched and of course I accepted the offer to expand on my original foreword!

Restoring the spine to its optimal shape and length, and the rest of the body to its optimal architecture, counteracts many negative consequences of aging such as loss of height, protruding belly, decreased bowel motility, increased urinary frequency and incontinence. For people of all ages the Gokhale Method improves body awareness, balance and appearance. I hope that the Gokhale Method will be taught in schools so that current generations can learn the benefits of healthy posture for mind, body and spirit. This truly is an antiaging program with no side effects to worry about.

I remain convinced that the dramatic postural changes that have occurred in our society over the last 100 years can be reversed and that we can return to a healthy, natural style with the help of Esther's insights and techniques. It has certainly worked for me and my patients, family and friends. Let this book be a guide to YOUR posture journey. The method's new tag line says it all:

"Move Like You Are Meant To"

Deirdre Stegman, M.D.,
Oakland, California, 2025

PREFACE

It is with great pleasure that I present this second edition of *8 Steps to a Pain-Free Back*. For many of us, a pain-free life is only a memory, but it doesn't have to be. The Gokhale Method emerged from my personal journey of healing my own back and has continued to evolve over more than 35 years of research and teaching. The method alleviates back pain by addressing its largely unrecognized root causes, rather than just its symptoms. It has been a privilege and a pleasure to help hundreds of thousands of people relearn to move the way we humans are meant to—gracefully, easefully, and pain free.

As a teenager I was encouraged to "stand up straight," as many of us are. I did this the only way I knew how—by thrusting out my chest and swaying my lower back. This looked like good posture, and I continued with it until it became a habit. My sway was exacerbated in gymnastics and in stints as a yoga model in Bombay.

It took my first pregnancy for the flaw in my architecture to show up as a problem. Between the extra weight of the pregnancy, the hormone relaxin coursing through my bloodstream, and my excessive lumbar curve, I severely herniated my L5-S1 disc in the ninth month of my pregnancy. The radiologist remarked that it was the worst herniation he had seen that year. The pain was searing, like an icepick in my buttock, and persisted after my daughter was born. I was unable to carry her without feeling electric jolts down my leg. I couldn't sleep for more than two hours at night without waking up with severe back spasms. After trying a lot of interventions without success, I decided to undergo surgery (a laminectomy and discectomy). This gave relief, but within a year I had re-herniated the same disc and was being offered another back surgery.

Around this time, I was fortunate to learn about L'Institut d'Aplomb in Paris, France, where Noëlle Perez-Christiaens taught an anthropologically based posture modification technique. Her theory is that we in industrialized countries don't use our bodies well, that this misuse can cause pain and damage, and that we have much to learn from people in traditional cultures. The theory resonated with my childhood memories from growing up in India. I remembered listening to my Dutch mother marvel at how gracefully our Indian maid went about her duties and how easily the laborers in the street carried their burdens. Classes in Noëlle's technique diminished my back pain significantly, and I spent five years training to become certified in Aplomb®. Spurred on by what I learned, I attended courses at Stanford University Medical School and the Department of Anthropology. I visited countries in Europe, Asia, Africa, and South America, where I observed, photographed, filmed, and interviewed people in communities where back pain is rare. I incorporated teachings from other disciplines, added elements from my field research, and created a unique, systematic method for helping people efficiently transform their posture and return to physically active lives.

I wrote the first edition of *8 Steps to a Pain-Free Back* for people who needed help and couldn't travel to see me in California. That book was a bestseller, selling over 250,000 copies in 12 languages. All the information you need to lead a pain-free life lies within these pages. However, I've come to realize that learning movement from a static medium is usually inadequate to help people change their habits. Since the first edition was published in 2008, I have trained a large number of Gokhale Method teachers who have been teaching people all over the world to transform their posture and reclaim their lives.

Then, in 2020, COVID-19 set us the challenge of teaching the Gokhale Method online. This proved surprisingly effective, and we have continued and developed our online offerings—now anyone around the world can access live coaching with a qualified Gokhale Method teacher.

Another development during COVID-19, which I had long wished for, is a robust, independent, objective test of the method's effectiveness. At the time of writing this preface, a randomized controlled trial—the gold standard for testing effectiveness—is underway, led by Professor Matthew Smuck, M.D., Chief of Physical Medicine and Rehabilitation at Stanford

University. The trial compares the Gokhale Method with physical therapy for patients with lower back pain. The Gokhale Method arm of the trial includes use of our recently developed PostureTracker™ wearable. This device consists of a pair of sensors placed on strategic locations of the body that provide real-time feedback when the user departs from a calibrated ideal. It enables students to learn and internalize new habits more quickly.

This new edition of *8 Steps to a Pain-Free Back*, includes these additions and improvements:

- New and updated instructions reflect how our teaching has evolved over the years. The step-by-step instructions for stretchlying on the side (Chapter 4), inner corset (Chapter 5), and glidewalking (Chapter 8), in particular, have been significantly altered and augmented for ease of learning.
- QR codes that connect with videos to enhance your understanding and practice of the techniques.
- Approximately 600 new, updated, and upgraded photographs and drawings.
- Clarification of the differences between the Gokhale Method paradigm of healthy posture (the J-spine) and that of conventional approaches, including how an anteverted pelvis is different from "anterior pelvic tilt."
- Guidelines for working with mobile devices without compromising your posture.

If you are familiar with the first edition, you may also notice that the step-by-step instructions in each chapter are accompanied by new photos of me demonstrating the techniques. The photographs were taken as placeholders after three months without exercise, owing to ear surgery followed by COVID-19. Later, my team and I decided to use the photographs for this edition, as an embrace of my state of fitness at that time and to emphasize the path of improvement rather than any particular ideal. I hope that you, dear reader, will also find it within yourself to embrace your current situation even as you work to improve it.

By practicing the techniques presented here, you can learn to carry yourself with ease, grace, and confidence—not by striving to change who you are, but by rediscovering the strength and beauty already within.

Warm wishes for your posture and health,

Esther Gokhale
Palo Alto, California, 2025

STUDENT EXPERIENCES

"Dear Esther,

I purchased your excellent book *8 Steps to a Pain-Free Back* around 9 months ago, after my younger brother recommended it to me. At just 18, he had back surgery to remove a herniated disc. I am 6'3" tall and up until the beginning of 2012 I had poor stooping posture, perhaps due to shyness and wanting to blend in. My posture caught up with me as since about 3 years ago I have had several episodes of back pain when I am barely able to move. In hindsight it is now clear this low back pain came on after heavy lifting with a rounded low back. I was concerned that at age 22 I was suffering this much. Then I read your book.

Through reading the chapters in turn and 're-learning' how to move and hold myself, I have quickly developed a general interest in the body and how it works; I have taken up athletics and bodybuilding. Your method is helpful with everything, and without wishing to tempt fate, I can definitely say my back pain has generally gone and when I do get an occasional twinge, I understand the anatomy and can work to fix the cause before it develops into something almost paralysing.

I have particularly enjoyed the hip-hinging and stretchsitting chapters, which I consciously implement in my daily life; my family and colleagues at work have noticed dramatic changes in how I move and stand, which improves my appearance. That is of course just one of the many advantages! I have even become a bit of a 'posture snob,' and I will be the first to recommend your book to people who think the human back is just 'dodgy' in its design...I am currently working on the glidewalking chapter, which I find more tricky than the others, however I am determined to implement it into my everyday life.

Thank you so much. For not only helping with my back, but inspiring a far more active and healthy life. I am grateful I discovered this knowledge now, hopefully before it is too late!"
— **Adam McStravick**, England

"Esther has changed my life. In 2006–2007 I was training seriously for running races and got a chronic foot injury (plantar fasciitis). This wasn't healed until late 2007, and by that time I'd been compensating so much for the foot injury that I had shifted the angle of my pelvis. This was pinching a nerve and I got shooting pains in my hip each time I ran even just two or three steps. I went to an orthopedist, had a cortisone injection in my spine, and did extensive physical therapy. These helped somewhat, especially the physical therapy. But even in 2010 I still couldn't run without shooting pain and sitting at my desk was making things worse. I couldn't run, play soccer or ultimate frisbee, nor ski or snowboard or hike. It was directly impacting my everyday life, my happiness, and my work as I have often used running as a way to create space, reflect, and think about the problems that I'm solving.

I took Esther's class in November 2010 and was amazed. It was eye-opening, and changed the way that I walked, sat, slept, and ran. Stretchlying was one of the most important elements to me. So was realizing that I shouldn't be trying to tuck my butt under me as I was taught as a gymnast when I was small, but could instead use those butt muscles to drive the way that I walked. Part of the key is that you apply what you learn with Esther to everything you do, until it comes naturally. While physical therapy is very important, it's hard for 15 minutes of physical therapy a day to compensate for the pain you may cause in the way that you walk, sit, and sleep the other 23.75 hours a day. Applying her principles meant that I could start running again and live without fear that if I did the wrong thing it would cause a shooting pain."
— **Zan Armstrong**, California

"I am a 76-year-old M.D., licensed physician and surgeon for 50 years, and practicing Diagnostic Radiologist for 41 years. I experienced four lumbosacral spine issues, in 1990, 2009, 2010 and 2011, three being disc extrusions and one being a nerve root trapped in a stenotic neural foramen. Following spine surgery (discectomy) in 2009, partial, permanent damage of the left L4-5 nerve root resulted in chronic, but bearable, pain, treated with daily Tylenol until that medication compromised my liver enzymes. In 2011, surgery involved removal of three discs, removal of bone from the spine from L3 to S1, and decompression of multiple neural foramina. That surgery put an end to my practice of Radiology due to 24/7 prominent low back pain, very slow progression in regaining ability to walk without a cane, inability to bend forward, and inability to sit for more than 20 minutes, in ANY chair, without severe back pain.

Physical therapy was extensive, but seemed to concentrate on strengthening the abdominis rectus muscles of the belly, which ultimately caused an inguinal hernia, but provided no relief of the back symptoms. My pre-op (hernia) evaluation at Palo Alto Medical Foundation included meeting my new primary care M.D., Dr. Santana. Once she heard of my low back situation she strongly suggested that I "check out" the Gokhale Institute for a proven "different" approach to my problem. From Amazon, I purchased *8 Steps to a Pain-Free Back*. Esther Gokhale's method was eye-opening to me. I quickly signed up for a preliminary evaluation, then a one-on-one course with Esther. Esther taught with scientific expertise, endless patience, describing each step, demonstrating it, then having me perform it until I got it right. The course taught me that I had been my own worst enemy, leaning toward, or over patients, doing gyn procedures or angiograms, and spending 10 hours each day in an uncomfortable chair, leaning forward and twisting left and right before a bank of computer monitors. At the end of each day I could barely walk…for years, and years. The Gokhale Method taught me to sit, stand, sleep (on my back or my side), bend with hip-hinging, rather than bending my spine, and to use the muscles of the "corset" in my mid-section to support and stabilize my spine. I learned to walk using the muscles of my feet/ legs/gluteus medius muscles. Esther was such an inspiring teacher that I incorporated her program into my life, and experienced rapid and progressive relief of my back pain, with my family complimenting me on my "new" posture, mobility, bending, and my "CAN DO" attitude. No more morning back pain and spasm, painful sitting or clumsy, uncomfortable walking.

The Gokhale Method has provided me with the TOOLS I needed to overcome my back pain, as well as to keep from causing further damage. It is up to me to use those tools so that they become second nature to me. Despite my age, and extensive medical/surgical history, Esther Gokhale's technique has been a blessing, and has restored quality to my life. IT IS A WHOLE NEW BALL GAME, NOW!!!

Thank you, Esther Gokhale, for the help you, and your technique, have given to me, and to so many other people."
— **Randolph M. Hall, M.D.**, California

"I am 53 years old. Looking back on photos of my childhood through adolescence and into adulthood, my posture was an absolute mess consisting of slouching, hunched shoulders, and swayback when encouraged to stand up straight or sit up. I further aggravated this baseline of poor body use with years of bodybuilding and powerlifting, followed by endurance running and biking. An MRI at age 47 demonstrated multilevel spinal stenosis, degenerative discs at all levels, and posterior bulging discs. The diagnosis my doctor presented me with was "messy spine" and added "you have the spine of a 90-year-old." I was advised to give up all exercise. About six months ago, I discovered the Gokhale Method after being forwarded a copy of a *New York Times* article. The shoulder roll and activation of my inner corset has become a daily activity of at least 20 times per day, the latter of which I see my dog perform at a similar frequency. As soon as I started everting my feet 15 degrees and walking in a line, my sciatica has completely resolved as has been my ability to walk longer than a couple of blocks without having to reset my spine."
— **Ralph Newman, M.D.**, North Carolina

"I am an orthodontist and in my job I spend many hours bending over to work on patients. I have had minor back problems in the past, but a few months ago I was overwhelmed by major back pain that was almost debilitating. I turned to every solution I could find. I ended up paying thousands of dollars in therapy. It did help, but it was horribly time consuming. My life seemed like an endless cycle of hurting myself while I worked during the day and at night coming home to hours of exercises in order to heal myself. With two orthodontic practices, two small children, work in nonprofit, well something had to give.

Then a good friend recommended Esther Gokhale's book, and it completely changed my life. I learned that I did not need to live in the cycle of daily injury and nightly healing. The key was healing myself in the way I live day *and* night. Esther's solution changes the way you live and thus it does not rely on exercises and gimmicks, it is about fundamentally changing the way we do everyday activities such as walk, stand, sit, sleep, bend, and lift. After "re-learning" how to do these actions correctly, the result has been extraordinary. Now I work pain free, have time when I come home to spend with my children (not doing exercises), sleep comfortably, and wake up without back pain. I am back to surfing and I can carry my heavy long board without any pain at all. This has been a truly life-changing experience. I cannot be thankful enough."

— **Sandra Kahn, D.D.S., M.S.D.**, California

"I am a 70-year-old woman. As a young woman I was tall (5'10"), slender, and active as I would ever be raising my six children. For the most part, my body and I had a good relationship, but, over time and with the demands of my life, something problematic happened. My body began talking to me: my knee, psoas, sacrum, and lower back hurt, and I also suffered a loss of balance. I mainly saw a chiropractor but also physical therapists, massage therapists, and acupuncturists…the list is long. When you want to function and feel halfway decent, you try everything.

By the time I was 60, I had three fractures in my spine and a diagnosis of osteoporosis. For 10 years I worked hard to control the osteoporosis and did well rebuilding my bones, but even so, I am now 5'6"—four inches shorter than I was. Perhaps it is vain to wish every day for the return of my stature, but to stand tall and straight has been a preoccupation. I tried to hide my posture under my clothes, but of course that doesn't really work!

In spite of the deterioration, I maintained hope of improvement. When I came across Esther Gokhale for the second time in a year, I paid attention. For all my efforts and the various things I had tried, nothing up to that point had worked for me. I was afraid that Esther's approach was not going to work either.

I started working with Esther and gave her my trust and commitment. I learned my new body awareness methodically through the 18 concise lessons of the Elements online program. At times I worried I would be disappointed again, but Esther's expectation of a good outcome—combined with her integrity and tenacity—kept me moving forward.

An important step for me was understanding the difference between a tucked pelvis and an anteverted pelvis, and that I could make it happen in my own body. Doing the "inner corset" also made visible changes. I wasn't bent over from fatigue by the end of the day. I was so grateful. I could be upright again, and I felt back to being myself. Previous to the Elements course, my body had become something to fear; it has now become something I take pleasure in.

So many things have gotten better. I had a tight psoas for decades, which caused pain in my groin. I don't feel that anymore. Before, if I fell asleep on my back, I would wake myself up snoring or run out of breath. That has gone. It had also been difficult to breathe when walking; now all of my breathing is much better. This entire journey of finding out how my body works has been transformative for me. Best of all, the Gokhale Method has shown me how I can once again live my life upright and pain free. What a gift!"

— **Susan Taormina**, Massachusetts

For more student stories,
visit gokhalemethod.com

FOUNDATIONS

Your body's way back to pain-free living

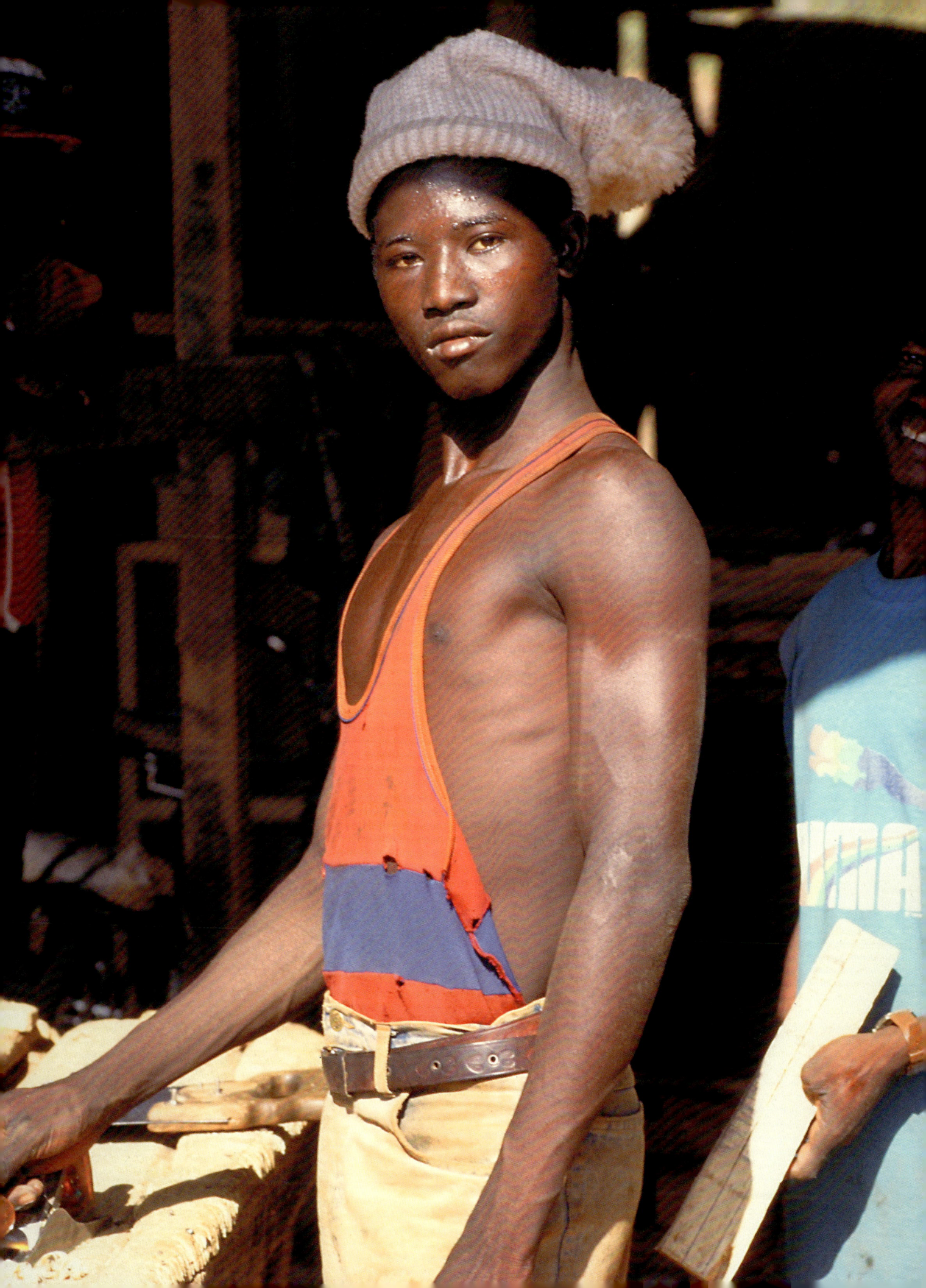

We are marvelously designed creatures. We have inherent grace and strength, like every other creature on the planet. We have evolved to sit, walk, run, jump, climb, carry, and even dance without pain. If we respect our natural design, our bodies heal spontaneously, and we can function well for close to a century. Indeed, there are many populations where most people live painlessly into old age (fig.F-1).[1-9]

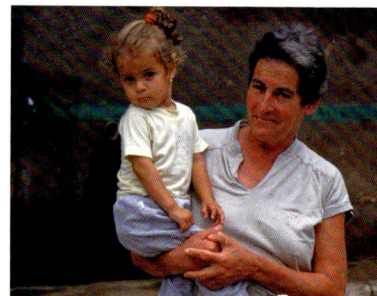

This grandmother carries her grandchild with ease (Brazil).

fig.F-1

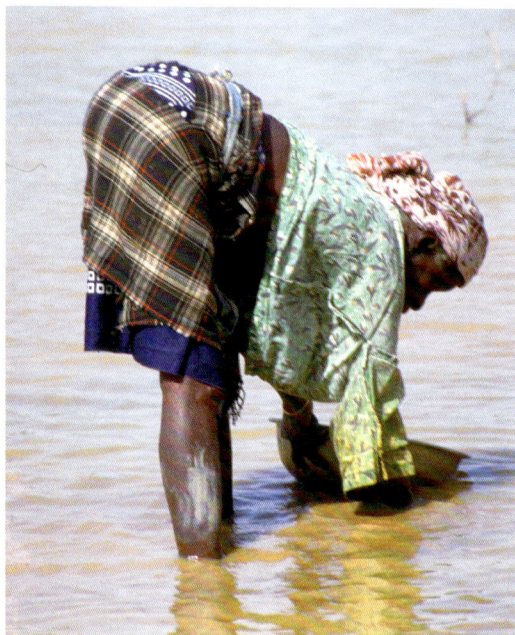

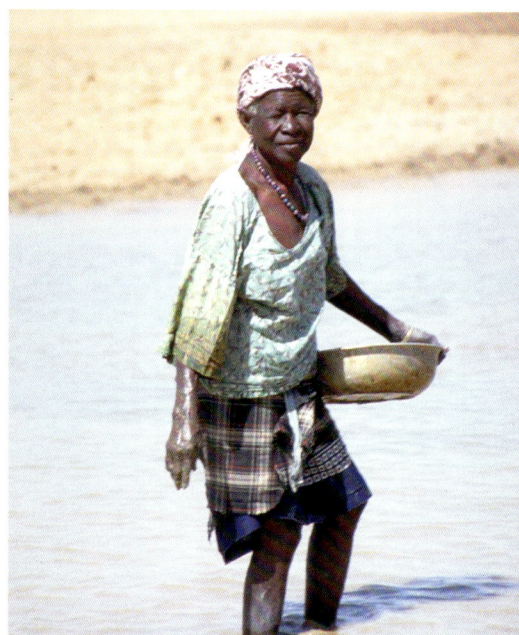

This older woman bends to gather water chestnuts for seven to nine hours a day, but reports no pain (Burkina Faso).

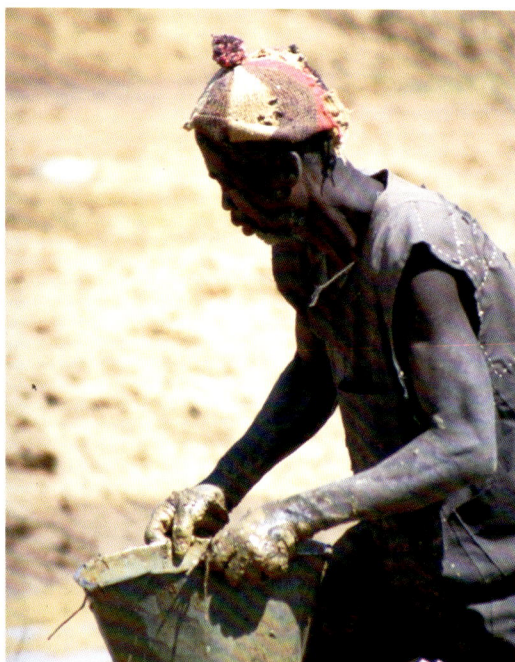

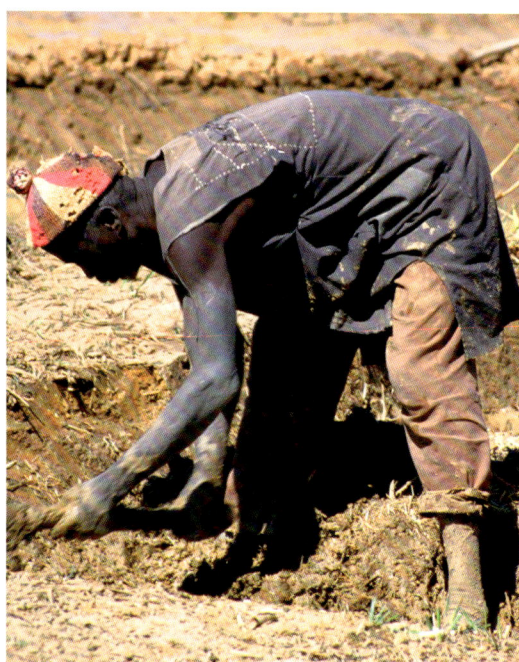

This man has molded clay bricks all day for most of his life with no negative physical impact (Burkina Faso).

Why, then, do so many people in our culture suffer back pain and other musculoskeletal ills? The problem is that we arrive on the planet without a user's manual. We depend on our culture to teach and support us. And the culture in industrialized societies has not been teaching or supporting us very well (fig.F-2). If we have pain and musculoskeletal problems, we need to look first at the laws of nature we are disrespecting, the blueprint for our skeletal structure we are disregarding, the pieces of our genetic code we are ignoring. This book introduces you to a method that teaches and supports you in a way that our culture no longer does, so that you can live a normal, pain-free life.

fig.F-2

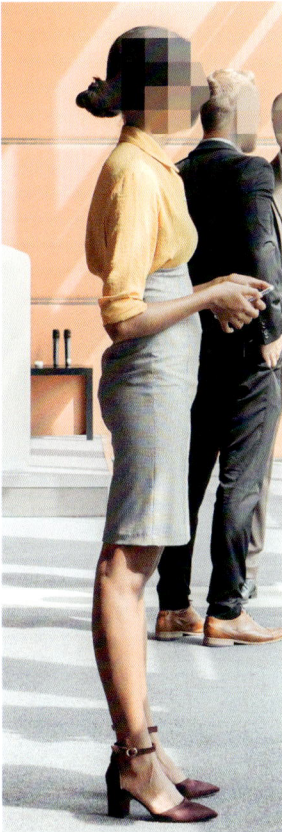

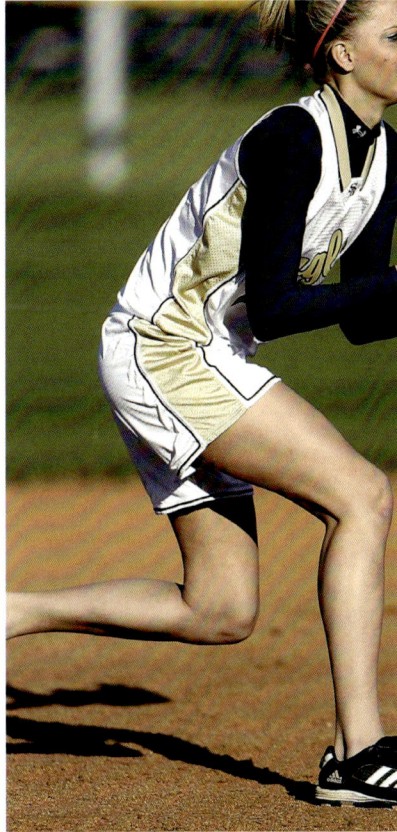

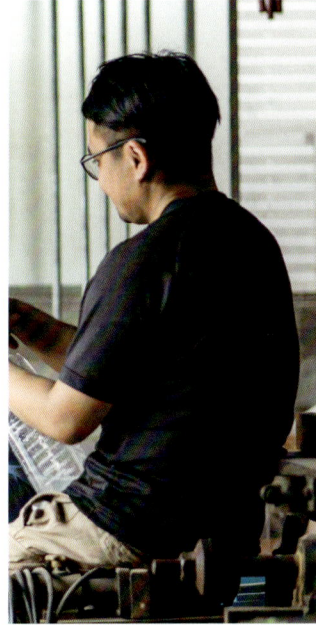

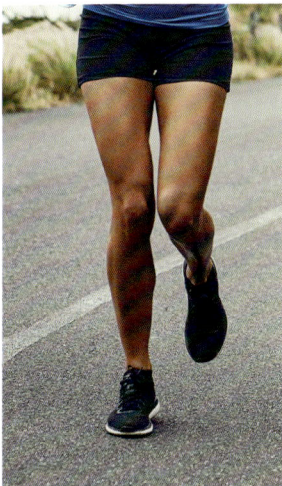

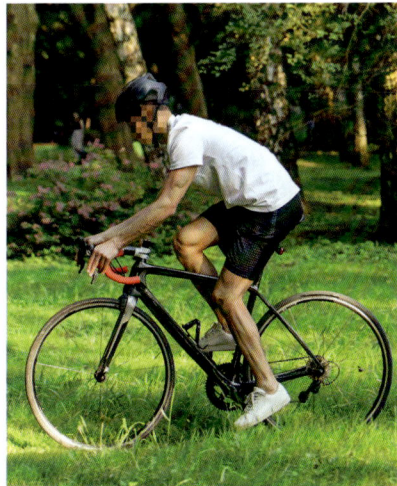

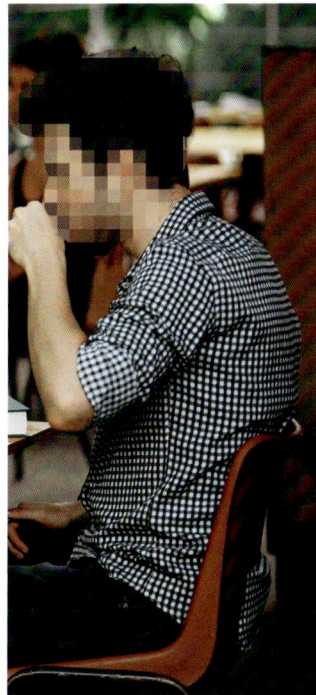

Years of working against the body's natural principles usually result in damage, pain, and dysfunction.

BACK PAIN

If you suffer back pain, you are not alone.
In industrialized societies, back pain has reached
epidemic proportions. Consider these statistics:

- Approximately 80 percent of individuals in the
  general population will have at least one episode
  of lower back pain during their lifetime.[10-22]

- In 2020, approximately 619 million people
  worldwide experienced lower back pain.
  Projections suggest that by 2050, this number
  will have risen by around 36%.[23]

- Back pain is the leading cause of disability
  globally.[24]

- Non-specific lower back pain (that is, back
  pain without an identifiable cause) is the most
  common type of back pain (~90% of cases).[25]

- The back is the most common site of pain in
  the body among adults in the United States.[26]

- Approximately 8% of all adults in the United
  States suffer from chronic severe back pain, and
  of these ~75% experience limitations in their
  daily activities.[27]

- By age 15, more than 60% of all adolescents in
  the United States have experienced back and/or
  neck pain.[28]

- Total direct and indirect costs for treatment
  of lower back pain in the United States are
  estimated to surpass $100 billion annually.[29]

> *After back surgery in 1991, I was still
> in excruciating pain and lived with
> prescription pain medication on a daily
> basis. Esther Gokhale changed all that.
> I no longer have any neck pain or back pain
> and I no longer use any pain medication.*
>
> Stacia Hurley,
> Concentric Network, CA

WHAT WE BLAME

Among the most commonly cited causes for
our high rates of back pain are that we are not
designed to stand upright, we are too sedentary,
we endure too much stress, we've grown too tall
or too heavy for our backs, and we wear out with
age. But are these factors really the problem?

STANDING UPRIGHT?

The argument goes that our spines have not
evolved sufficiently to carry the weight of our
upper bodies, necks, and heads without strain
or damage.[30] By this reasoning, we should all
be suffering back pain. Yet there are whole
populations where the incidence is very low.[1-9]

Five and a half million years of being upright is
plenty of time—even by evolutionary standards—
for our spines to adapt and accommodate the
"new" burden of our upper bodies. I believe that
the problem is not an evolutionary flaw, but a
cultural one. The cause of our pain is not *that*
we stand upright, but *how* we stand upright
(fig.F-3,fig.F-4).

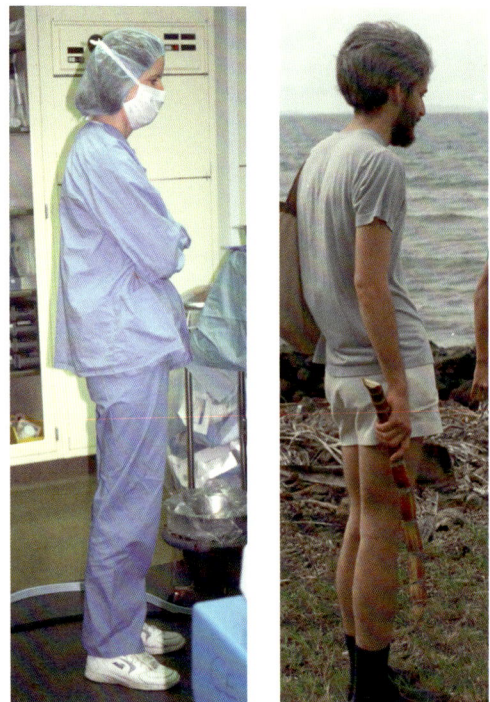

fig.F-3

Our problem is not that *we stand upright,
but* how *we stand upright.*

fig.F-4

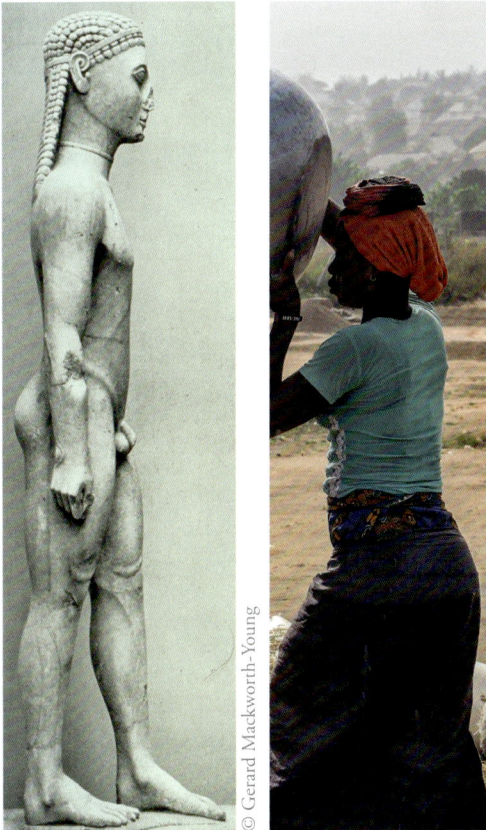

© Gerard Mackworth-Young

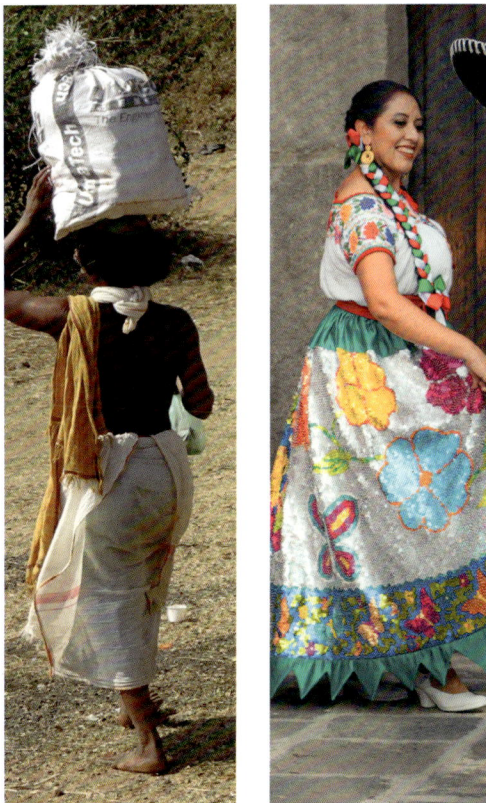

People from diverse cultures exhibit healthy upright posture (Greece, Nigeria, India, Mexico).

SEDENTARY LIVES?

Another frequently cited excuse for our back pain is our sedentary way of life: unlike people in many parts of the world, most workers in industrialized societies earn their living sitting down. Yet statistics show that in industrialized societies manual laborers have an even higher incidence of lower back pain than sedentary workers.[31] This suggests that switching from sedentary jobs to more physical ones would not solve our back problems.

In my travels in Burkina Faso, Ecuador, and India, I encountered numerous sedentary workers including potters, basket makers, and weavers, who spend long hours sitting and yet do not suffer from nearly as many back problems as we do (fig.F-5). In our culture as well, some people manage long hours in front of computer screens without negative consequences to their backs. In fact, medical statistics call into question the agreed-upon philosophy that static sitting at work is a risk factor for lower back pain.[32] Again, I believe that it isn't *that* we sit but *how* we sit that causes our problems (fig.F-6).

My students, after they have learned a few simple relevant techniques, usually find sitting extremely comfortable, even if it previously caused them pain.

STRESS?

While stress is a risk factor for back pain,[30] it is possible to address physical pain independently from stress. Stress correlates with pain, but doesn't have to cause it. If you have stress-related back pain, you can lessen your pain by learning physical relaxation even if you are not able to resolve your stress. In fact, learning positions that are physically relaxing can help you deal better with mental and emotional stress.

WEIGHT AND HEIGHT?

Extra weight challenges the entire skeleton and enormous extra weight is certainly unhealthy. A moderate amount of excess weight, however, need not cause serious musculoskeletal problems (fig.F-7).[33] It is when an individual lacks good alignment that even a small amount of extra weight can be disproportionately damaging because it torques the spine. A building that is built true is not unstable, even if it is bulky; but if it is even slightly skewed, the extra bulk

fig.F-5

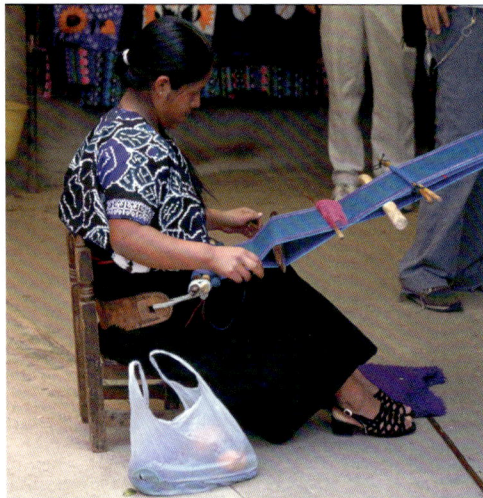

Weaving cloth (Mexico)

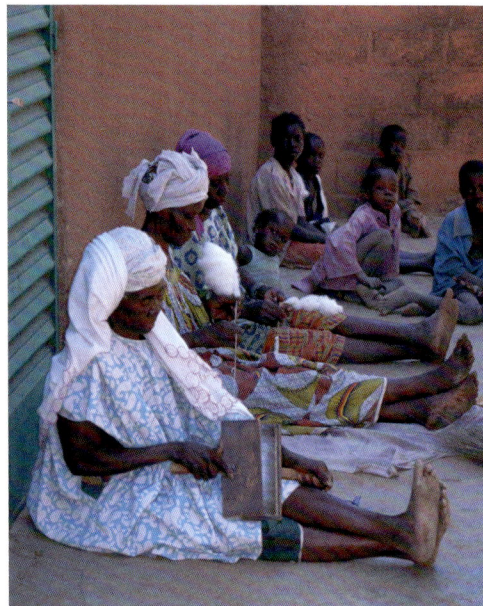

Spinning cotton (Burkina Faso)

These sedentary workers have healthy posture and report no back pain.

I no longer must quietly accept my condition and continue to watch my world become smaller and smaller. [Using Gokhale Method techniques], I was immediately able to sleep longer and with less pain. This has given me much hope and confidence.

Joan Northway,
Chelsea, MA

fig.F-6

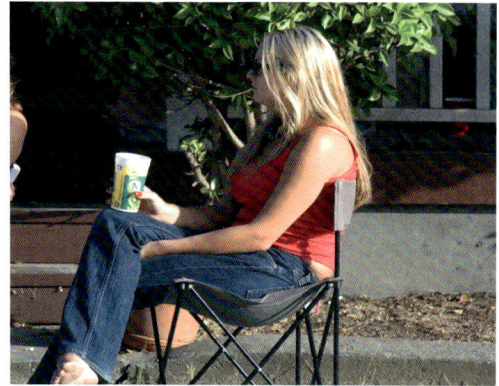

Hunched sitting (USA)

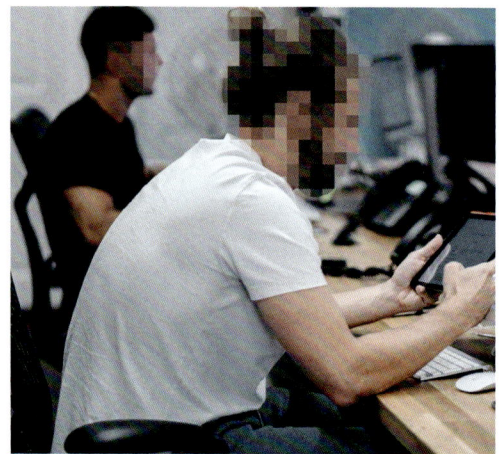

Hunched sitting (UK)

It isn't that we sit, but how we sit that causes our problems.

exerts great strains on the underlying structure. Similarly, if the spine is properly aligned, it will tolerate moderate amounts of extra weight without damage; if the spine is poorly aligned, every degree of misalignment causes a large increase in stress. For people who carry extra weight and experience back pain, learning proper alignment may provide a faster and more direct solution to their back pain than losing the extra weight.

Just as excess weight can challenge the skeletal system, so can unusual height. Similar logic applies: on a poorly aligned skeleton, extra height significantly stresses the spine; on a well-aligned skeleton, extra height need not cause damage.[34] Consider the Masai, who are usually well over six feet tall, but are spared our epidemic of back pain.[35]

AGE?

Many people think that age is the biggest contributor to back pain. Certainly with age our bones and muscles weaken; however, the same is true for all humanity. If we use our bodies wisely, normal wear and tear should not incapacitate us. The Burkinabè brickmaker in figure F-8a shows what is possible even in advanced age. He spends numerous hours every day digging clay, mixing it with straw, and fashioning it into bricks using a wood mold. In some low-income, rural communities, 80–90% of workers are laborers who often carry heavy weights on their backs and heads and may work well into old age. Yet their rates of lower back pain are 50–75% less than in higher-income, industrialized populations.[1]

fig.F-7

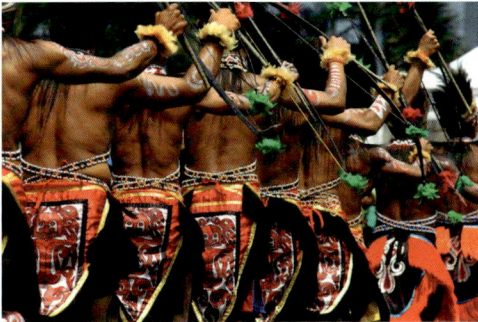

(Papua New Guinea)

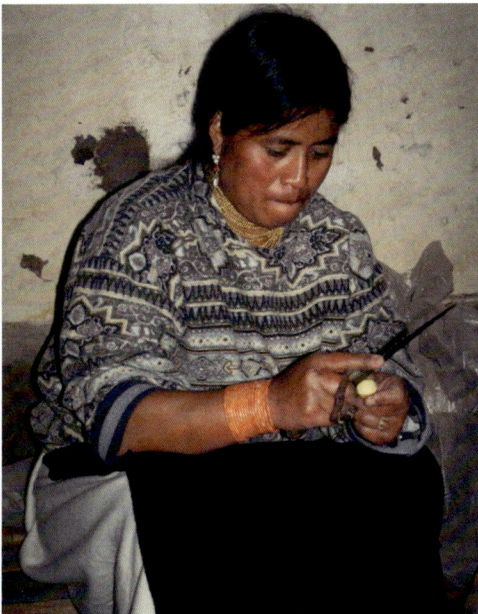

(Ecuador)

Extra weight does not condemn people to back pain. In many cultures, full-bodied people carry their extra weight without great difficulty.

THE REAL CAUSE

Scientific research substantiates the following risk factors for back pain: genetics,[36, 37] psychosocial stress, exposure to vibration, inadequate physical fitness, strenuous body positioning (bending, twisting, static standing), age,[30] height (only in the case of sciatica),[34] smoking,[38] and other health conditions (such as arthritis, infections, tumors, and osteoporosis).[39] I believe that the biggest risk factor for back pain, as yet unidentified and underappreciated, is posture.

fig.F-8

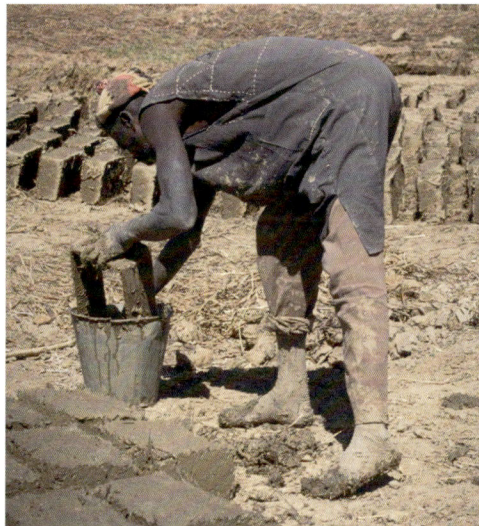

a. This brickmaker works long hours making bricks from straw and clay despite his age (Burkina Faso).

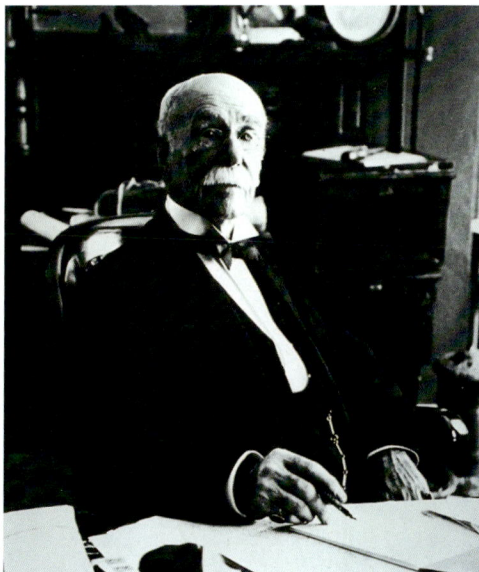

b. The clerk in this photograph from the turn of the century is not young but works from "sunup to sundown six days a week" (USA).

9

Many of these known risk factors can be mitigated by healthy posture. People with healthy posture can better withstand the effects of whole-body vibration, strenuous body positioning, weight, height, age, and even genetic predisposition to disc degeneration. Without healthy posture, however, some of the above factors, especially genetics, become very significant.

Much of our back pain results from how we hold ourselves and how we move. We have lost sight of what constitutes healthy posture; in fact, many popular guidelines for "good posture" do more harm than good. To find a model for healthy posture, we need to return to the ways of moving that were normal for us in earlier times and that are still normal for people in many cultures.

Until the 20th century, debilitating back pain was not common in our society. By the turn of the 21st century, back pain was more than twice as common as it was in 1950.[40] Shortly after World War I, a confluence of trends began a vicious cycle that continues today. Compare the pictures of individuals taken at the end of the 19th century (fig.F-9) with that from the mid-20th century (fig.F-10). The change is dramatic. Notice that, compared with the people in the earlier images, after the 1920s, people began to tuck their pelvises, thrust their pelvises and necks forward, and hunch or round their shoulders. It became fashionable to slouch.

Even more startling is a comparison of spine illustrations from two medical textbooks, one published in 1911[41] (fig. F-11a), the other in 1990[42] (fig.F-11b). The 1911 illustration shows gently curved, elongated lower back (*lumbar*) and upper back (*thoracic*) spinal contours, such that the overall shape of the spine is similar to a calligraphic letter J or a hockey stick. The later drawing shows significantly increased curvature both in the lumbar and thoracic spine, resembling more of an "S" shape. The shape of the spine in the 1911 illustration is shared not only by our ancestors, but also by adults in traditional cultures today (fig.F-3), and young children the world over (fig.F-12).

The consistency across generations, cultures, geography, and age provides compelling evidence that this is indeed the natural shape of the human spine. Here is a dramatic clue to the cause of our current back pain epidemic. Clearly, a mere 80 years

fig.F-9

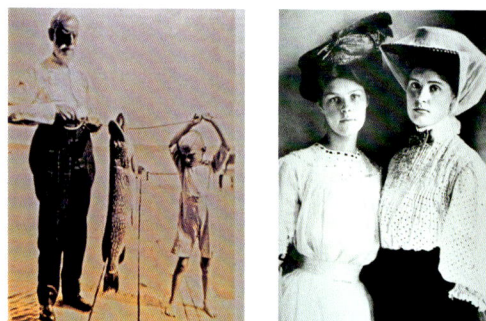

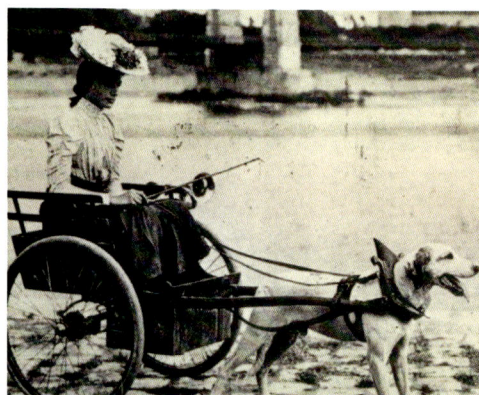

Healthy posture was typical in Western societies until the late 19th and early 20th centuries (USA).

fig.F-10

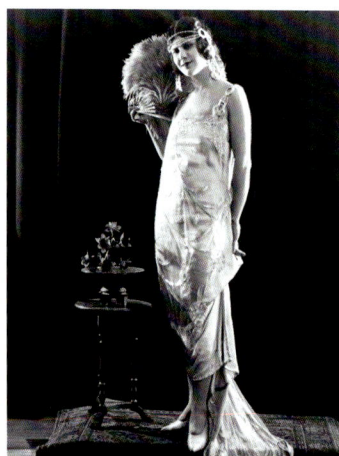

Beginning in the 1920s, it became fashionable to slouch.

of human history is not sufficient to account for any substantial genetic alteration of something as basic as the shape of our spines. What we are seeing is a cultural drift away from our natural design and an ancient and widespread kinesthetic tradition—the tradition of movement and posture handed down through earlier generations.

10

fig.F-11

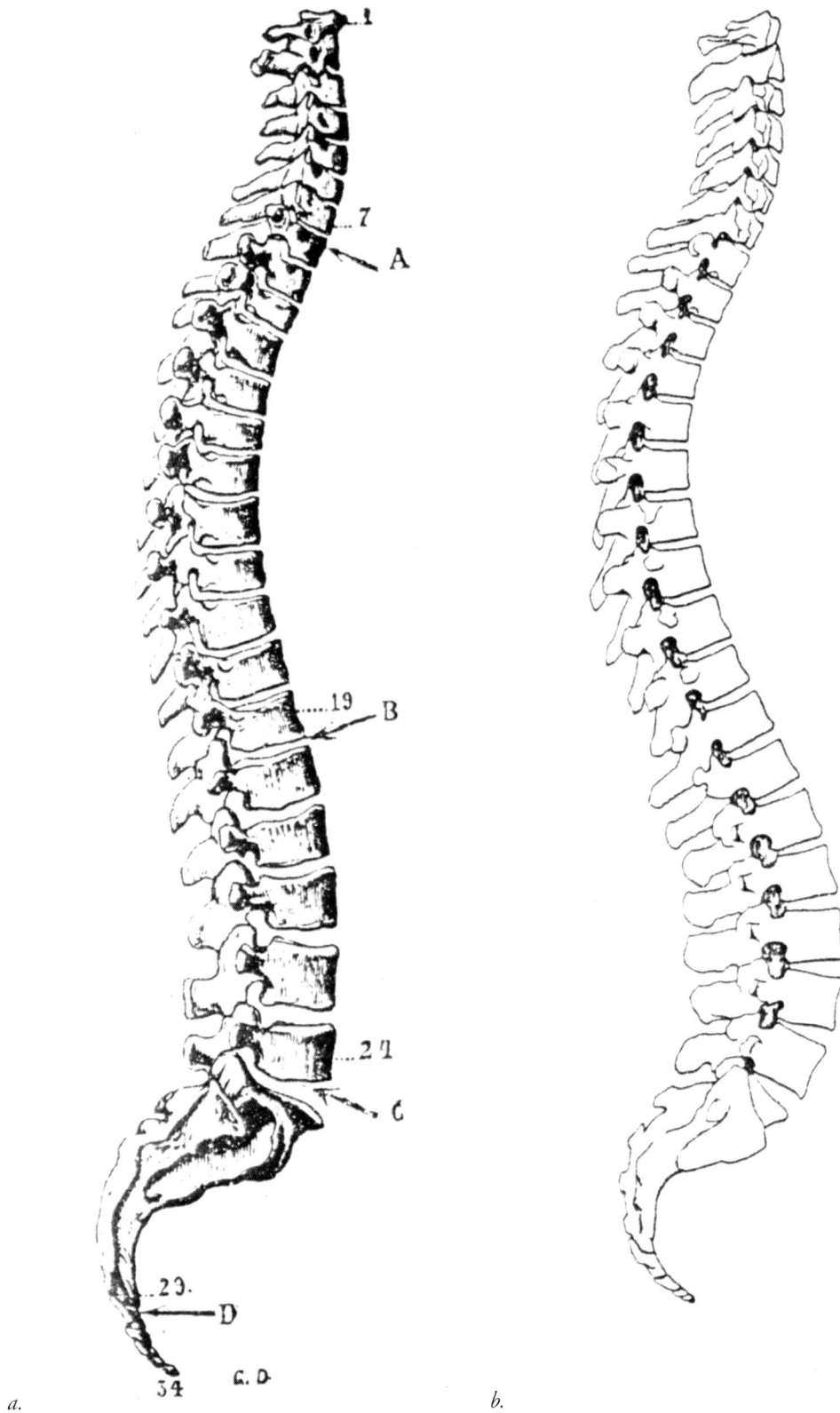

a.

b.

The spine on the left is from an anatomy book published in 1911[41] and shows what was considered normal then. The spine on the right is from an anatomy book published in 1990[42] and shows what is considered normal spinal curvature today. Notice the marked shift in the degree of curvature throughout the spine and especially in the lower back (lumbar) area, more similar to an "S" shape than a "J" shape.

fig.F-12

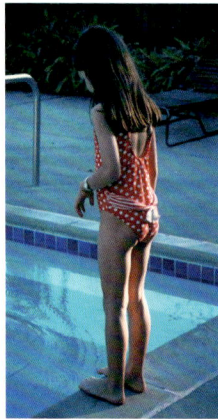 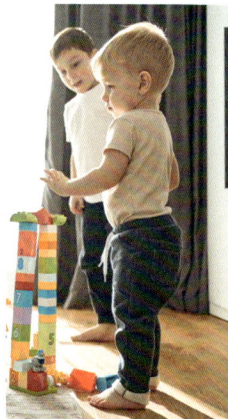

(USA)   (Ukraine)

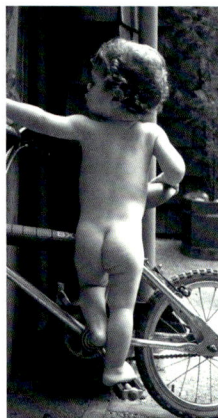 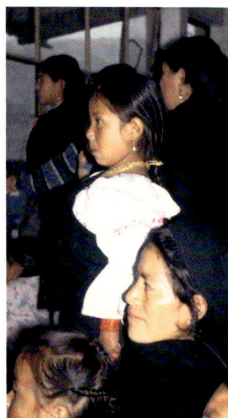

(USA)   (Ecuador)

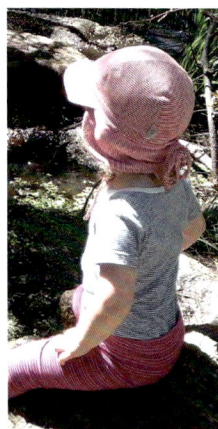 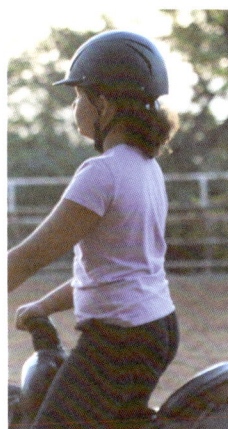

(Australia)   (Israel)

Young children the world over share a similar, healthy posture, and provide compelling evidence that this is our natural posture.

fig.F-13

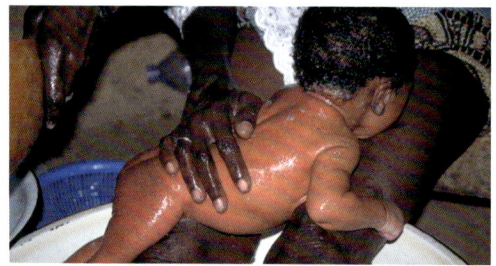

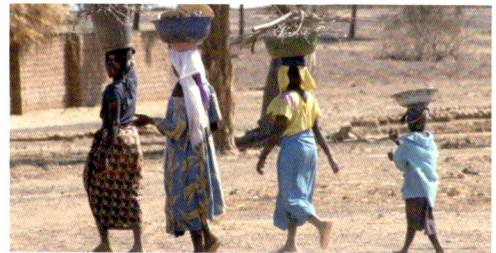

Cultural transmission occurs through formal training, physical handling, and mostly mimicry (Burkina Faso).

LOSS OF KINESTHETIC TRADITION

In modern industrial societies, many families have become geographically dispersed, with couples raising their children far away from parents and grandparents. This has led to a break in cultural support and the handing down of kinesthetic tradition. By contrast, in rural communities in Africa, Portugal, India, and other traditional societies, families are not dispersed and kinesthetic traditions remain intact. Though human beings share a fine blueprint for physical well-being, it takes cultural support, especially in the formative years, to pass body wisdom from one generation to the next. Cultural support comes in the form of grandparents showing parents how to carry their children, of teachers guiding their students to sit well in class, of children mimicking parents as they bend to gather food, or walk, etc. (fig.F-13).

Whereas certain cultural knowledge is easily transmitted by modern means of communication, kinesthetic knowledge needs physical proximity and repeated visual cueing. When the kinesthetic line is broken, we improvise each action rather than draw on the wisdom of thousands of generations.

Especially important among our kinesthetic traditions are those relating to children, since it is during the crucial early years that posture and movement patterns are etched into the brain. These traditions include how to hold a child while

So, what is the cause of this cultural drift? This is a matter for research, but I conjecture that two forces play an important role: a disruption in the link between generations in our culture, and the influence of the fashion industry.

fig.F-14

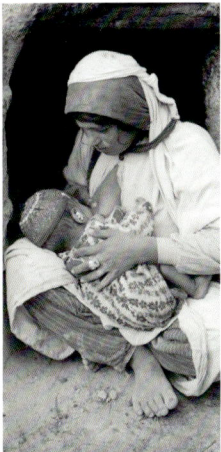 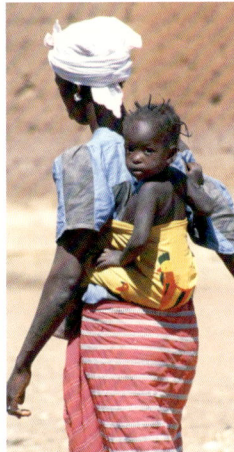

(Syria) *(Burkina Faso)*

Skillful handling and modeling help children learn healthy posture and movement patterns.

fig.F-16

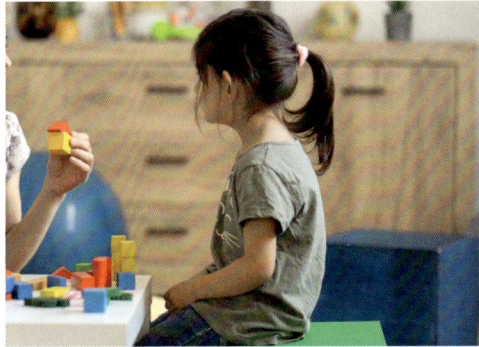

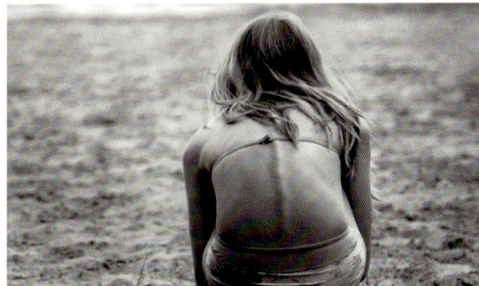

Children who were not handled skillfully as babies tend to retain poor posture habits later (USA).

fig.F-15

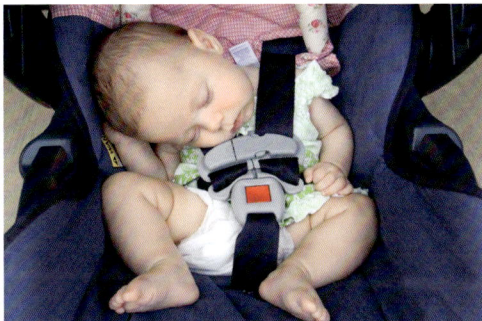

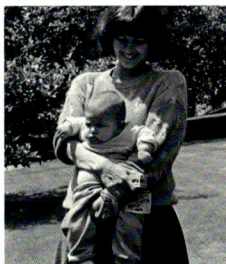 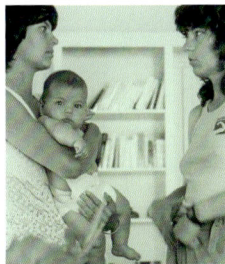

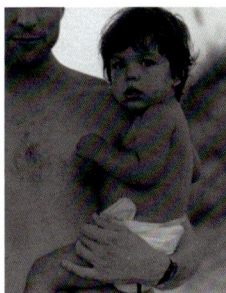 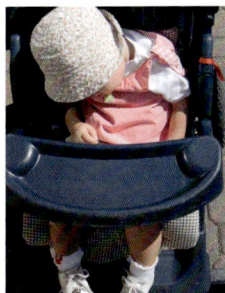

© Sandra Starkey

These photos show babies in unhealthy positions (USA).

nursing, how to carry a child, and how to teach a child to sit well (fig.F-14). Today's parents and grandparents have lost the generational wisdom for performing these actions well (fig.F-15) and today's children are the worse for it (fig.F-16).

Often, the only posture guideline children receive today is an occasional admonition to "sit up straight." Not knowing how to sit well, most children briefly adopt a stiff pose with tension in the lower back, but quickly tire of it and revert to slouching. Our popular knowledge no longer includes postural wisdom.

Even our medical experts are not well-informed about the elements of good posture and how to implement them. The medical establishment has lost sight of what truly ideal posture is, and mistakes the current average for normal or even ideal. Medical recommendations, interventions, and devices such as lumbar support cushions (page 51), cervical pillows (page 66), and TLSO body casts (page 125) reflect and perpetuate this cultural drift. They tend to accentuate excessive curvature in the small of the back (upper *lumbar spine*) and the neck (*cervical spine*), and flatten the natural *lumbosacral curve*.

INFLUENCE OF THE FASHION INDUSTRY

Another major contributor to our posture drift is the fashion industry. Around World War I, fashions in clothing and furniture converged to transform the conception of the human figure. In a matter of a few years, French fashion magazines moved from showing models with natural posture (fig.F-17) to showing ones with severely distorted frames, tucked pelvises, slouched shoulders, and protruding necks (fig.F-18)—much like the runway models of today.

The fashion industry in the 1920s promoted this posture as relaxed, casual, and new, as opposed to classical posture, which was reframed as stiff, rigid, and passé. Furniture styles also shifted in the 1920s (fig.F-19,fig.F-20), reinforcing the trend towards slouching in the name of comfort and ease. The Mies van der Rohe chair in fig.F-20 is an early example of furniture that tucks the pelvis and strongly distorts the spine. Many modern chairs do the same (fig.3-15 on page 90).

fig.F-17

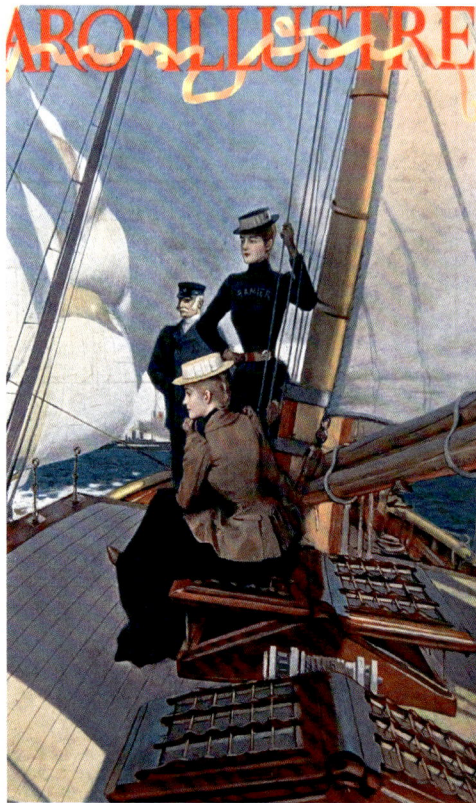

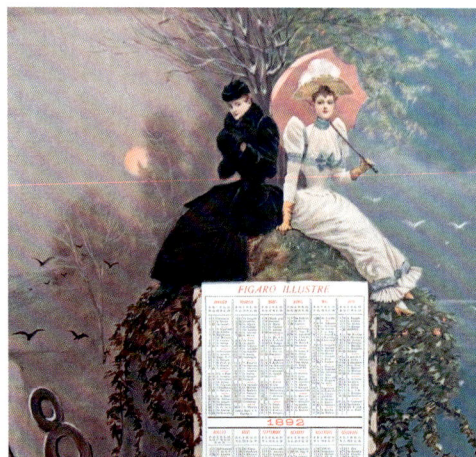

French fashion magazines from before World War I depict healthy posture.

fig.F-18

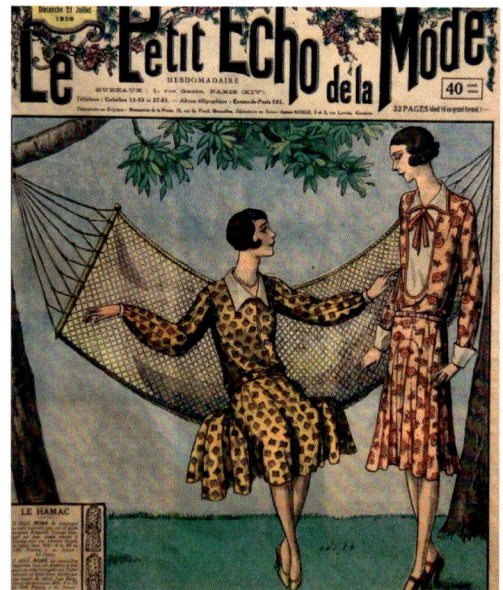

French fashion magazines from the 1920s and later show slouching as chic.

fig.F-19

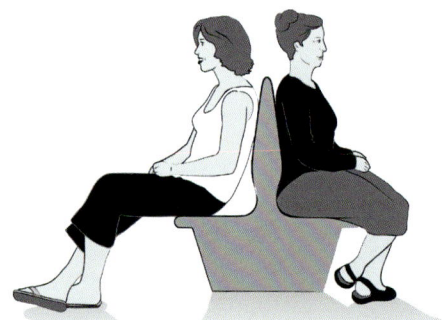

This sketch of passengers on a Portuguese barge shows a seat constructed when the average person had healthy posture—a "J" shaped spine. Notice how the older woman uses the seat to support a healthy pelvic position while the younger woman tucks her pelvis in spite of the favorable contours of the seat.

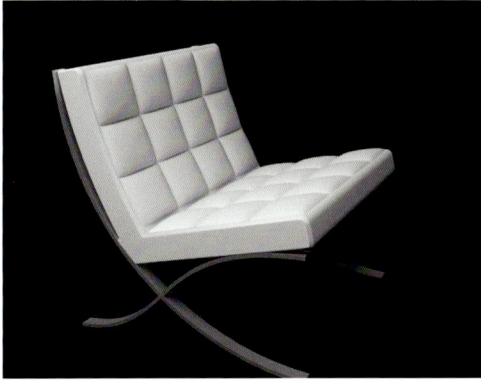

fig.F-20

The Mies van der Rohe Barcelona® Chair, first exhibited at the World Fair in Barcelona in 1929, reflects and perpetuates the trend of its day, forcing a tucked pelvis in the name of casual comfort.

THE EFFECT ON OUR BACKS

Whatever the cause, many of us are faced with the reality of a distorted and compressed spinal column. This may be fairly benign, but it usually gets worse over decades until the cumulative compression crosses a threshold. Beyond that threshold lies the potential for real damage to nerves, bones, and discs, with accompanying pain. Sometimes the pain does not arise directly from the damaged tissues, but rather from muscle spasms in the back that are a protective response to the worsening situation. Pain, whether from damage or muscle spasms, is what drives most people to seek relief. It is very likely why you are reading this book.

MOVING OUT OF MISERY

In your efforts to reduce or eliminate your back pain, you may have tried well-established interventions that physicians typically recommend: anti-inflammatories, muscle relaxants, physical therapy, injections, and even surgery. You may also have tried such alternative therapies as chiropractic, acupuncture, massage, yoga, or the host of specialized techniques popular today.

At last you have come to the right place! By reestablishing natural posture and movement patterns, you will be addressing the root cause of your pain, regaining and maintaining a pain-free back.

As you will discover, the Gokhale Method is quick to learn and effective from the beginning. Equipment can be as simple as a good chair, a few cushions, and good shoes. Once you have learned the key principles, the method puts almost no demands on your time. You integrate the basic principles into all your everyday positions and movements, and your physical activities become effective exercises to stretch and strengthen your body, rather than hurt it (fig.F-21).

fig.F-21

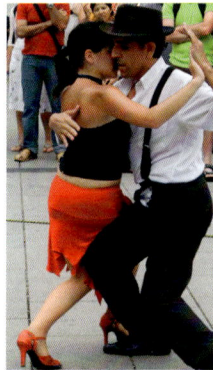

(Argentina)

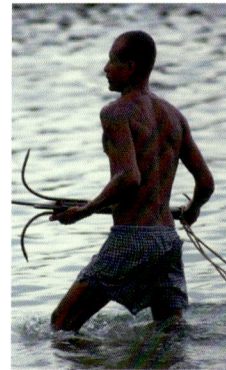

(Brazil)

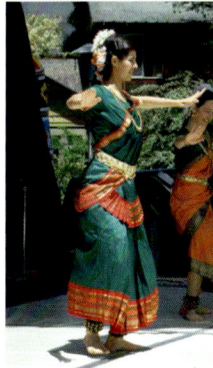

(USA)

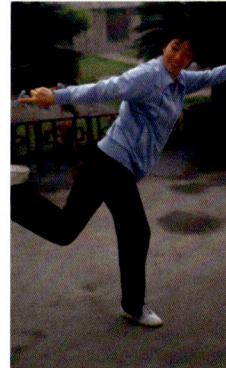

(China)

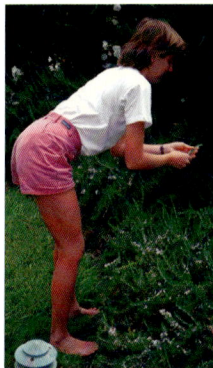

(USA)

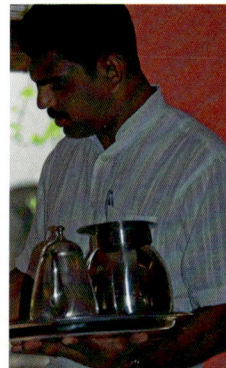

(India)

Everyday movements serve as therapeutic stretching or strengthening exercises.

As you learn the techniques in this book, you can also expect to:

- Reduce or eliminate other muscle and joint pain
- Prevent further muscle and joint degeneration and injury
- Increase your energy, stamina, and flexibility, and reduce stress
- Improve your appearance

HOW IT WORKS

You will learn to sit, sleep, stand, walk, and bend in ways that protect and strengthen your bones and muscles, in ways for which the body was designed.

- Sitting will be comfortable, either with a backrest when you place your back in therapeutic traction (stretchsitting) or without a backrest, when you stack your spine on a well-positioned, *anteverted* pelvis (stacksitting).
- Sleeping will be comfortable and provide hours of restorative traction, whether lying on your back or side (stretchlying).
- Standing will be a resting position for most of the muscles of the body with the weight-bearing bones vertically stacked over the heels (tallstanding).
- Bending will involve hinging at the hip rather than the waist, exercising the long back muscles and sparing the spinal discs and ligaments (hip-hinging).
- Actions that challenge spinal structures, such as carrying or twisting, will use particular muscles of the abdomen and back (inner corset) to protect the spine.
- Walking will be a series of smooth forward propulsions, challenging the muscles of the lower body and sparing the weight-bearing joints throughout the body (glidewalking).

In relearning these everyday actions, you will reposition and reshape your shoulders, arms, neck, torso, hips, legs, and feet the way they were designed to be. You will develop a high level of confidence in and sense of control over your well-being.

- Because of the emphasis on lengthening and decompressing the spine, you will remove some of the stresses that cause disc degeneration and certain arthritic changes.
- Because you will spend so many hours a day

decompressing your spine through gentle "traction," you may regain as much as an inch (2.5cm) in height.
- Because of the emphasis on correct stacking and alignment, you will increase the deposition of bone where needed and help to prevent osteoporosis.
- Because your muscles can relax at rest, your circulation will improve. This enables your system to efficiently nourish and heal your tissues and clear waste products.
- Because of altered alignment, your breathing mechanism will change, with more action in the rib cage. Over time, this enlarges the rib cage and allows for greater lung capacity, improved processing of oxygen, and extra energy.
- Because you are using your muscles and sparing your joints, you will be less prone to injury and joint degeneration.

WHAT DOES UNHEALTHY POSTURE LOOK LIKE?

Let's begin by training your eye to recognize the hallmarks of unhealthy versus healthy posture. Refer to fig.F-22 as you read the following description. The most common unhealthy posture traits include:
- a tucked pelvis
- an arched (or "*swayed*" or "*lordotic*") lower back
- a rounded (or "*kyphotic*") upper back and/or rounded shoulders and/or forward head
- a "C" shaped spine (rounded everywhere)
- internally rotated legs, usually accompanied by pathology including flat feet, bunions, and knock knees
- pelvis parked forward, usually accompanied by locked knees, locked groin, collapsed metatarsal arches, hammer toes, Morton's neuroma, and other foot pathology.

As a weekly air traveler who has tried cortisone shots, massage, acupuncture, and physical therapy, I had almost come to accept my constant back pain. [Now], my pain has almost completely disappeared. As an unexpected plus, strangers comment on my great posture.

Maggie Kuhlmann, Chicago, IL

fig.F-22

a.

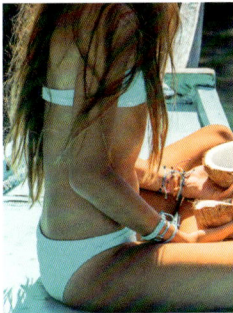

Pelvis tucked

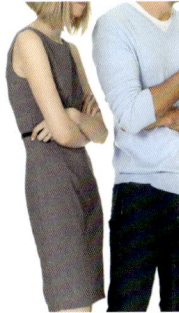

Pelvis tucked and spine "C" shaped

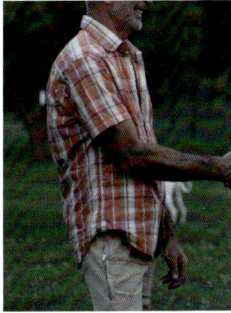

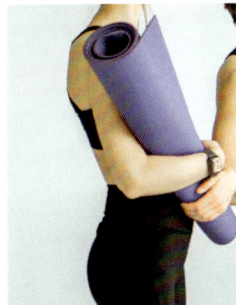

b.

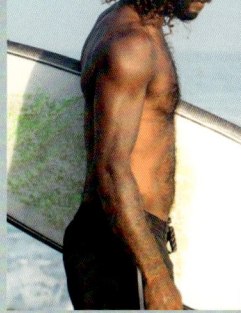

Pelvis not tucked and spine relatively straight

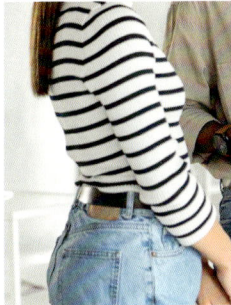

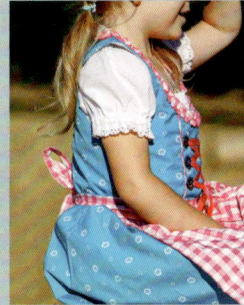

Lumbar spine swayed

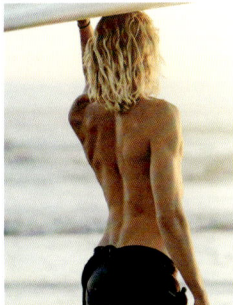

Lumbar spine relatively straight

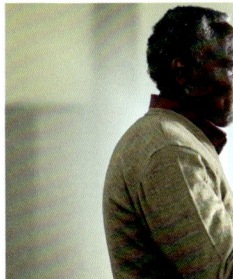

Rounded upper back and shoulders, forward head

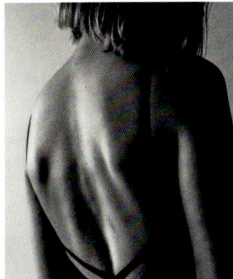

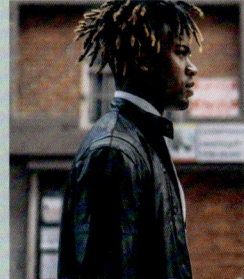

Upper back relatively straight, shoulders and head back

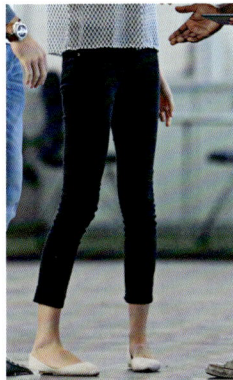

Internally rotated legs

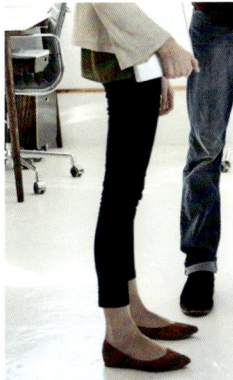

Pelvis parked forward, knees and groin locked

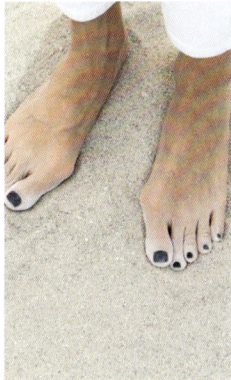

Flat feet, bunions

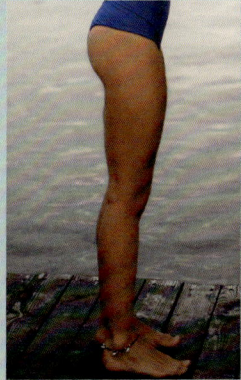

Pelvis stacked over heels, groin and knees soft

Note the differences between unhealthy postures (a) and healthy ones (b).

WHAT DOES HEALTHY POSTURE LOOK LIKE?

If you lived a hundred years ago or in a village in Southeast Asia or Africa today, you would have a good sense of what healthy posture looks like. Since you likely live in a modern industrialized society, and are surrounded by people who have poor posture, it is helpful to articulate some of the characteristics that constitute healthy posture. Refer to fig.F-23 and fig.F-24 as you read the following description.

The spine is "J" shaped.

The pelvis is tipped forward or *anteverted*. An easy way to see this is to imagine a belt line and notice that it angles downward toward the front. Pelvic anteversion is accompanied by a pronounced angle low in the spine (between the L5 vertebra and the sacrum), the *lumbosacral arch*. This is distinct from a swayback, in which an unhealthy lumbar curve occurs higher than at L5-S1.

There is an even groove over the vertical midline of the back. The groove is not especially deep in any location (for example, the lower back), nor are the vertebrae prominent in any location (for example, the upper back). The entire spine above the lumbosacral arch has relatively little curvature.

The shoulders are positioned posteriorly relative to the torso, with the result that the arms align with the back of the torso. The arms are somewhat externally rotated so that the thumbs, or even the palms, face forward.

The lower border of the rib cage does not protrude from, but rather is flush with, the abdominal contour. The front contour of the torso is dome-like and smooth. The chest is full with a raised sternum as a result of the chest expanding with every breath.

There is a soft angle at the groin between the front of the torso and the legs that permits the femoral arteries, veins, and nerves, and *lymphatic vessels* to function without compromise.

The chin rests downward and the cervical spine is elongated as a result of relaxed muscles at the back of the neck.

The buttock muscles are well developed because they are in a position of mechanical advantage and are used in walking.

The muscles throughout the body have a healthy amount of tone rather than being flaccid or bunched up with long taut tendons.

The main weight-bearing bones in the body are vertically aligned over the heels.

The feet point 10–15 degrees outwards and the arches of the foot are muscular and pronounced.

fig.F-23

© Gerard Mackworth-Young

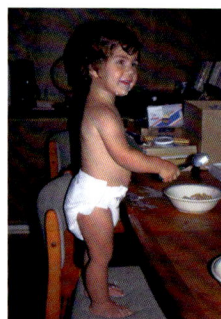

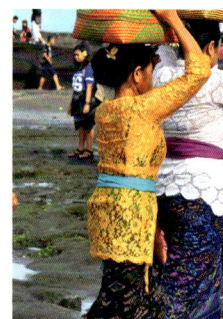

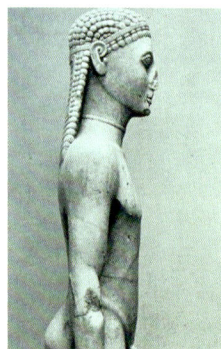

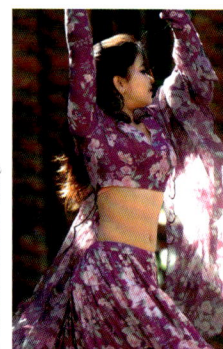

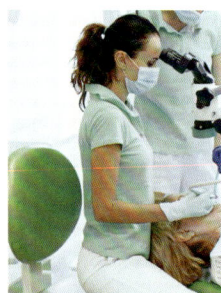

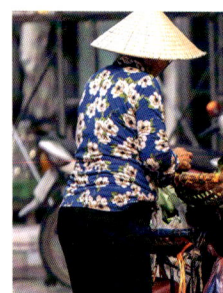

In these images, notice the pronounced lumbosacral angle and the relatively flat upper lumbar spine, the chin angled down, the posterior shoulders, the lower border of the rib cage flush with the contour of the abdomen, and the soft angle at the groin. The image of my one-year-old daughter shows the vertebrae and leg bones stacked over the heels.

fig.F-24

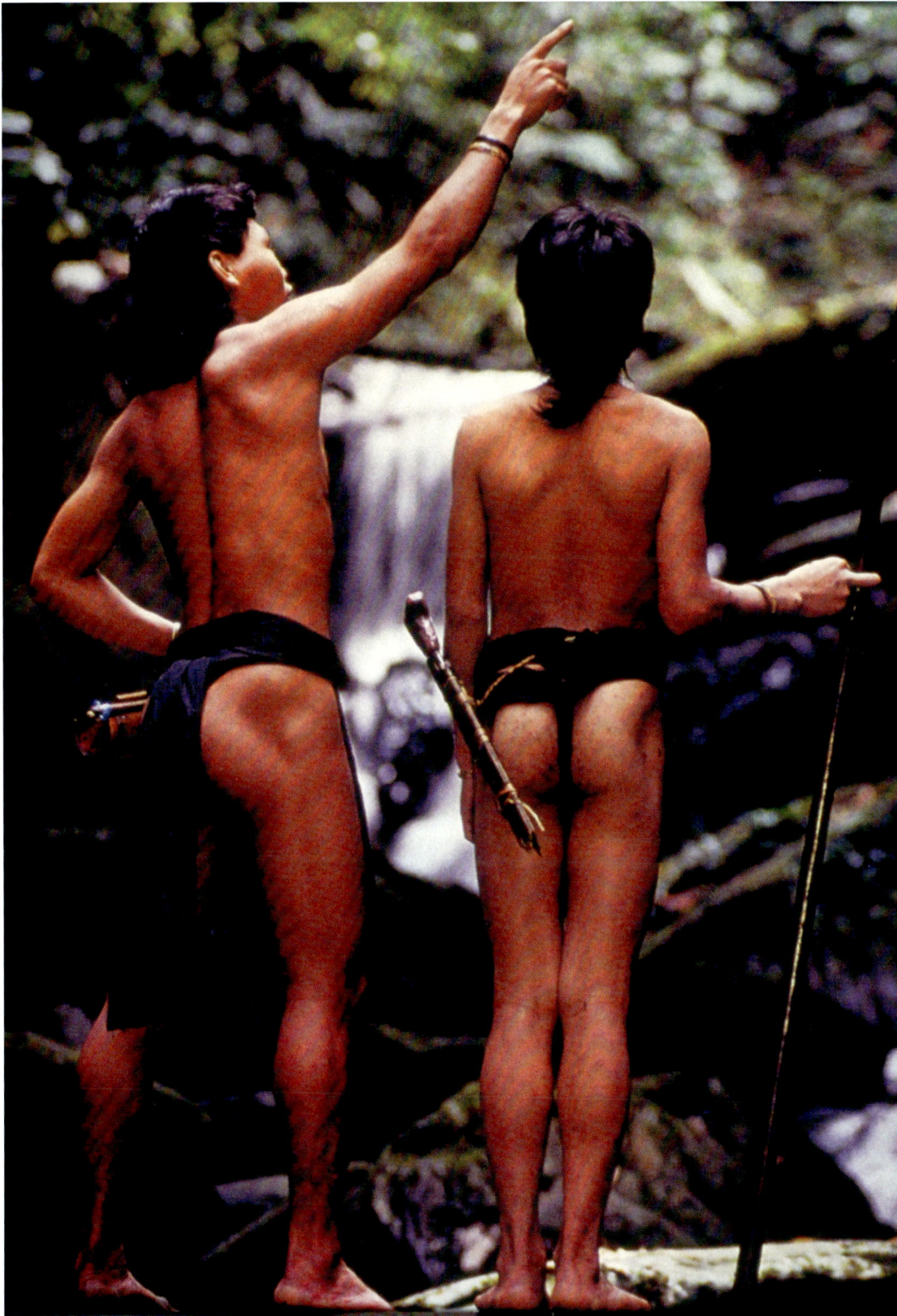

This duo of Ubong tribesmen was photographed by Ian Mackenzie (published in Nomads of the Dawn*).*
He generously agreed to let me use the photograph which, more than any other, lives in my mind's eye and reminds
me of the beauty, strength, and grace that is natural to our species. Notice that the buttocks are positioned well
behind the spine and are well-developed, the shoulder blades are also positioned behind the spine, the groove over
the midline of the back is even, the feet point slightly outward and have well-developed arches, and the muscles in
general are toned but not taut.

19

ANTEVERTED PELVIS

Pelvic anteversion is the foundation of a healthy human frame, affecting the placement of every other part of the body.

Today, many medical and fitness experts advise a "neutral" pelvic position.[43,44] Compared to a J-spine pelvis, the "neutral" pelvis is tucked or *retroverted*. A retroverted pelvis leads you into one of two postures: upright but tense (in the back muscles); or relaxed but slumped (fig.F-25a,b). Neither of these postures is healthy; both cause damage.

In this book, you will learn how to position your pelvis in the natural way seen in babies, indigenous peoples, and your ancestors. This ideal, anteverted position includes a significant lumbosacral angle (between L5 and S1) created by a forward rotation of the pelvis and a relatively straight upper lumbar spine (fig.F-25c). (Note, "ante" means "forward" and "vertere" means "rotated" in Latin.)

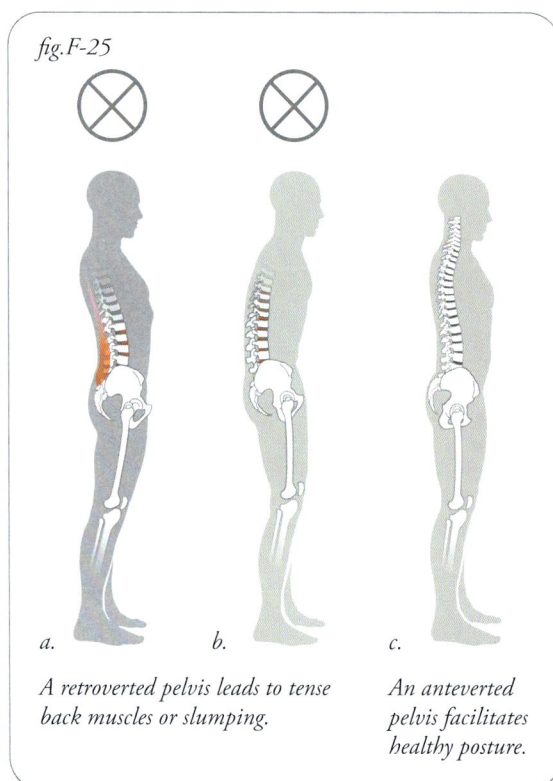

fig.F-25

a.   *b.*   *c.*

A retroverted pelvis leads to tense back muscles or slumping.

An anteverted pelvis facilitates healthy posture.

Now I know how to protect the spine, stand tall, and even stretch the spine while I am sleeping!

Ellen Anderson, Atlanta, GA

An anteverted pelvis allows for natural stacking of the vertebrae and an upright posture that does not require muscle strain. Anteversion also allows for healthy alignment of the spine over the leg bones in standing and walking and puts the buttock muscles in a position of mechanical advantage. In this way, the weight-bearing bones in the body get the healthy level of stress they need to prevent osteoporosis and not the unhealthy stress they don't need that creates osteoarthritis. Since the hamstring muscles attach to the sitz bones (*ischial tuberosities*), an anteverted pelvis also maintains a healthy baseline length in these muscles; a retroverted pelvis permits the hamstring muscles to adapt to a shorter-than-normal resting length, increasing their susceptibility to injury.

The natural amount of anteversion is something that varies by race, family, and—most importantly—by individual. It is a mistake to try to copy someone else's baseline lumbosacral angle. Students of the Gokhale Method discover by degrees over time what their natural lumbosacral angle is through techniques including stretchlying on the side and stacksitting.

Note that an anteverted pelvis is different from a "forward pelvis" or a pelvis with "anterior pelvic tilt." These names are typically used to describe the angle of the pelvis relative to the ground, without any heed paid to where the curve in the lumbar spine occurs. This confusing nomenclature, and the biomechanical philosophies that use it, makes no distinction between a healthy curve (occurring at L5-S1) and unhealthy curves (occurring higher in the lumbar spine). The usual recommended fix for "forward pelvis" is to tuck the pelvis; this causes a problem, even if there wasn't one to begin with.

One difference between bipedal mammals (that would be us humans!) and quadrupedal mammals is that our L5-S1 disc is wedge-shaped. An anteverted pelvis preserves the wedge-shaped space that accommodates the L5-S1 disc perfectly (fig.F-26a). Retroverting or "tucking" the pelvis compresses the anterior part of this wedge-shaped disc. The contents of the disc are forced posteriorly (fig.F-26b). Over time, this compression can lead to degeneration of the fibrous exterior of the L5-S1 disc, with damage ranging from *bulging* to *herniation* to *sequestration*. Since the nerve roots at this level contribute to the sciatic nerve, disc-related impingement here is a common cause of sciatica.

In addition to affecting the bones, spinal discs, and muscles, the position of the pelvis also affects the pelvic organs. An anteverted pelvis allows for ample space in the pelvic cavity and optimal circulation in the pelvic organs; a retroverted pelvis compresses the pelvic organs into an unnaturally small space, compromising their shape, orientation, and function. On learning to antevert their pelvis, many of my students report improvement in conditions such as irritable bowel syndrome and constipation, menstrual irregularities like painful cramps and bloating, prostate problems, and fertility issues. I look forward to research studies done in these areas.

An anteverted pelvis places the pubic bone and supportive connective tissues in an ideal configuration under the pelvic organs; a retroverted pelvis leaves much of the support of the pelvic organs to the relatively flimsy "Kegel" (*pubococcygeus*) muscles (fig.3-9 on page 73). In my clinical experience, a tucked (retroverted) pelvis predisposes for organ prolapse and urinary incontinence; restoring pelvic anteversion helps with these conditions if they are not too advanced. Again, a research study in this area would be valuable.

ANCHORED RIB CAGE

It is common for people in modern industrialized cultures to arch the lumbar region of their spine (fig.F-27a). In such a "swayback," the rib cage (which is attached to the thoracic spine) is pulled into a backwards lean; the lower front border of the rib cage flares out beyond the contour of the abdomen. With a well-aligned lumbar spine, the lower front border of the rib cage is flush with the abdomen, rather than jutting out (fig.F-27b).

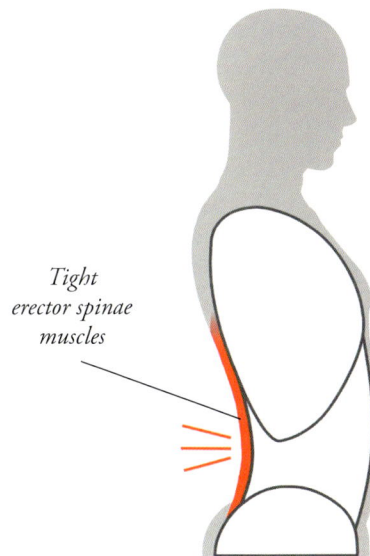

fig.F-27

Tight erector spinae muscles

a.

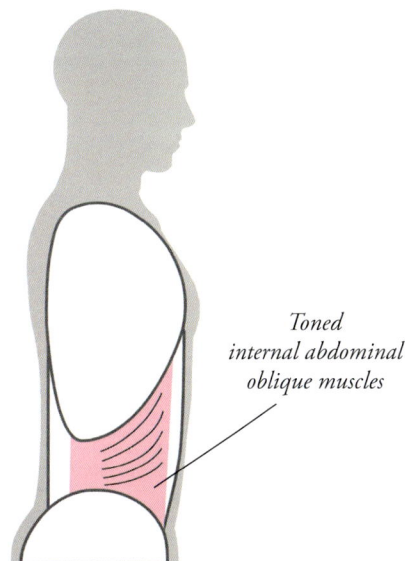

Toned internal abdominal oblique muscles

b.

With a swayed back, the lower back muscles are tight and the front lower border of the rib cage is flared outwards (a). In a J-spine, the lower back muscles are relaxed and healthy tone in the abdominal muscles holds the front lower border of the rib cage flush with the abdomen (b).

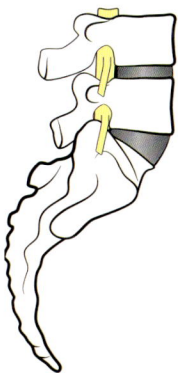

fig.F-26

a. An anteverted pelvis preserves the wedge-shaped L5-S1 disc.

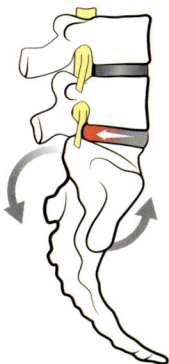

b. A retroverted pelvis can cause the L5-S1 disc to bulge, herniate, or sequestrate posteriorly, potentially causing sciatic pain.

A swayback may help people feel and appear upright but is actually an unhealthy compensation for rounding in the thoracic spine (kyphosis) and forward head and shoulders. The two wrongs don't make a right. A swayback involves chronic contraction of the erector spinae muscles, resulting in compressed spinal discs, nerves, and vertebral edges (fig.F-28a).

In this book, you will learn to draw the front of the rib cage downwards using deep layers of muscle in the abdominal wall (mainly the *internal abdominal oblique* muscles). We call this technique "rib anchor." As the lower front border of the rib cage rotates inward and downward relative to the torso, the lower back border of the ribcage moves upward and outward. Since the back of the ribs attach to the thoracic vertebrae, the vertebrae are pulled upward too, straightening out and lengthening the often curvy "necklace" of lumbar vertebrae.

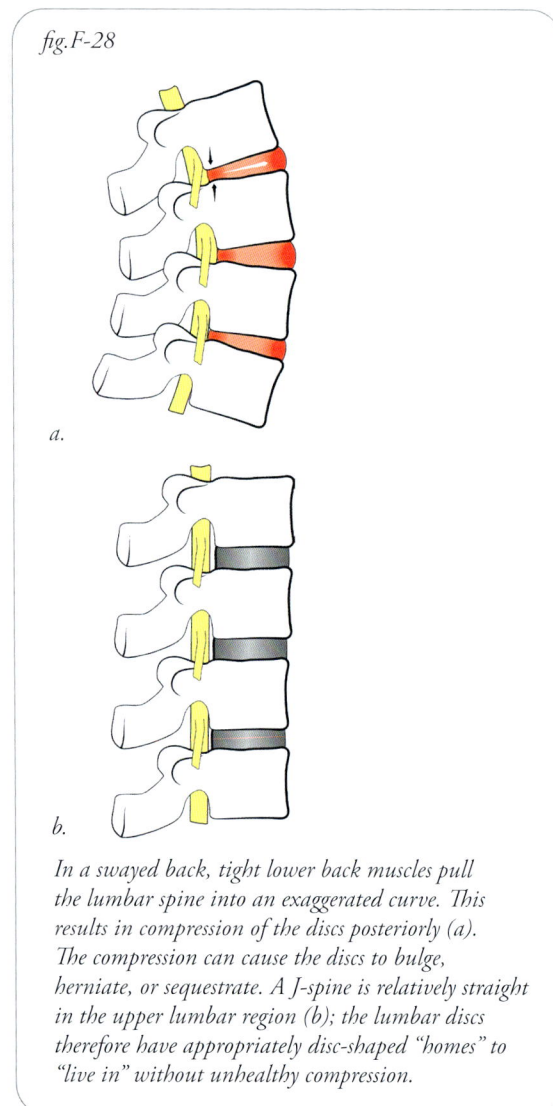

fig.F-28

a.

b.

In a swayed back, tight lower back muscles pull the lumbar spine into an exaggerated curve. This results in compression of the discs posteriorly (a). The compression can cause the discs to bulge, herniate, or sequestrate. A J-spine is relatively straight in the upper lumbar region (b); the lumbar discs therefore have appropriately disc-shaped "homes" to "live in" without unhealthy compression.

This lengthening decompresses the lumbar discs and nerves (fig.F-28b), and stretches the erector spinae muscles. It also has a positive effect on the position of the upper spine, shoulders, and head. Over time, you will develop a healthy baseline tone in your abdominal muscles and healthy baseline length in your erector spinae muscles. Your rib cage will then settle in this healthy position without effort.

AN ELONGATED "J" SHAPED SPINE
The ideal shape of the spine is a gentle, elongated curve, not an exaggerated "S" curve. Pronounced curvature should occur only at L5-S1 at the base of the spine.

In current lay and medical thinking, a normal spine curves significantly forward in the lower back (lumbar spine), backward in the upper back (thoracic spine) and forward again in the neck (cervical spine). "Chin up and chest out," a directive many people follow when trying to have "good posture," results in exaggerated spinal curves. A lot of modern furniture and clothing reflects and perpetuates exaggerated spinal curvature. Lumbar cushions and cervical pillows, for example, are designed to support and even create these "natural" curves.

Medical research, on the other hand, establishes that reducing spinal curvature can alleviate compression, reduce pain, and increase comfort.[45,46] Though most research on curvature in the lumbar area does not distinguish between lower and upper lumbar curvature, one paper reports on the radiographic examinations of upper and lower lumbar curvature in subjects with and without lower back pain. The results are consistent with my claims: the back pain patients had more upper lumbar curvature and less lower lumbar curvature, whereas the subjects without pain had more lower lumbar curvature and less upper.[47]

TRAINING YOUR EYE
Now that you know the basics of healthy versus unhealthy posture, you can hone your skills through observation. People-watching is a great way to train your eye to recognize posture features. Do your best to judge whether the people pictured in fig.F-29 have healthy or unhealthy posture (or a combination) before reading the captions.

fig. F-29

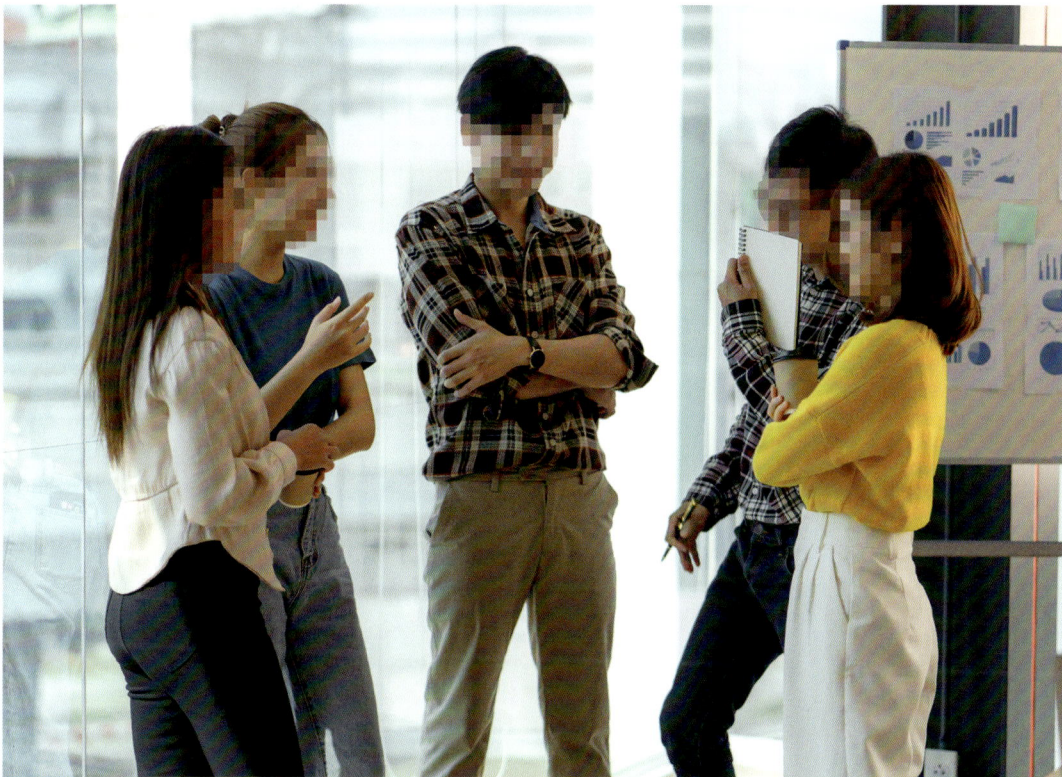

The woman on the left has healthy posture, with a J-spine and posterior shoulders. The others show less desirable posture: forward head (woman in blue), pelvis parked forward (man in center), and swayed lower back (woman in yellow).

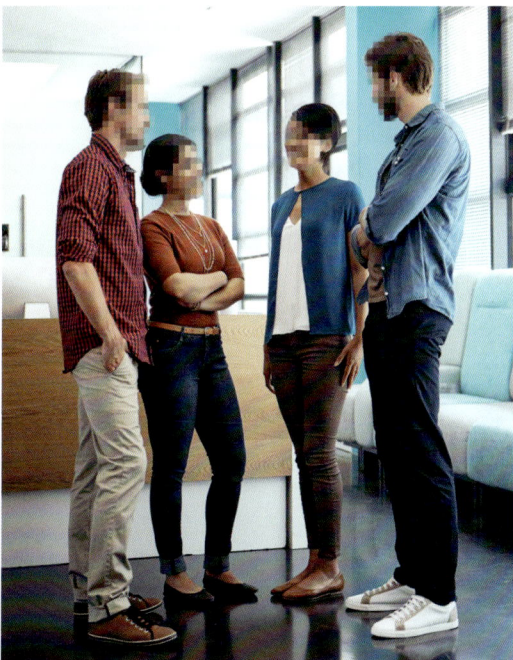

The man on the left has healthy posture, with a J-spine, posterior shoulders, and weight stacked over his left heel. The others show less desirable posture: the woman on the left is slightly swayed; the woman on the right has forward head and internally rotated legs; the man on the right has a rounded upper back, forward head, his pelvis is tucked and parked forward, and his lower back is swayed.

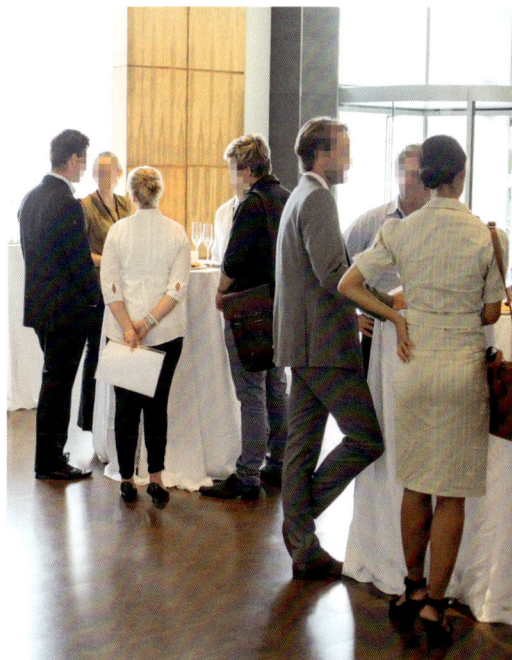

The woman on the right has healthy posture, with a J-spine, posterior shoulders, and externally rotated legs. Each of the other people have "forward head," pelvis parked forward, swayed lower back, rounded shoulders, and locked knees.

EVERY BONE IN ITS NATURAL PLACE

The particular arrangement of the human skeleton is a product of the demands of upright living and the constant force of gravity over the span of human existence. Each bone has a natural place relative to its neighbors. Adjacent bones are designed to fit together in a certain way.

Our weight-bearing bones need stress to remain strong. Without this stress, calcium leaches from the bones or is inadequately deposited, leading to osteopenia and osteoporosis. Weight-bearing exercise provides the healthy stress that keeps bones strong. However, stress on the wrong part of the bone, caused by misalignment, can lead to arthritic changes such as bone spurs (*osteophytes*). In this book, you will learn how to restore your bones to their proper places, reducing harmful stress while restoring healthy stress in the bones.

Our spines are not the only bony structures that suffer from misalignment. Our feet, knees, and hips are also subject to problems from poor alignment.

Foot problems

When we evolved from being quadrupedal to bipedal, the heel became reinforced to bear most of the weight of our upright structure. By comparison, the bones in the front of the foot are delicate. Today, instead of carrying most of the weight on their heels, many people displace their weight forward to the middle or front of the foot, putting undue stress on bones that are not designed to bear such weight. Doing so increases the chances of having bunions, sesamoid bone fractures, and plantar fasciitis.

Knee problems

Rotating the knees inward, a common problem, correlates with pronation of the foot and under-use of the buttock muscles. If the legs are misaligned as they bear the body's weight, they are subject to increased wear and tear, especially when bending, and make the knee joint more prone to injury. Rotating the knees inward increases the chances of torn ligaments, frayed menisci, and arthritic changes in the knee.

Another common knee problem is hyperextension or "locking the knees," a classic element of unhealthy posture, causing muscles to be tense and inhibiting good circulation. Locked knees are usually accompanied by improper hip position, which has its own set of problems.

Hip problems

In our culture it is rare to find good alignment in the hip joint. People tend to "park" their hips forward, significantly misaligning the head of the femur in the hip socket (*acetabulum*). The muscles that bridge the area become tense in this misalignment. This tension reduces the natural gap between the ball and socket and can result in bone-to-bone contact. Over time, the unnatural stresses can lead to arthritic changes and possibly even the need for hip replacement surgery. Hip misalignment can also occlude the femoral arteries, veins, and nerves, affecting circulation to and from the legs and feet. Symptoms of this condition include cold feet, Raynaud's Syndrome, and slowed healing of leg injuries. In "Tallstanding" (Chapter 6), you will learn the natural alignment of your pelvis on the heads of the femurs. In "Glidewalking" (Chapter 8), you will learn to reestablish the natural gap between the head of the femur and the hip socket.

USE THE MUSCLES, SPARE THE JOINTS

In many daily activities, people underuse their muscles and overload their joints. This has a doubly negative effect: muscles do not get enough healthy stress to remain strong; joints get too much stress, leading to wear and tear. For example, walking poorly, as most people do, is hard on the weight-bearing joints of the knees, hips, and spine, and jolts the frame with every step. It may also leave the buttock and leg muscles underused. As you will learn in this book, walking well uses muscles in the legs and buttocks to propel the body forward smoothly to a soft landing, sparing the joints from the stress of significant impact. The muscles gain strength; the joints remain undamaged.

You will also learn how to bend in a way that uses your muscles more and your joints less. Rounding the back to bend is hard on the spinal discs and ligaments, and leaves the muscles of the back largely unchallenged. On the other hand, bending with a straight back engages the long muscles of the back and spares the spinal discs and ligaments. Again, muscles gain strength while joints remain healthy.

In Chapter 5, you will learn to use your "inner corset" in the face of threatened spinal compression or distortion. Again, this is a technique that takes the burden off the joints (the spinal discs), where it would be harmful, and puts it on the muscles (abdominal and intrinsic back muscles), where it is beneficial.

MUSCLES FULLY RELAXED WHEN NOT WORKING

When something goes wrong with our musculoskeletal systems, we are often directed to muscle-strengthening exercises as a solution (as in most physical therapy regimens). While we are keenly aware of the need for muscle strength, we may not adequately appreciate the importance of muscle relaxation.

To maintain strength, a muscle must be allowed to relax. Thorough muscle relaxation facilitates good circulation, delivering nutrients and clearing waste products. Many people spend hours tensing their muscles unnecessarily. Often the tension is initiated through poor alignment; then it becomes habit. Reorganizing skeletal structures can break the cycle, enabling muscles to be relaxed when appropriate and to be tense only when needed.

BREATHING AS A THERAPEUTIC EXERCISE

Breathing does more than oxygenate the system. The physical action of breathing has its own therapeutic value: it exercises the key tissues of the chest and spinal area, keeping the area well circulated and healthy. Breathing is nature's way of exercising the area around your spine even when you are not engaged in aerobic activity. The natural elastic movement associated with the breath includes mild lengthenings and settlings of parts of the spine with every inhalation and exhalation, and provides a gentle massage-like action that stimulates good circulation to support healthy tissues 24 hours a day.

As your vertebrae become better stacked, the muscles around your spine will relax, which will facilitate the elastic action of breathing. In general, you will find that as your posture improves, all your muscles of respiration will both engage and relax more appropriately, and your lung capacity will increase.

Instead of getting weaker as I've gotten older, I've experienced surprising strength, flexibility, and balance. Whenever the inevitable happens, and I bend or lift or sit or move in a way that tweaks a muscle or joint, I have the tools to recover using Gokhale principles that have become a way of life. For several years now, I've made it a priority to attend the daily online offerings [Gokhale Active]. The lovely community of participants and teachers from around the world provides a warm and enjoyable environment in which to hone my J-spine. I'm deeply grateful to Esther for making the fundamentals of good posture and movement so accessible, and for infusing this work with such contagious joy.

Jean Weininger, Ph.D., Berkeley, CA

I have significant structural problems with my spine (scoliosis, spondylolisthesis, degenerative disc disease, facet arthritis, spinal stenosis, and rotation of the spine). I recently received an outstanding report from my doctor (an osteopathic physician). It was the first good news I have had regarding my spine in a very long time. After a year when I was unable to see him for routine visits and manipulation, he informed me that I had changed the architecture of my spine! Specifically, he told me three things: that I had improved my lumbar lordosis; corrected the angle of my pelvis; and my leg length discrepancy was gone (it had been 3/8 inch, requiring modification of my extensive shoe wardrobe, including my ballroom dancing shoes and ski boots!). I attribute this dramatic change to working with the Gokhale Method techniques.

Mary Rajala, M.D., Green Bay, WI

ORIENTATION

How to use this book

My ex-husband had hunched posture as a teenager and into his twenties. He developed an interest in my work and attended classes occasionally over the years, resulting in some profound changes in his appearance and muscle health. On the left he is 28 years old; on the right he is 48.

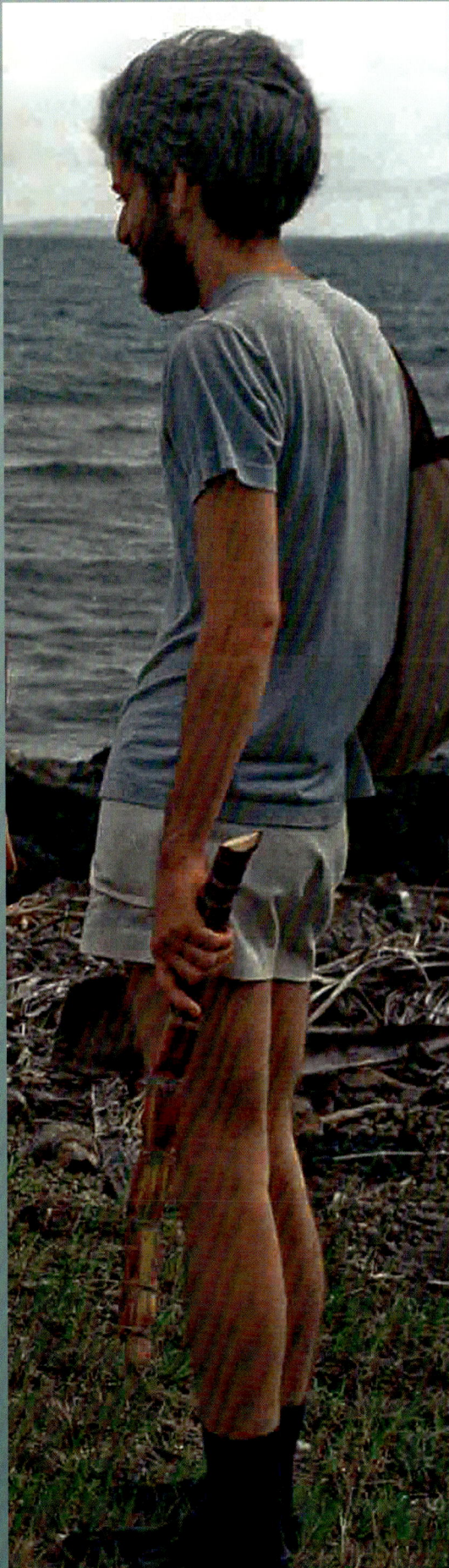
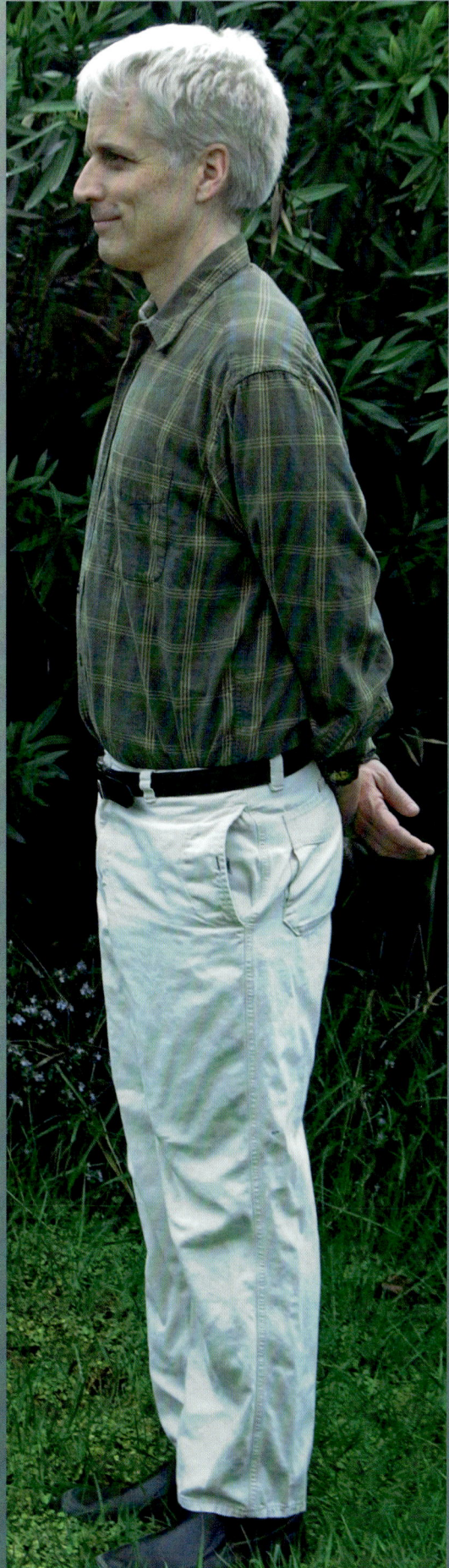

This book is intended to start you off on your Gokhale Method journey. By following the chapters, you will gain a foundational knowledge of the principles of healthy posture. The chapters combine background information, supporting visuals, and precise step-by-step instructions. Just as a travel guide can lead you safely through the byways of a foreign city to introduce new sights and sounds, this book can guide you safely through the route to acquire improved, more healthful posture and ways of moving.

FOLLOW THE CHAPTER SEQUENCE

People new to the Gokhale Method may feel impatient to skip or hurry through some chapters and proceed to those that seem to address their area of concern. Based on my experience teaching this technique for 30 years, I encourage you to follow the chapters in sequence. By doing this, you will:

- Realize substantial postural improvement with the very first chapter, easing the pain and discomfort you may be experiencing.
- Learn to support and protect delicate structures, ensuring that you can learn each technique safely.
- Build skills in early chapters that are used in later ones, reducing the effort required to master the more complex skills.

I encourage you to trust that the seemingly disparate parts within and across chapters will soon connect. Performing an architectural remodel of your frame is much like working a puzzle: most of the time, you work on isolated areas, not necessarily seeing how they will later fit together. For example, for most people it is not apparent that working on foot position will help resolve back pain. Because it is important occasionally to see the big picture, I have included explanations with each chapter to help provide that overview.

Some situations require that you modify your route through this material. The following are exceptions to the recommendation that you complete the chapters in sequence.

HERNIATED DISC
Caution:
If you have a diagnosis, or any suspicion, of a herniated disc in the lower lumbar area (L5-S1), you should be working with a medical professional as you learn the techniques in this book. It is extremely important that you not proceed to Chapters 3 (Stacksitting), 4 (Stretchlying on Your Side), and 7 (Hip-hinging) until you have mastered the ability to maintain extra length at the site of the injury. Gaining additional length in the back is therapeutic and safe for everyone. Chapters 1, 2, and 5 teach you to lengthen your spine, which will make you more comfortable and can accelerate healing of the injured disc. The recommended chapter sequence, then, is 1, 2, 5, 6, 8, 3, 4, 7. From the exercises in Appendix 1, focus especially on those that strengthen the muscles of the torso.

HIGH IMPACT ACTIVITIES
Activities that involve high impact (such as running or impact aerobics), if done incorrectly, carry a significant risk of damage to spinal discs. If you participate in such activities, you may want to begin immediately to protect your back. I recommend you read over Chapter 5 (Using Your Inner Corset). You will gain insights that have immediate value, although you will understand them better after having completed Chapters 1–4.

BENDING ACTIVITIES
If your everyday activities involve a lot of bending (for example, gardening), be aware that, of all actions, bending technique correlates most closely with back health. People who bend well usually enjoy good back health; people who bend poorly often develop back pain. If currently you have no back pain, read Chapter 7 (Hip-hinging) to begin exploring a better way to bend. (Stop if you experience any discomfort.) Then proceed through the chapters in their normal sequence. When you encounter the bending chapter a second time, you will refine your technique and transform your bending activities into healthy exercise.

ALLOW TIME TO CHANGE

People often ask how long it will take to learn this approach. There is no pat answer to that question.

Changing the way we move requires repatterning the brain, as it discards an old set of habits and replaces it with a new one. We need to "rewire" how we sit, lie, stand, and move, changing these basic movements. People learn and integrate our techniques at different speeds.

In general, a person who is engaged in a variety of physical activities and sports tends to readily absorb new kinesthetic input. Yet sometimes very sedentary people surprise me with their kinesthetic acuity for this particular training. These people may experience quick success because the training is so basic. And sometimes a person with extensive physical training must work hard to unlearn certain ingrained ways. However, most people are pleasantly surprised at how quickly they learn the techniques. Perhaps it is because they are returning to a more natural way of moving, one that was familiar to them in their early years. As they relearn these forgotten habits, the "new" ways of sitting, lying, and moving become natural and automatic.

As with any physical transition, you might experience some initial difficulty. While you are learning a new posture or way of moving, be sure to explore the change gradually. Don't force your body to achieve the ideal result immediately, as that may strain your muscles. Instead, let your body gradually adapt to the ideal over time.

Common wisdom holds that you must repeat an action at least 20 times for it to become habit. Be patient as you work to integrate the techniques into your daily movements. You will create these new habits more from a sustained awareness over time than from an infrequent but heroic effort. The only requirement is that you not let your awareness slip away.

KNOW WHAT TO EXPECT

HOW QUICKLY CAN I EXPECT RESULTS?
Most people enjoy immediate benefits from the very first chapter, in which they learn the technique of "stretchsitting" to lengthen the spine. Not only is this the safest posture modification for a compromised spine, it also is simple to understand and easy to execute. Some of the subsequent chapters may take a bit longer, but should provide tangible benefits.

The method blends intellectual, visual, and kinesthetic cues. As you learn each new postural shift, you will simultaneously understand it, see it, and feel it. Because the learning occurs on three levels, it accelerates and deepens the process of turning these shifts into new habits.

HOW LONG SHOULD EACH CHAPTER TAKE?
Hurrying through the chapters offers no advantage and, in fact, reduces your chances of success. You should expect to spend 30 to 45 minutes on each new chapter. Subsequently, as you integrate the material into your daily activities, it will take at first a few minutes, and later a few seconds, each time. For example, when you first seat yourself at your desk or in your car, you should take some time to concentrate on the fine points of positioning yourself well. Then forget about your posture and enjoy a period of relaxation, allowing your body to gain muscle memory from this pose.

Allow enough time between chapters that you can incorporate your new learning into your everyday life, as your brain repatterns each new physical skill. That said, as with language learning, it's ok to move on to a subsequent technique without having fully mastered a previous technique.

HOW DIFFICULT ARE THE TECHNIQUES?
Although the steps in each chapter are simple, they are not necessarily easy. Certain steps tend to be difficult for everybody; other steps are easy for some people and hard for others. Sometimes the difficulties are caused by physical limitations associated with age, pathology, or obesity. Sometimes the necessary repatterning in the brain is extensive and therefore challenging. During the repatterning, a particular position or movement will likely feel peculiar because it is not yet habitual. The brain needs time to adjust to the "new normal."

Learning new movement patterns is similar to learning a new language, which ideally alternates periods of immersion and usage with periods of attention to detail. In learning the language of movement, you will benefit from a mix of focusing on large-scale movements and on finer points. And don't expect to become fluent overnight!

UNDERSTAND HOW THE CHAPTERS ARE ORGANIZED

Each chapter is organized into three sections:
- An introduction provides background and discusses the importance of the posture or movement, describes its benefits, and includes specific caveats where necessary.
- Instructions provide detailed step-by-step instructions with accompanying photographs. Photographs marked with an ⊗ show what not to do. Page sidebars include lists of required equipment, anatomical drawings, schematics to help you understand the material, and photos of good technique to inspire you.
- Wrap-up includes indications of improvement, troubleshooting, further information, and a recap.

RECOGNIZE YOUR PROGRESS

When learning any new skill, you will move through four stages of mastery. As you are working on a new posture or movement, try to recognize the stage you are in.

STAGE 1
UNDERSTANDING THE MOVEMENTS INTELLECTUALLY
Each chapter teaches a posture or movement through discussion and demonstration. By carefully reading and studying the material, you should be able to achieve Stage 1.

STAGE 2
PERFORMING THE MOVEMENTS WITH GUIDANCE
Using each chapter as your guide, you should be able to imitate the posture or movement. Remember that you may be unable to achieve the ideal result at first, but you can work towards it.

STAGE 3
PERFORMING THE MOVEMENTS WITHOUT GUIDANCE
Stage 3 is the ability to step yourself through the process of sitting, lying, or moving without referring to the book. You should be able to remember the steps to position your body appropriately.

STAGE 4
PERFORMING THE MOVEMENTS WITHOUT CONSCIOUS THOUGHT
This is, of course, the goal of your training, and may take some time. Regular practice (Stage 3) is the secret to reaching this stage. Eventually, you will have moments of awareness when you realize you are indeed using the technique but have not used conscious thought to do so.

GENERAL HEALTH IMPROVEMENT
In addition to reducing or eliminating back pain, most students experience other health improvements. These may be physical, physiological, or psychological. Students over the years have reported improvements in muscle and joint problems, sleep, digestion, respiration, menstrual ease, urinary function, sex drive, mood, energy level, self-esteem, and athletic performance.

PHOTOS
Consider asking someone to take photos of you in various positions and angles—sitting, standing, bending, etc.—so you have a baseline to compare your progress with.

> At age 72, I was wondering how well I would be able to enjoy gardening in my retirement. Arthritis caused pain in my neck, back, and hands and both hips had already been replaced. I was horrified when a friend emailed me a recent photograph of myself revealing a very hunched back. That is when I resolved to do something to improve my posture. On the surface, the concepts of the Gokhale Method may seem simple. However, they have profoundly affected my awareness of my posture and given me the tools to dramatically improve it. My back pain has diminished and I feel confident that I will be able to enjoy a very active and happy retirement.
>
> Linda Grass, Sherwood, Oregon

30

BARRIERS TO SUCCESS

MUSCLE SORENESS

Be aware that you might experience some muscle soreness as you transform your posture. Underused muscles may complain at their new, more demanding role. Surprisingly, overused muscles that now relax may also cause some discomfort, due to the release of lactic acid into the surrounding tissue. In both cases, this soreness is temporary and can be relieved by hot baths, massage, rest, or acupuncture. Take a little more time with the lessons, be careful as you practice new techniques, and soon the soreness will pass.

"IT FEELS WEIRD"

At first, you may feel awkward in these new poses and movements. Some people describe this feeling as "weird but comfortable." As the strangeness diminishes, many people report that the new ways now feel "right"; the old ways of moving no longer feel comfortable. What they are feeling is valid, in two senses. They are returning to kinesthetic ways that are genetically encoded, and that were natural in their early years before they learned our culture's bad habits.

"IT STILL HURTS"

The techniques won't work if you just go through the chapters and forget about them. You need to apply what you learn to your everyday life and everyday movements. If you simply complete the chapters, but don't work to integrate what you've learned, you will easily slip back into your old habits—the ones that caused much of your back pain.

"MY CLOTHES DON'T FIT"

It would be unfair not to mention the only downside to learning this method: over time your body shape may change enough that your more tailored clothing no longer fits. Current fashions are cut for today's average posture, which includes rounded shoulders and a tucked pelvis. Your new carriage may require you to alter or replace some of your fitted clothing. However, this seems a small price to pay for your improved health and appearance.

BACKSLIDING

Whenever you learn something new, there is a tendency to backslide to your old habits. In this case, the tendency is aggravated because you are surrounded by people with poor posture. We are natural mimics and unconsciously replicate the posture and movements we see. Therefore, after studying the techniques in this book, most people find it helpful to refresh their learning. Here are some suggestions:

- Review the techniques you found most transforming, or the ones that gave you the most trouble.
- Tour a museum to observe and critique how artists have rendered human posture.
- Observe a culture with intact posture traditions.
- Do something that reinforces the technique you have learned, such as taking yoga or dance classes taught by an informed instructor, or practicing a sport with an informed coach. (Posture and movement training is not a substitute for physical activity; I encourage you to pursue your favorite activities and incorporate the principles in this book.)
- Communicate with other people working on their posture.

All of these are incorporated into our online Gokhale Active offering (visit gokhalemethod.com for more information).

GOKHALE

ACTIVE

The Gokhale Method has led me not only to reduced pain, but also a much greater awareness of how posture and body movement can either reduce or increase pain. One of the best features of the method for me, is that Gokhale is not a workout or therapy session. It is proper standing, sitting, bending, and even sleeping, which is incorporated into the whole day.

Sarah Doyi, Cowen, TN

1
STRETCHSITTING

Sitting with a lengthened back

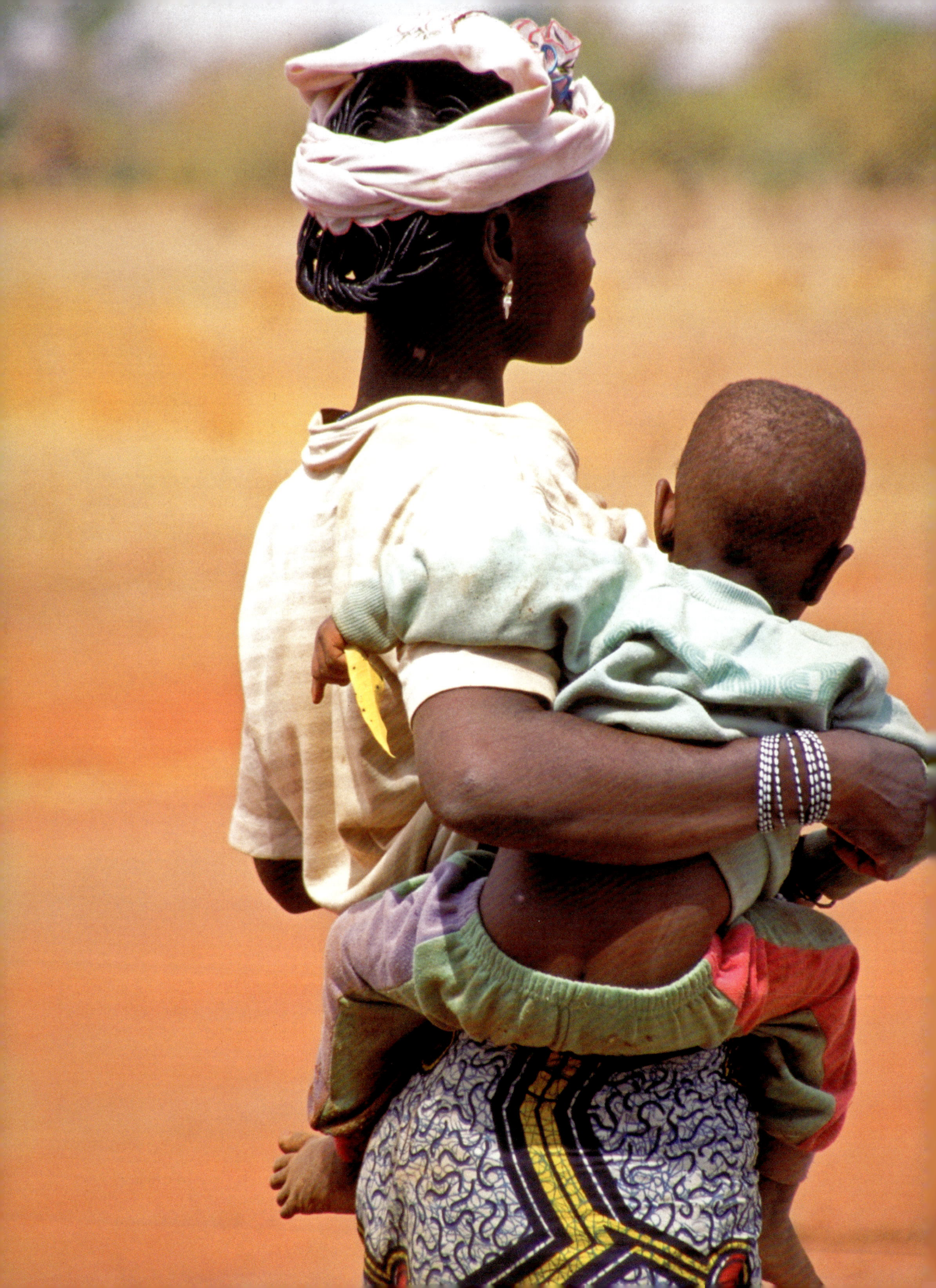

In this chapter, you will learn to put your back into gentle traction when seated, a technique I call "stretchsitting." This simple but powerful technique will not only give you a comfortable way to sit, but also help undo some of the damage caused by years of hunching (fig.1-1) or swaying (fig.1-2).

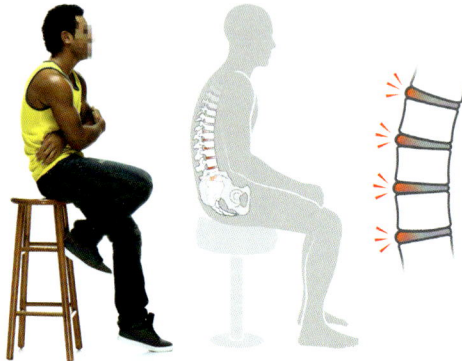
fig.1-1

Hunching compresses the spinal discs anteriorly, causing degeneration and related problems.

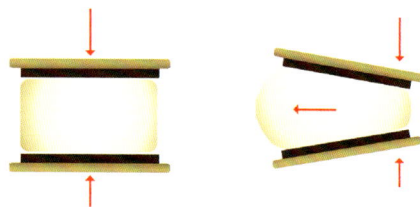

The effect of hunching is similar to what happens when pressure is applied to one side of a S'more.

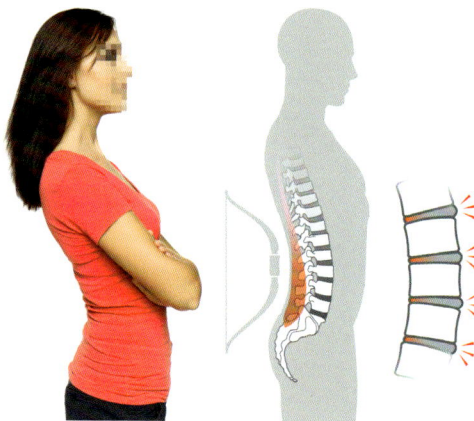
fig.1-2

Swaying arches the spine excessively, compresses the discs posteriorly, and compromises circulation around the spine. The result is similar to a tightly strung bow.

When you stretchsit, you lengthen your spine against the back of a chair. This immediately decompresses your discs (fig.1-3), preventing further damage and allowing them to heal. The long muscles of your back get a significant and sustained stretch, helping them adjust to healthier, longer baseline lengths. Over a period of months, you can expect to become 1/4" to 1" (0.5–2.5 cm) taller, depending on how much height you have lost to extra curvature or compression in your spine. The additional length in your spine may also result in related health benefits, such as improved circulation and nerve function around the spine.

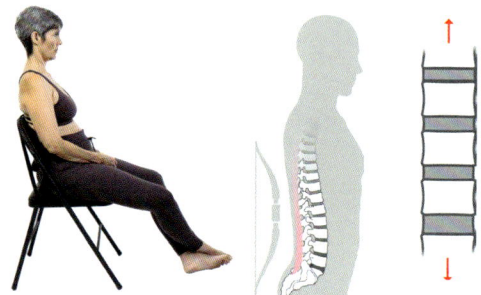
fig.1-3

Stretchsitting lengthens the long muscles of the back in an action similar to relaxing a bow. Stretchsitting also decompresses the discs, allowing them to heal and preventing further damage.

As part of stretchsitting, you will restore your shoulders to a natural baseline position by doing a "shoulder roll." This will augment the blood circulation to and from your arms, accelerating repair of any damaged tissue and preventing injury. If you have arm problems such as carpal tunnel syndrome or a repetitive stress injury, it is especially important that you learn to reposition your shoulders. Hunching your shoulders while placing demands on your arms—such as when using a device, typing, playing a musical instrument, using a game console, pushing a wheelbarrow, or playing a racket sport—is especially problematic (fig.1-4a). While the activity increases the demand for blood, the compromised shoulder architecture reduces the supply. Positioning your shoulders well allows you to work and exercise longer without pain or injury (fig.1-4b).

As part of stretchsitting, you will also learn to lengthen and align your neck. Not only will your neck feel more comfortable, but the nerves that

fig.1-4

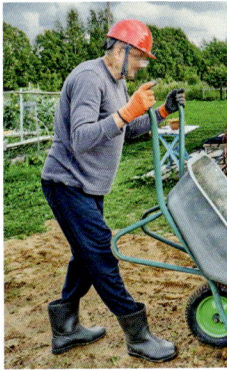

a. Hunched shoulders compromise circulation to and from the arms and predispose people to injury.

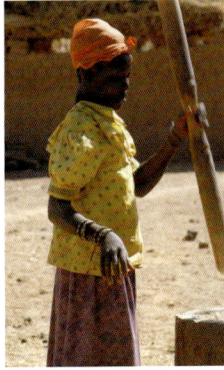

b. Well-aligned shoulders allow for good circulation to and from the arms, and protect against injury.

fig.1-5

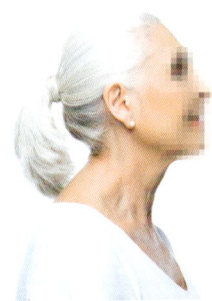

a. Compression in the neck can result in cervical disc and nerve damage.

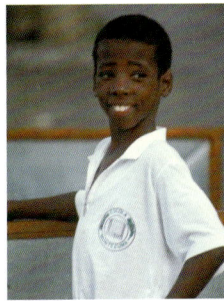

b. A well-aligned neck allows the cervical discs and nerves to remain healthy.

they already have the necessary length in their spines to optimize disc and nerve health (fig.1-8 on page 37).

Note some important differences between stretchsitting and other common ways of stretching the back:

- Stretchsitting is beneficial for muscles and discs alike; many conventional back stretches compromise the discs as they stretch the muscles (fig.1-6).
- Stretchsitting avoids further stretching of the ligaments in an already rounded upper spine (kyphosis).
- Stretchsitting trains our muscle memory to align the spine optimally.
- Stretchsitting takes no time out of your schedule and yet provides hours of therapeutic effect; conventional back stretches take time and can realistically be done for only a few minutes a day.

There are several reasons why stretchsitting is the first technique you will learn. It is safe (if your back and neck muscles spasm easily, be sure to lengthen your spine very slowly and gently). It is easy to learn. It helps protect your spine from injury as you prepare for later techniques. And it will likely produce benefits immediately, especially if you have compression in your spine.

emanate from your cervical spine will function better (fig.1-5). If you have tingling or numbness down your arms, for example, the techniques taught here are crucial to your recovery. Since every nerve that distributes to the arms originates in the neck, restoring healthy neck architecture can help alleviate arm nerve problems.

In this chapter you will also learn the basics of healthy foot alignment. (Chapter 6 explains more about how foot shape relates to posture: the goal here is merely to gain familiarity with this new foot position.)

Stretchsitting may strike you as a little contrived. In a way, it is. People in traditional cultures do not need to actively stretchsit in this way because

fig.1-6

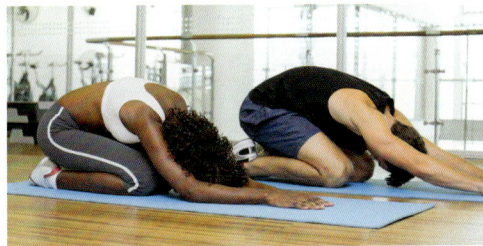

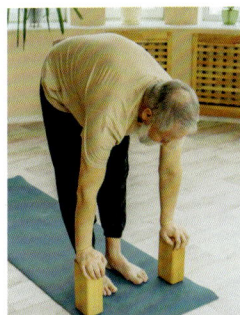

These common ways of stretching the back muscles are harmful to the discs, bones, and ligaments of the spine.

BENEFITS

- Resets the baseline length of the long back muscles, reducing muscle pain

- Decompresses the spinal discs, preventing further disc damage and reducing disc pain

- Decompresses the spinal nerves, facilitating normal nerve function and reducing nerve pain

- Improves circulation around the spine and to the arms, supporting better tissue health and repair

- Reduces stress on other spinal structures

- Increases the safety margin for everyday movements that distort the spine (fig.1-7)

fig.1-7

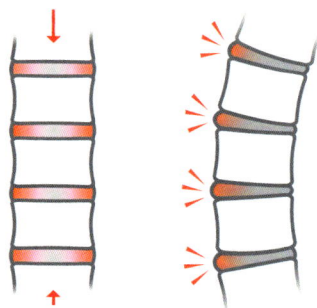

A compressed spine is especially prone to injury when distorted.

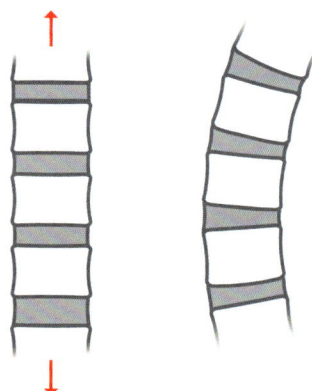

Decompressed discs remain healthy even with moderate spinal distortion.

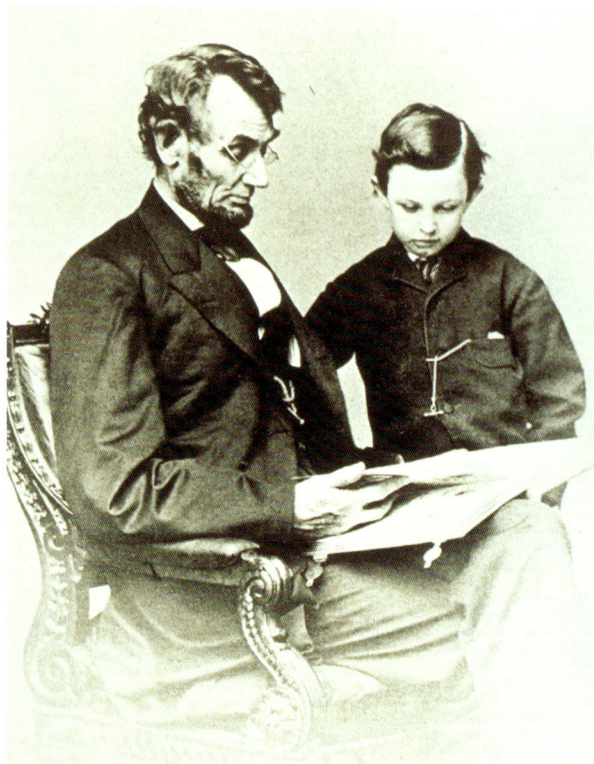

I no longer suffer pain and discomfort when at home, at work, or traveling. No more fidgeting when the seatbelt sign is on for a long time; no more compression during turbulence. What a difference stretchsitting makes—I now arrive rejuvenated and a little taller at my destination.

Barbara Beasley, Belmont, CA

I experienced back pain on a daily basis. After sitting at my computer all day at work, I would come home and lay on the floor to relax my back and then start begging for a back rub. Also, during family outings (museums, theme parks, etc.), I often had to take breaks to stretch or sit down to rest my back. It took effort to learn the [Gokhale] techniques but once I did, suddenly good posture became natural and comfortable instead of feeling like an impossible amount of work. The back pain is now gone, and the posture compliments from strangers are fun too!

Jenny Price, Atlanta, GA

fig. 1-8

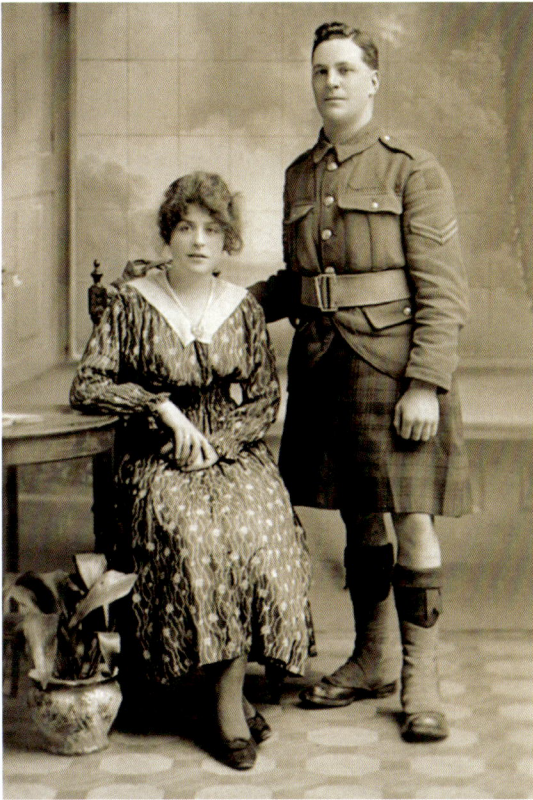

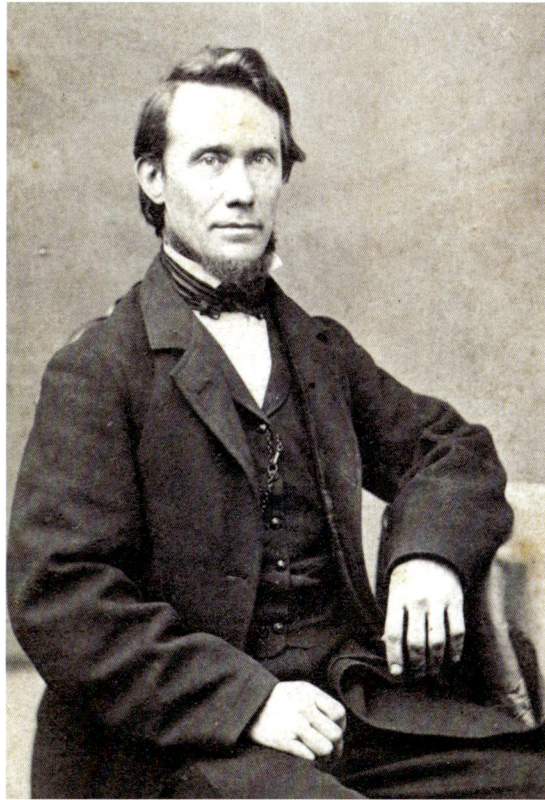

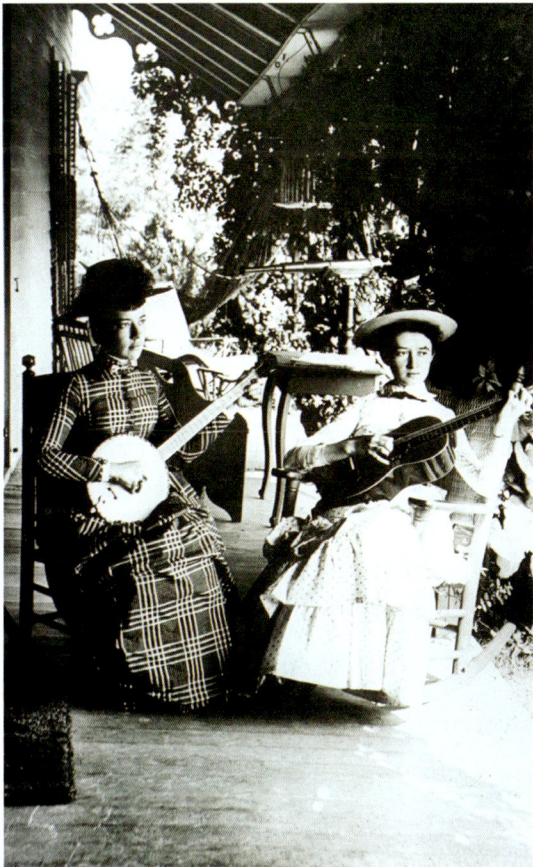

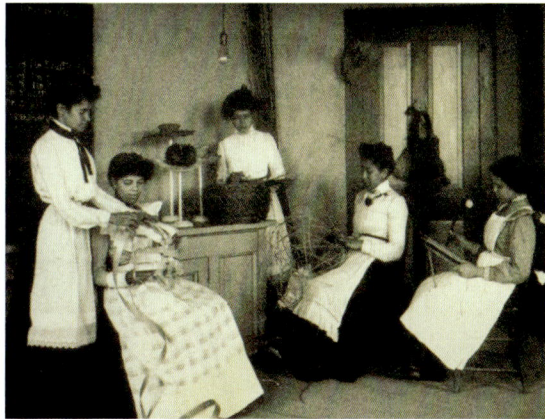

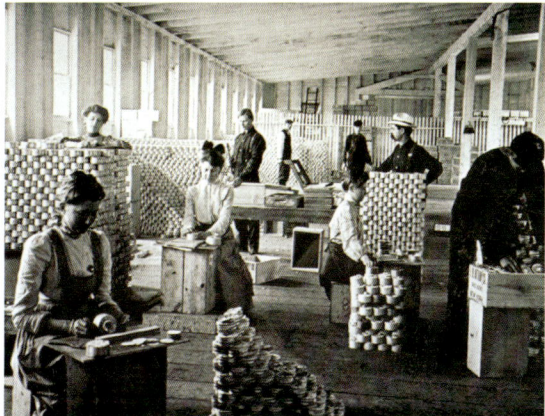

Examples of people from former times sitting with a healthy baseline length in their back muscles (USA).

EQUIPMENT

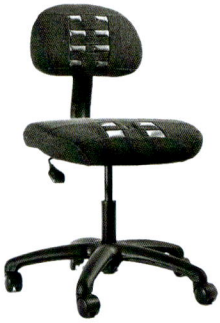

You will need a suitable chair, such as an office chair or padded folding chair. The ideal is a chair with:
- *A firm seat*
- *A low, straight backrest that, if adjustable, can be locked into position*
- *An outcropping at the mid-back level to which you can "hitch" your spine*

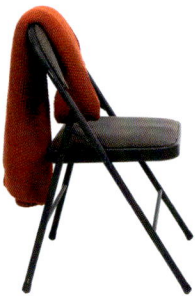

If your chair lacks an outcropping, you can fashion one from a folded towel, flannel sheet, or sticky yoga mat that you place just below your shoulder blades.

The folded material:
- *Offers a place to hitch your mid-back*
- *Gives your buttocks space to settle behind you in the chair*
- *Provides enough clearance to let you perform a shoulder roll*

1 SIT DOWN, PLACING YOUR BUTTOCKS TOWARDS THE BACK OF THE CHAIR

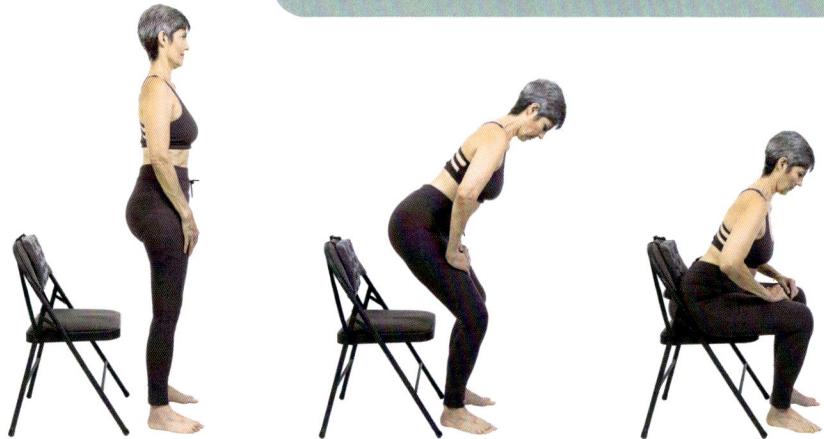

If the chair has a gap between the seat and the back, be careful not to place your buttocks too far back. If you do, your back will sway in later steps.

2 PLACE YOUR FEET ABOUT HIP-WIDTH APART AND RELAX YOUR LEGS

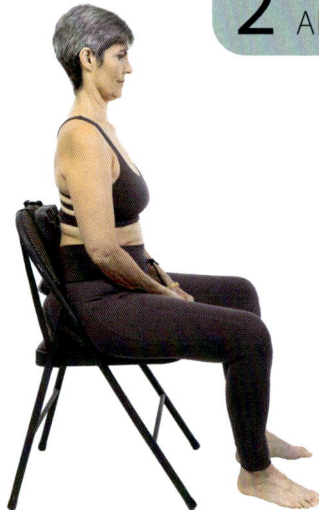

3 LENGTHEN YOUR SPINE

Bend at the waist to curve forward slightly. This lengthens and straightens your lumbar spine, eliminating any sway you may have.

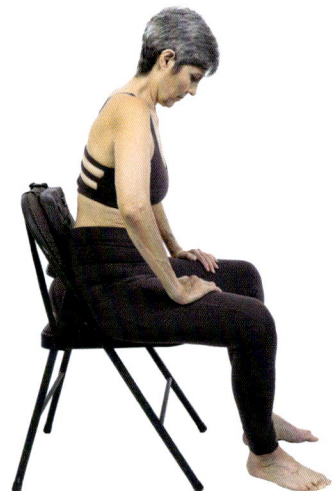

4 FURTHER LENGTHEN YOUR SPINE

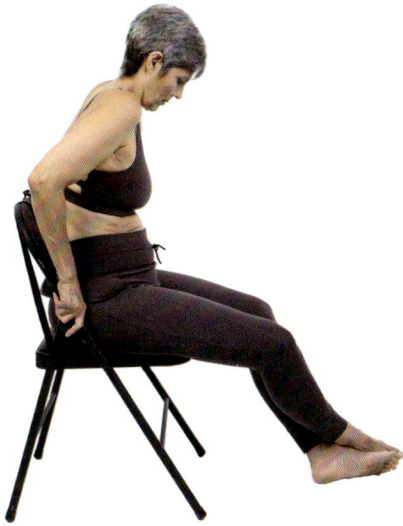

Leave your buttocks anchored to the chair and your torso curved forward to avoid reintroducing a sway as you perform the following actions. With both hands, hold on to some part of the chair (armrests, backrest, or seat). Relax the muscles of your torso and straighten your arms, allowing your lower back to lengthen. The distance between the back of your rib cage and your buttocks will increase.

A very common mistake is to arch backwards, which actually compresses the spine instead of lengthening it.

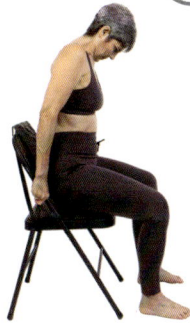

Another common mistake is to raise the buttocks out of the chair.

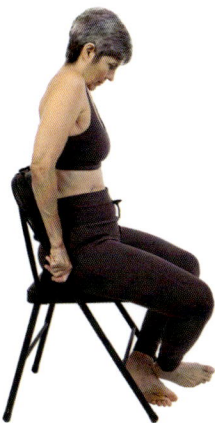

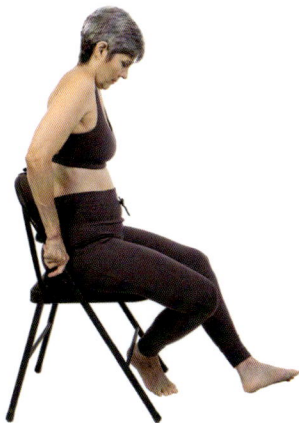

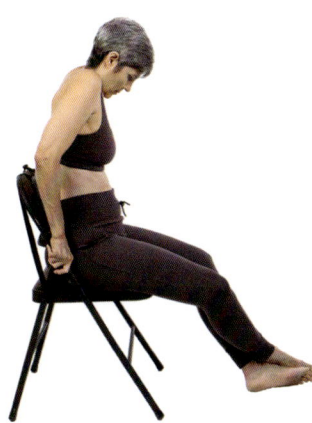

Be sure you are not engaging your leg muscles in this step. If you find they are tense, stretch your legs forward, fold them under your chair, or use any relaxed position.

ROTATING THE RIB CAGE FORWARD TO LENGTHEN THE LOWER BACK

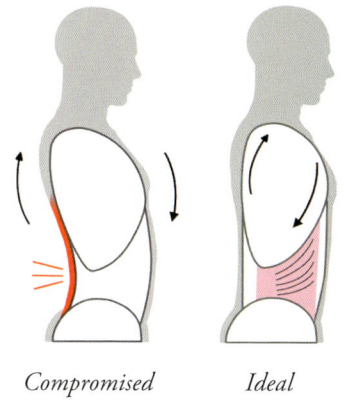

Compromised   *Ideal*

EXAMPLES OF STRETCHING THE SPINE IN EVERYDAY LIFE

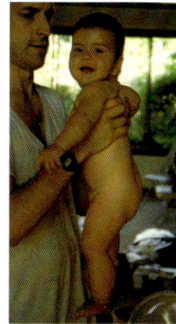

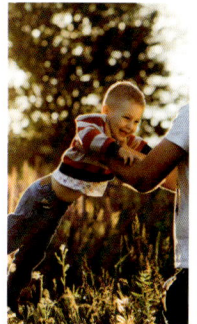

These photos show a maneuver familiar to us all: lifting or swinging a child, helping to lengthen its spine.

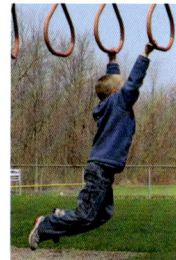

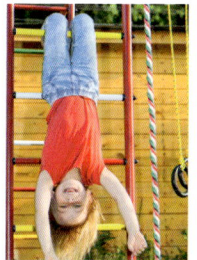

Many common childhood activities lengthen the spine.

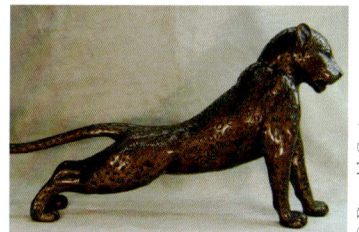

We often see animals stretching their spines.

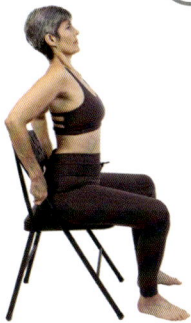

© Donald Greig

39

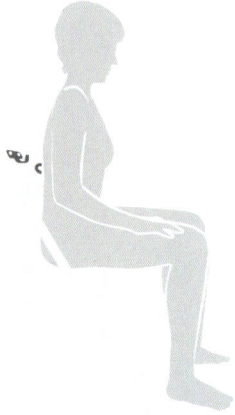

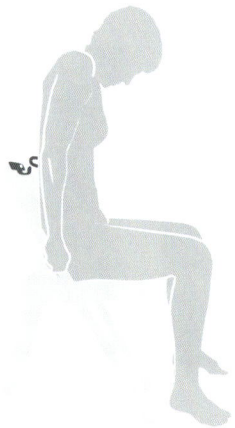

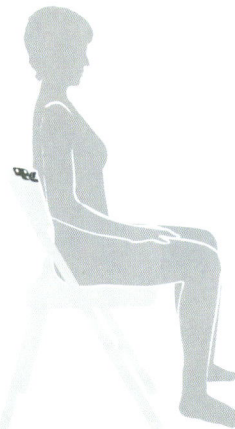

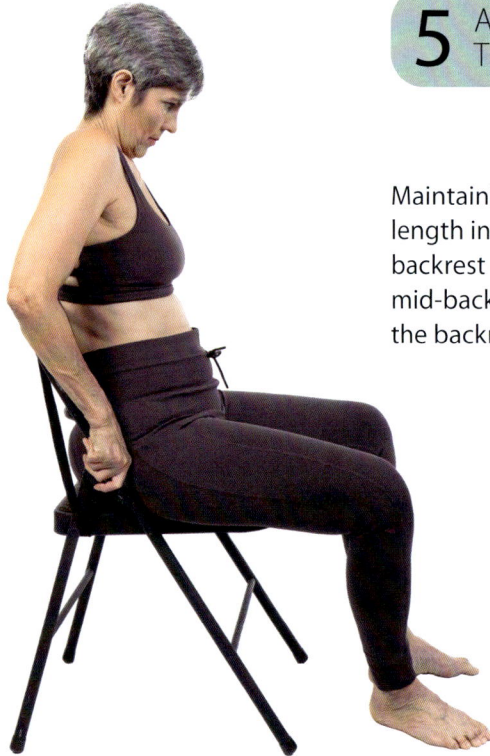

5 ATTACH YOUR MID-BACK TO THE BACKREST OR CUSHION

Maintaining the curl forward and the extra length in your spine, "hitch" your back to the backrest of the chair. Think of pinning your mid-back to a point higher than usual on the backrest.

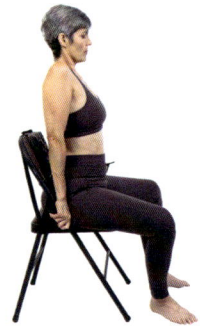

A common mistake is to straighten out or arch your back before it touches the cushion.

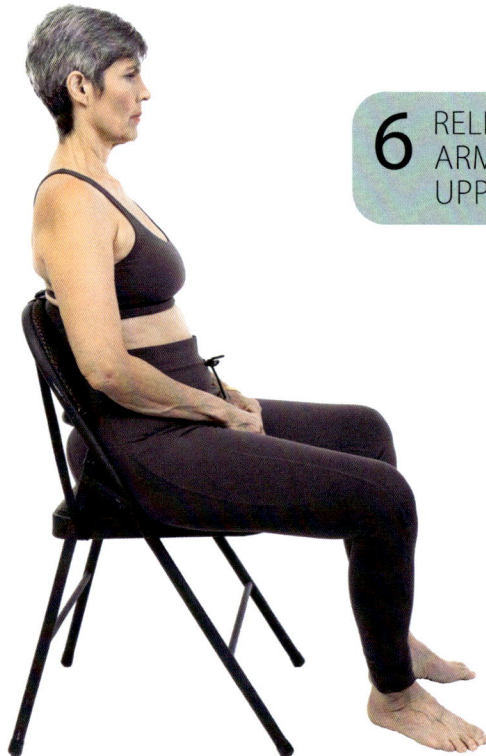

6 RELEASE THE TENSION IN YOUR ARMS AND STRAIGHTEN YOUR UPPER BACK

Feel the chair take the weight as you release your arms. Now your lower back is in traction.

It may help to imagine that you hang from the point of contact with the chair like a picture hangs from a picture hook; you lengthen your back to reach the hook.

7 CHECK FOR RELAXATION; ADJUST TRACTION IF NECESSARY

Stretchsitting should be a very passive pose, where the back muscles can completely relax. Let friction with the chair hold you upright; there is no need to press backward into the cushion. Check in every now and then to be sure you are not pressing back, or arching backward over the backrest.

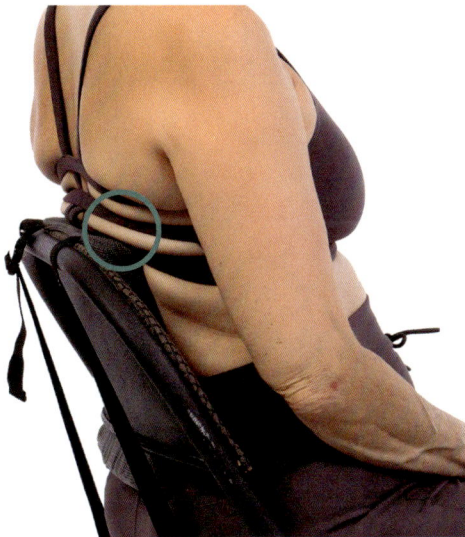

If your lower back feels stretched out, you are right on track even though it feels strange at first. If you are not sure that you have succeeded in stretching your lower back, place a hand on your back just above the point of contact with the chair. You should feel a roll of skin there. The chair stretches your skin, which stretches your flesh, which eases your vertebrae apart.

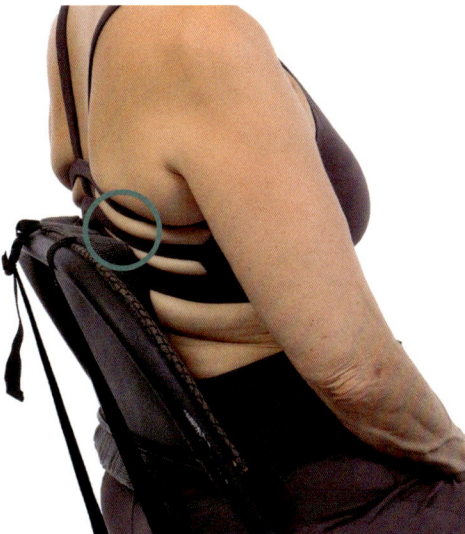

If you are uncomfortable, try backing off a little so as to lengthen in a more subtle manner. It is important that you lengthen, but not that you achieve an ideal length overnight. Proceed gently.

TRADITIONAL WAYS OF CARRYING BABIES HELP TO STRETCH THEIR SPINES

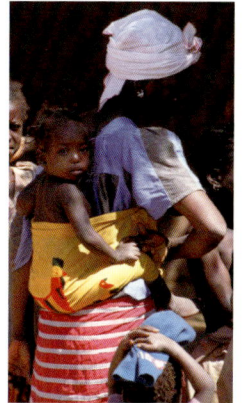

Mother carrying baby. Fabric stretches baby's back (Burkina Faso)

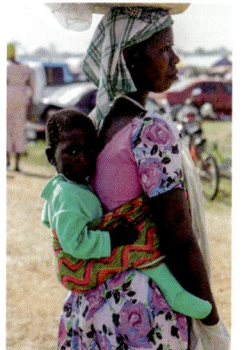

Woman using traditional African technique to carry baby (Ghana)

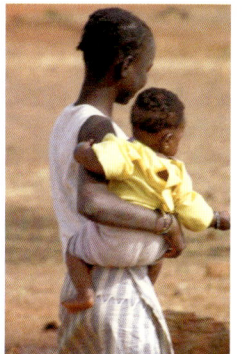

Teenager carrying baby on hip, stretching the baby's back with forearm (Burkina Faso)

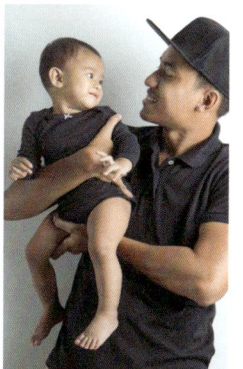

Man facilitating baby's mild spinal stretch (Indonesia)

MECHANISM OF A SHOULDER ROLL

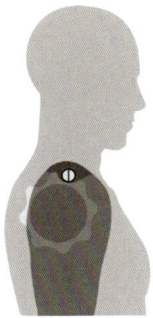

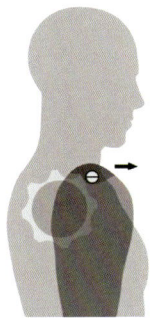

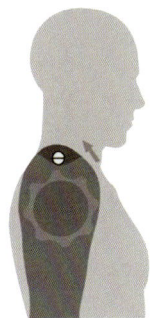

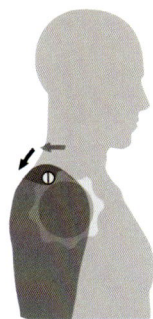

8 PERFORM A SHOULDER ROLL

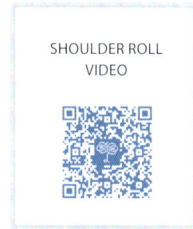

SHOULDER ROLL VIDEO

(You will need a free gokhalemethod.com account to access this video.)

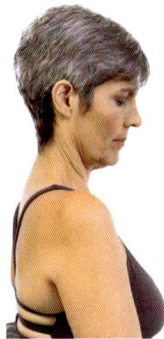

Take one shoulder forward.

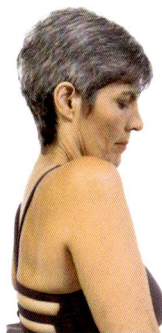

Lift the shoulder toward your ear.

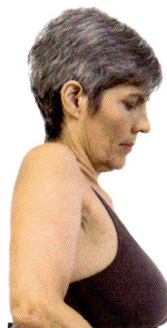

Roll the shoulder back as far as you comfortably can.

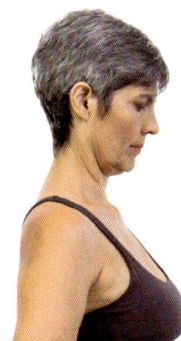

Let gravity settle your shoulder blade gently down along your spine.

When doing a shoulder roll, imagine the shoulder's soft tissue ratcheting back one notch on a cogged wheel. Unless the pectoral muscles are very tight, the shoulders tend to remain in this position without any sustained muscular effort. (See Appendix 1 for exercises to help stretch tight pectoral muscles.)

As with all the movements you will learn in this book, the shoulder roll may feel exaggerated and awkward at first, something you wouldn't be comfortable doing in public. With practice and time, the movement becomes subtle, and you can easily incorporate it into seating yourself at a company meeting, in a restaurant, or on your sofa.

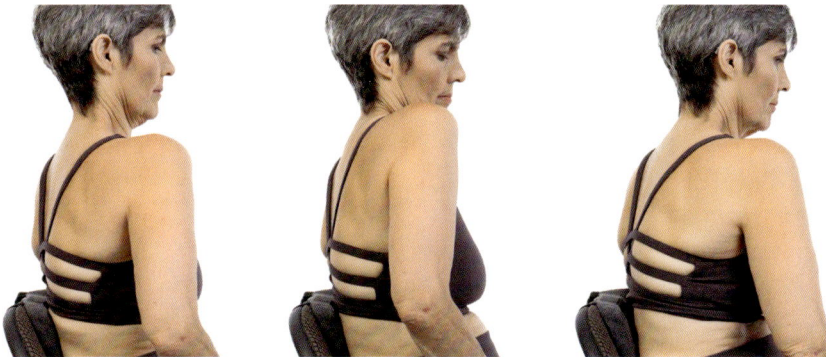

Common mistakes are to exaggerate the movement, do it too abruptly, or move the arm more than the shoulder blade.

Pushing the shoulder too far forward

Raising the shoulder too high

Moving the arm excessively

After performing a shoulder roll, you may notice that your reach is shorter. This is because your arms now originate further back than before. This is a healthy home base position that you don't want to compromise during normal activities. If you have difficulty reaching your task, try moving closer to it. For example, when working at a computer, you may need to move the keyboard closer. When driving a car, you may need to move your car seat closer to the steering wheel (but keep a safe distance from the airbag).

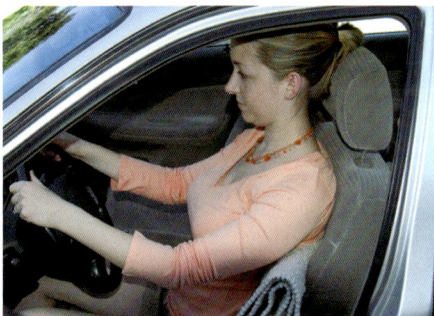

Driving with shoulders well-positioned

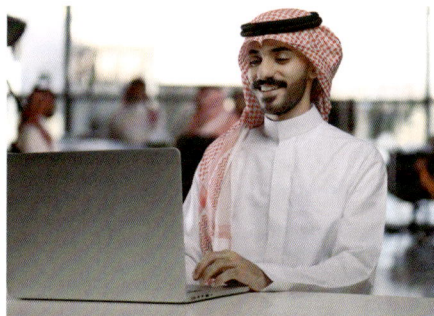

Typing with shoulders well-positioned

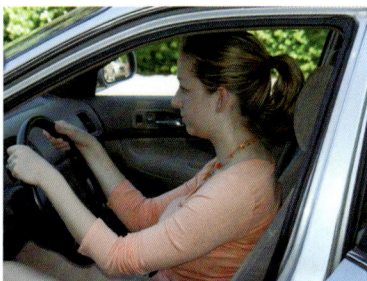

Driving with shoulders too far forward

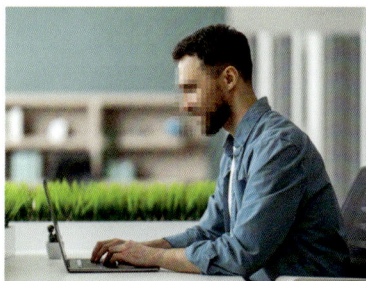

Typing with shoulders too far forward

EXAMPLES OF GOOD SHOULDER ALIGNMENT

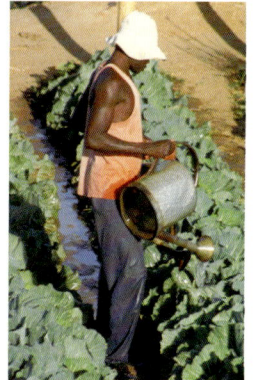

Farmer (Burkina Faso)

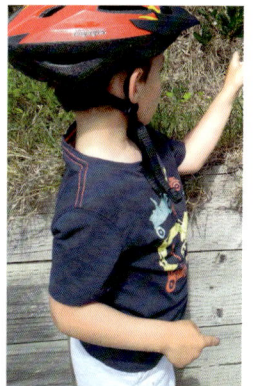

Young boy (Australia)

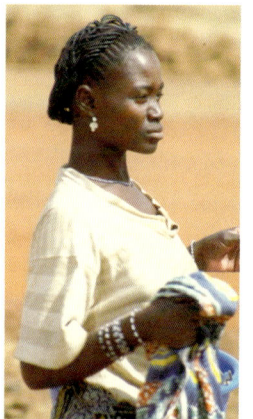

Young mother (Burkina Faso)

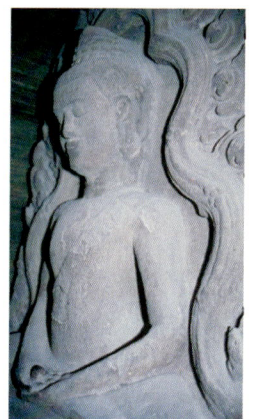

Buddha figure (Thailand)

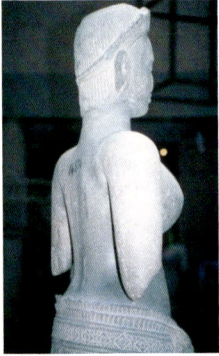

Bodhisattva figure (Cambodia)

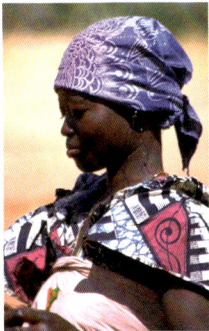

Young mother (Burkina Faso)

ROTATING THE HEAD FORWARD TO LENGTHEN THE NECK

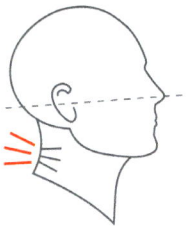

Compromised

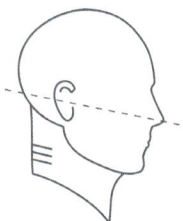

Ideal

9 LENGTHEN THE BACK OF YOUR NECK

Though you have lengthened your back, your neck may still be compressed. There are many ways to lengthen the neck. If your neck is injury-prone, choose Option A. If you are looking to make fast progress, use Option E occasionally. Otherwise, choose according to what is comfortable for you. The goal is a vertically aligned neck position with the head gliding back and up and the chin angled down.

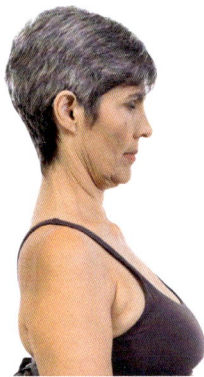

Option A. Imagine a helium balloon inside your head. Consciously release any tension in your neck muscles that prevents the balloon rising.

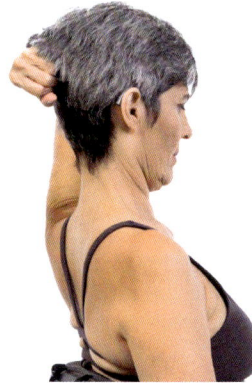

Option B. Grasp a clump of hair at the base of your skull and gently pull it back and up.

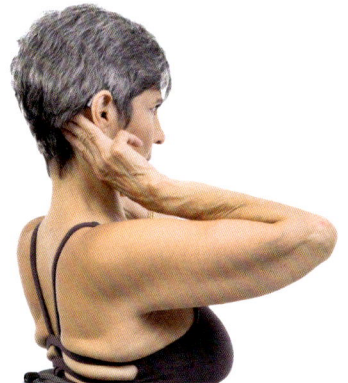

Option C. Position your fingertips in the two side indentations at the base of your skull (the *occipital grooves*) and move your skull up and away from your body.

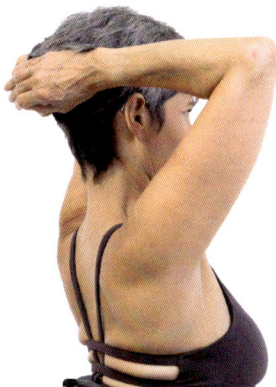

Option D. Grasp the base of your skull with both hands and gently pull upward while lowering your shoulders.

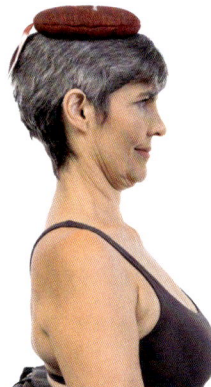

Option E. Place (or imagine) a light object on the crown of your head. Push up against it.

HAIR PULL VIDEO

If there is some rigidity in your neck or upper back, your head and neck may still crane forward. See Appendix 1 (page 217) for exercises to help stretch muscles in this area.

⊗

Try to avoid these common mistakes:

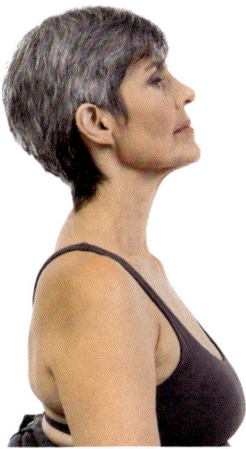

Do not lengthen the front of your neck instead of the back.

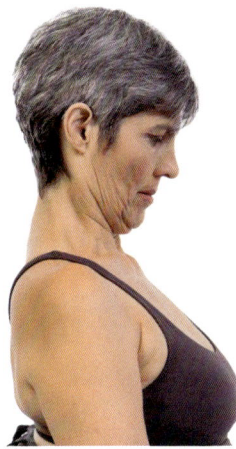

Do not tuck your chin into your neck as you lengthen the back of your neck.

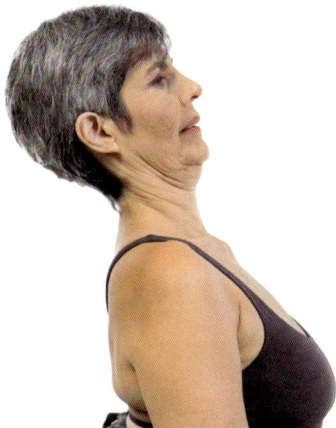

Do not tilt your head back in an attempt to lengthen the neck.

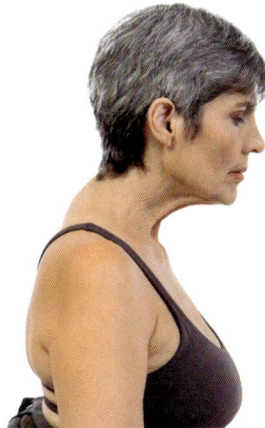

Do not jut your head forward as you lengthen the back of your neck.

HEALTHY NECK POSTURE FROM AROUND THE WORLD

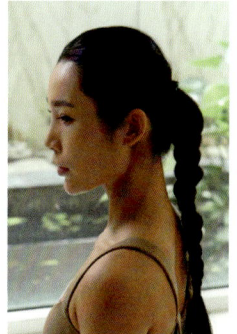

Yogini (Vietnam)

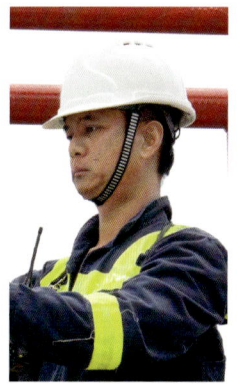

Cargo ship operator (Ukraine)

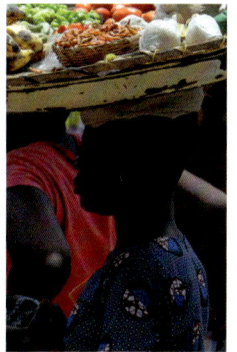

Woman carrying produce (Benin)

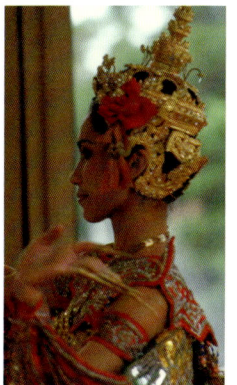

Dancer (Thailand)

HEALTHY FOOT SHAPE FROM AROUND THE WORLD

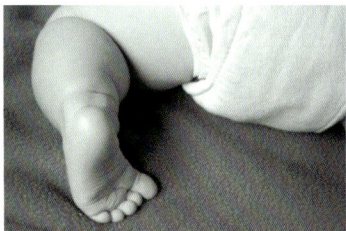

Six-month-old infant with pronounced kidney bean-shaped foot (USA)

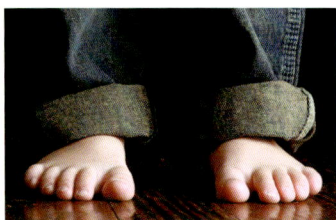

Young child showing healthy toe spacing (USA)

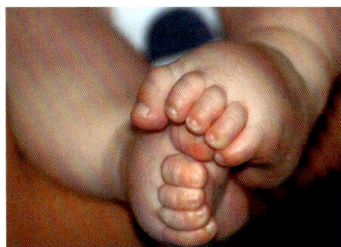

Baby with pronounced transverse arches in the feet (USA)

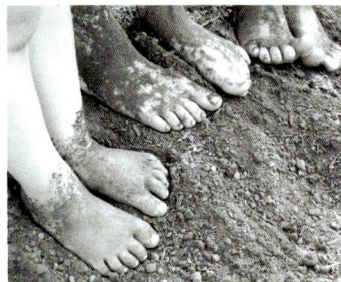

Children with sturdy feet from walking on natural surfaces (India)

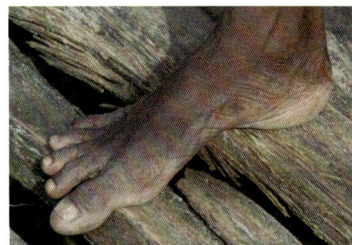

Laborer with muscular, healthy feet (India)

10 KIDNEY BEAN SHAPE ONE FOOT

While continuing to stretchsit, lift the heel of one foot just high enough that it clears the floor.

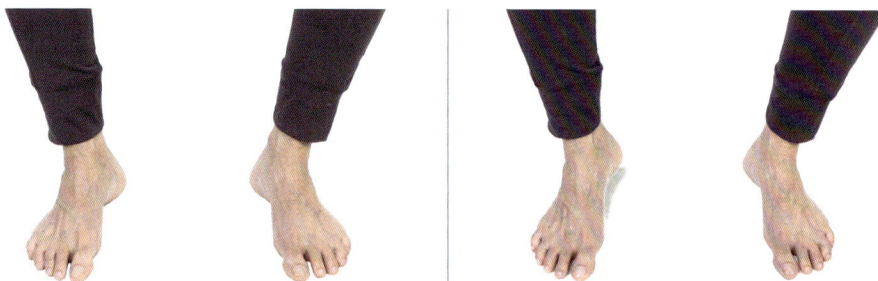

Keeping the toes and ball of the foot fixed to the floor, twist and pivot the heel inward, then plant it firmly on the floor.

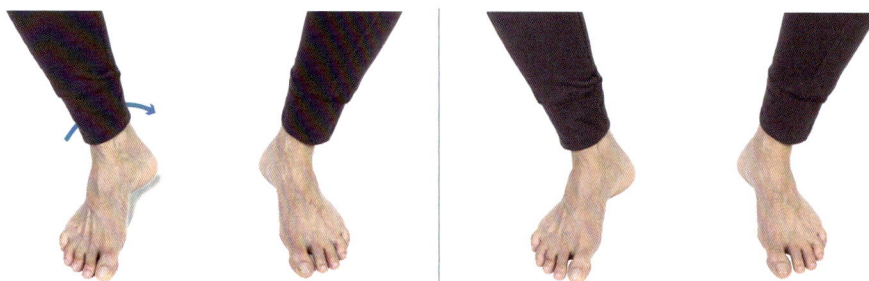

Your goal is to create a "kidney bean" shape with your foot.

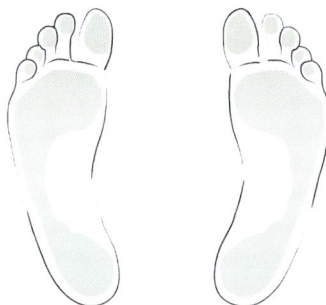

A common mistake is to lift the heel too high, tensing the foot muscles and making the heel pivot step difficult.

46

11 REPEAT THIS ACTION WITH THE OTHER FOOT

Notice that your knees are wide and point outwards, in the same direction as your feet.

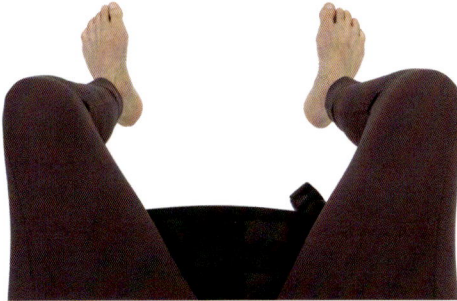

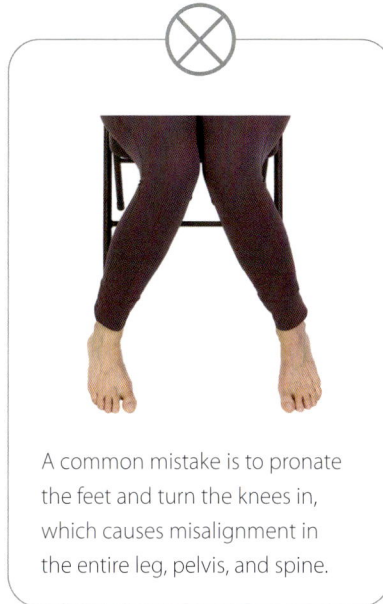

A common mistake is to pronate the feet and turn the knees in, which causes misalignment in the entire leg, pelvis, and spine.

12 RELAX YOUR WHOLE BODY

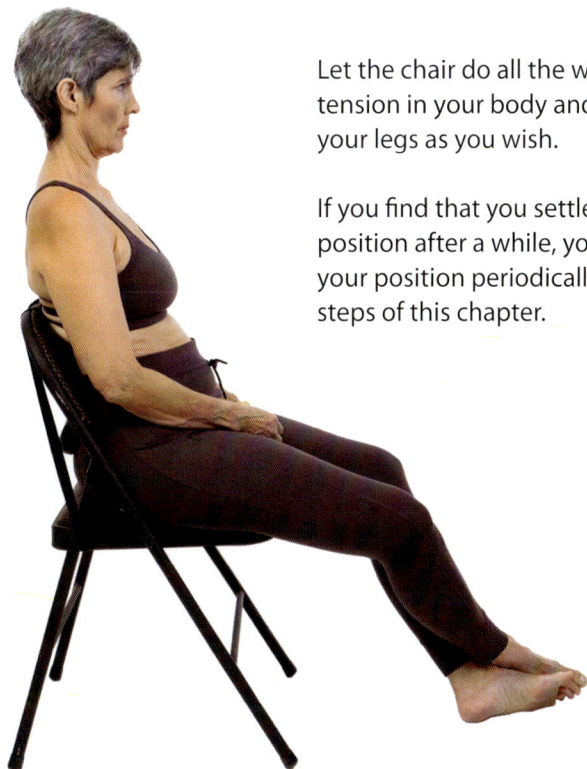

Let the chair do all the work. Try to locate any tension in your body and release it. Reposition your legs as you wish.

If you find that you settle back to your habitual position after a while, you will need to reset your position periodically. Simply repeat the steps of this chapter.

STRETCHSITTING VIDEO

STRETCHSITTING CAN HAPPEN AT MANY ANGLES

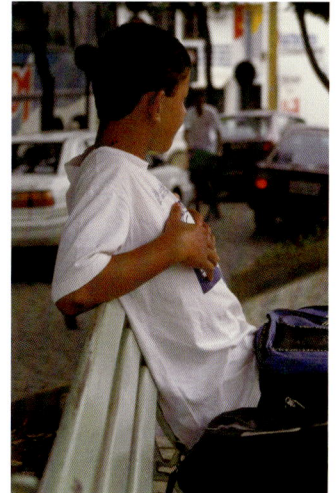

Schoolboy sitting slightly reclined while lengthening his back (Brazil)

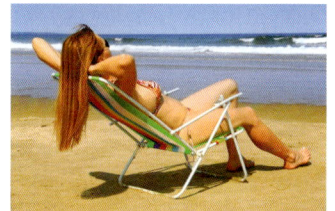

Woman reclining on a beach chair while elongating her neck (USA)

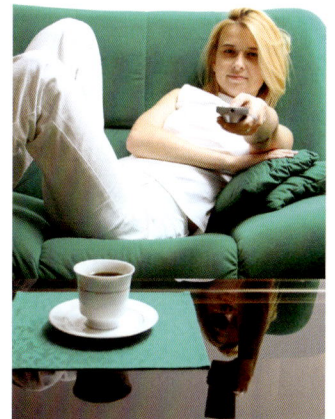

Woman propped on sofa with cushions supporting her spine (USA)

Stretchsitting does not oblige you to sit bolt upright. As long as your spine is in an elongated J shape, you will be comfortable and protected in a variety of positions ranging from upright to reclining.

INDICATIONS OF IMPROVEMENT

With practice, you will learn how to stretchsit quickly and easily. Usually this sitting position, though unfamiliar at first, becomes very comfortable. It allows you to sit for extended periods without squirming. Eventually, the resting length of your back will change, your height will be measurably taller, and you will be more comfortable even when you are not in traction.

Over time, your lengthened back muscles will contribute to improved circulation (which in turn hastens healing of damaged areas), and will help to decompress discs and nerves—all with the result of increased comfort and function. Because most nerves in the body originate in the spinal column, normalizing this area will improve your general well-being.

You may also notice gradual changes in your breathing pattern. Pay attention to which parts of your body move during a breath cycle. Place one hand on your chest and one hand on your abdomen to check the relative movement in these two areas (fig.1-9). When you have lengthened your spine and opened your shoulders, you will probably notice the possibility of more expansion in your chest and less in your abdomen.

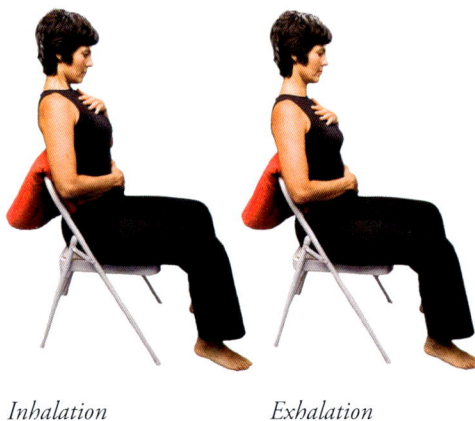

fig.1-9

Inhalation   Exhalation

With stretchsitting, the chest moves more than the abdomen during breathing.

TROUBLESHOOTING

FEELING OVERLY STRETCHED

If you feel as though you are on a rack, you have stretched yourself too severely. Ease the stretch by moving slightly away from the backrest and letting your upper back slide down the backrest just a little (fig.1-10).

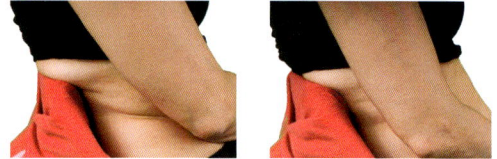

fig.1-10

If a large stretch (with a pronounced roll of flesh) feels uncomfortable, back off a little.

UNABLE TO STRETCH THE SPINE

If after following the directions in this chapter you don't feel a stretch in your spine, check for a telltale roll of flesh above the point of contact with the chair. If you find it, you are actually stretchsitting but just not feeling it yet. In time, you will probably begin to feel the stretch.

If your arms are weak or injured, you may not be able to push with them effectively to lengthen your torso. Instead, reach your hands around to your mid-back, and stretch the skin on your back upwards before hitching yourself to the backrest (fig.1-11). Alternatively, if your chair is stable, you can use your legs to help push your back higher up against the backrest.

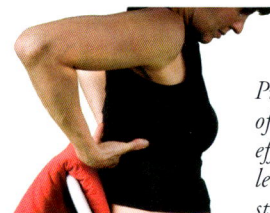

fig.1-11

Pulling up on the skin of the back is another effective way to lengthen the back for stretchsitting.

If you are still unable to lengthen your spine, you may be having difficulty relaxing your abdominal and back muscles enough to allow any separation between your upper body and your lower body. As you stretch your back, try consciously to relax the muscles in your torso (except those you need for maintaining your slight forward curve), and proceed very slowly. You may need to spend more time suspending yourself by your arms in Step 4 to give your tissues time to "let go."

If your muscles feel very tight, you may benefit from some supplemental bodywork, such as yoga, massage, acupuncture, and stretching exercises.

DISCOMFORT AT POINT OF CONTACT

If the place where your back contacts the chair feels sore, you may have some inflammation there. Arrange your back support object a little higher or lower to avoid this spot. If you still have trouble, you may want to skip to the next chapter until you can perform this exercise comfortably. Consider massage or acupuncture to help resolve the inflammation.

SORENESS IN THE LOWER BACK

Check that your sacrum (the triangular bone at the base of your spine) is not so far back as to force your lumbar spine into a sway. Without tucking your pelvis, shuffle your bottom forward until your lower back is comfortable.

MUSCULAR SPASM

Muscles can behave somewhat like frightened animals, stiffening if they feel threatened. Progress slowly. Underdo each step of the stretchsitting process, allowing your muscles to gradually get used to being longer.

SORENESS IN THE NECK

If you have kyphosis (rounding) in your upper back, your neck has to work harder to stop your head dropping forward when you are sitting. You can reduce strain on your neck by sliding your bottom forward a little to sit at a more reclined angle. Until your upper back is less rounded, continue to "stretchrecline" like this.

INADEQUATE CHAIR

Some chairs are difficult to modify. Try different combinations of chairs and back supports. Don't settle for anything less than an extremely comfortable sitting position. One way to modify almost any chair is with the back support I have designed specifically for stretchsitting (fig.1-12).

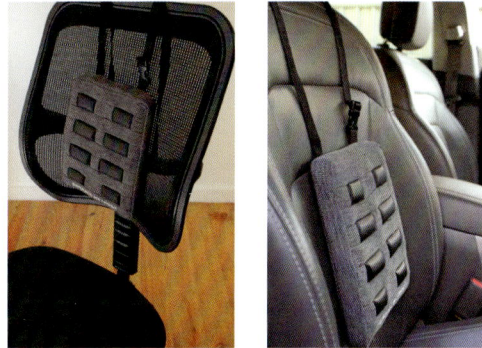

fig.1-12

The Stretchsit Cushion facilitates stretchsitting in almost any chair. For more information, see gokhalemethod.com

FURTHER INFORMATION

SHOULDER REPOSITIONING

Most people who recognize they have poor posture know that their shoulders hunch forward. Unfortunately, the ways they know to fix the problem are either ineffective or harmful.

A common approach to correcting hunched shoulders is to pull them directly back (fig.1-13). People usually hold this position for a few seconds before they again slouch their shoulders—until the next time they become aware they are hunching. The movement of pulling the shoulders back involves contracting the *rhomboid* muscles, which is a good exercise but a bad way to correct one's posture. It is just as well that people don't hold this position for long: If they did, they would suffer inflammation from overuse of the rhomboids.

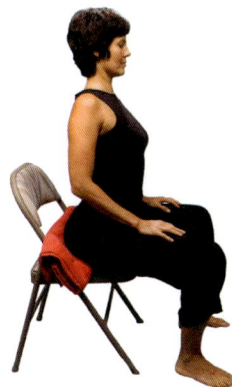

fig.1-13

Correcting for hunched shoulders by pulling the shoulders back is neither effective nor desirable.

Another common, and worse, compensation for hunched shoulders is to sway the lower back (fig.1-14). This approach creates two problems in place of one. The original hunching remains unresolved, and the lower back is compromised as well. Sometimes this combination of excessive curvatures is mistakenly perceived as good posture, because the upper body appears upright.

fig.1-14

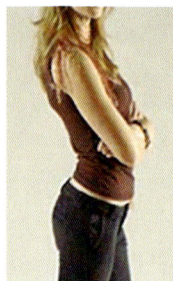

Correcting for hunched shoulders by arching the lower back results in two problems instead of one.

Performing careful shoulder rolls is the best way to remedy hunching. Shoulder rolls influence the architecture of the area just beneath the pectoral muscles (fig.1-15). This area, which includes the *brachial plexus*, is a major thoroughfare for nerves and blood vessels supplying the arms. Hunching the shoulders compromises the architecture of this area, affecting blood supply to and from the arms, and nerve function in the arms. Symptoms range from cold hands and dry skin to arm pain and dysfunction.

Shoulder rolls are relatively easy to learn and perform. If you have extremely tight pectoral muscles, you should proceed gently with shoulder rolls. Otherwise, your overstretched muscles may press down and impinge on underlying blood vessels and nerves. For exercises to help you progress faster towards well-aligned shoulders, see Appendix 1.

fig.1-15

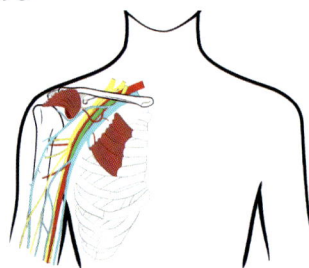

Numerous blood vessels, nerves, and other structures traverse the area directly under the pectoral muscles.

READING OR USING A DEVICE

It has become common for people to protrude their heads forward and downward, curving the neck, while looking at their devices (fig.1-16a,b,c). This compresses the cervical discs and other important structures in the neck. A conventional postural recommendation is to lift the device to the level of your eyes such that your neck can remain in line with your upper back. This can be tiring for the arms over even short periods. In fact, our species is well-equipped to look downwards for extended periods—to avoid thorns, sharp stones, and scorpions, forage for berries, and nurse our babies. Our problem is not *that* we look down at the devices or books in our laps, but *how* we look down. It's entirely possible to look downwards while maintaining a healthy neck and head position (fig.1-16d); depending on the angle required, you will need to look down with your eyes, pivot the head downwards, and/or hinge forward from the C7-T1 juncture (keeping the neck straight and elongated).

fig.1-16

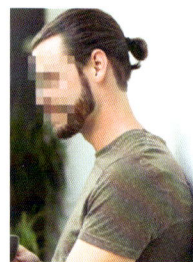

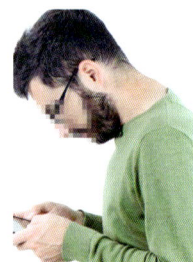

a.

b.

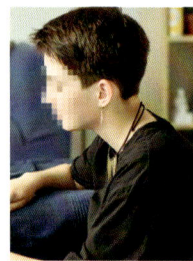

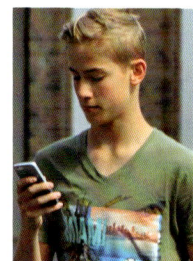

c.

d.

Curving the neck (a), putting excessive pressure on the C7-T1 juncture (b), and protruding the head forwards and downwards (c) are unhealthy ways to look down. To protect your cervical spine when looking at a book or device, use a combination of holding your object closer to your eyes, and adjusting your eyes and head without curving your neck (d).

COMMENTS ON LUMBAR CUSHIONS

A common solution for an uncomfortable chair or seat is a lumbar support cushion that supports and even exaggerates lumbar curvature (fig.1-17a). The design of these cushions is based on misguided notions about ideal spinal curvature. Even when placed above the lumbar spine, most lumbar cushions do not work for stretchsitting, as they don't have the appropriate firmness or texture for "hitching" the spine.

I designed my Stretchsit® Cushion for effective hitching, and for easy attachment to most seats at the appropriate height (fig.1-17b). Its design helps to lengthen the lumbar spine, making sitting a comfortable and therapeutic position.

fig.1-17

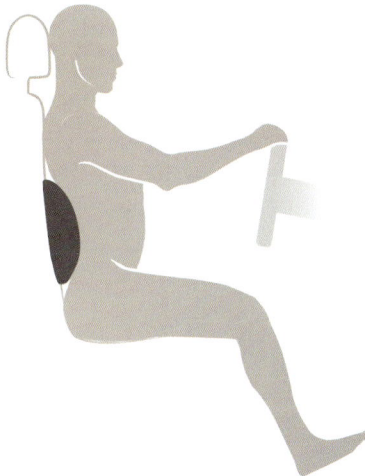

a. A lumbar support cushion exaggerates lumbar curvature.

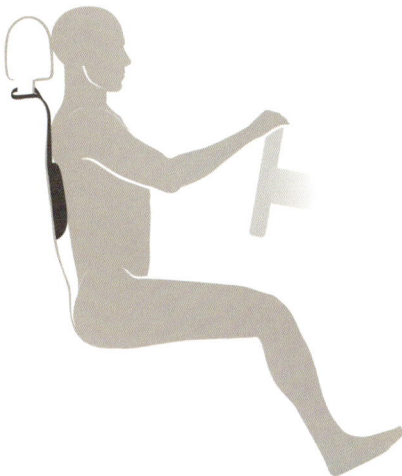

b. The Stretchsit Cushion straightens and lengthens your lumbar spine.

SITTING IN A CAR

This chapter would be incomplete without describing how to sit in a car. Because so many of us sit for hours every week in our cars, it is essential to spend those hours sitting well. You may remember a time when riding in a car was so comfortable that we called it "joy riding." With age, too many of us find that even a short road trip causes discomfort or pain. When you succeed in positioning yourself well, you will again find that driving is a pleasure, and you will no longer arrive at your destination feeling pain or stiffness.

Stretchsitting is especially important when driving. Using the instructions in this section will enable you to elongate your spine in your car. The extra space you gain between the vertebrae acts as a buffer against the motions of the car. It also counteracts the extra compression that can result from muscle tension when driving in stressful conditions.

Most car seats are poorly designed, including those with numerous adjustments. This is because they are made to reflect the average posture of the people using them. Unfortunately, they also perpetuate this average posture. The seats are too concave both vertically and horizontally. They push the driver's shoulders forward, causing the back to hunch (fig.1-18). They offer no place to hitch the thoracic spine and no possibility of doing a shoulder roll. However, you can remedy these problems by placing a support so that it rests at the level of the mid-back, just below the shoulder blades.

fig.1-18

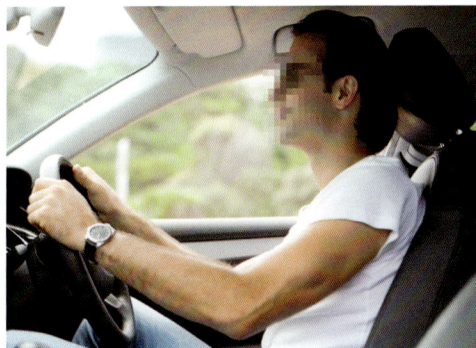

Most car seats cause your shoulders to hunch and your head to protrude forward.

FASHIONING A SUPPORTIVE BACKREST

The trick is to fold a piece of fabric into the appropriate shape for your back (fig.1-19a). The exact dimensions will depend on the contours of your car seat. The more curved your car seat, the thicker the cushion should be. In cars with slippery leather seats, position the folded material vertically, jamming one end between the headrest and the back of the seat (fig.1-19b). The rest of the material should drape down the seat to the level of the mid-back in a strip that fits between the shoulder blades. Be sure that your head still reaches the headrest. Or use my Stretchsit Cushion, which works by fastening around the headrest in all car seats (fig.1-19c).

fig.1-19a

Folded fabric can modify a car seat for healthy posture.

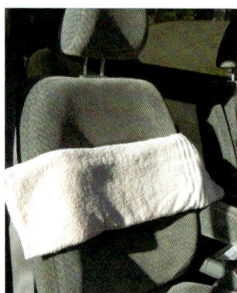

fig.1-19b

Some ingenuity is needed to modify leather seats for healthy posture.

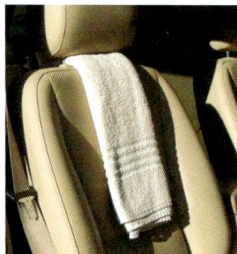

fig.1-19c

The Stretchsit Cushion has a strap that attaches around the headrest.

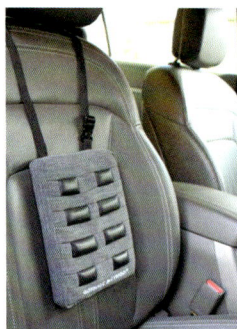

Once you have modified your car seat, the steps are similar to those for stretchsitting in a chair:

1. Shift your buttocks back into the seat relative to your upper body.
2. Lengthen your back and place it in traction by hitching to the back support you are using.

Rather than using just your arms to hoist your torso onto the outcropping, you may find it helpful to push with your legs. This works in a car because the seat is fixed and stable.

3. Perform a shoulder roll to move your shoulders back and down. Be sure your back support is thick enough that our shoulders are not impeded by the poor contours of the seat.

4. Check and adjust your distance to the steering wheel. You should be close enough to comfortably reach the wheel without rounding your shoulders. Note: Be sure to follow the manufacturer's guidelines for maintaining a safe distance from the air bags.

5. Lengthen your neck. Just as you can place your torso in traction against the back support, you may be able to place your neck in traction against the headrest (fig.1-20). If you find the headrest is pushing your head forward, increase the thickness of your back support.

Note: All adjustments should be made when your car is stationary, before driving.

fig.1-20

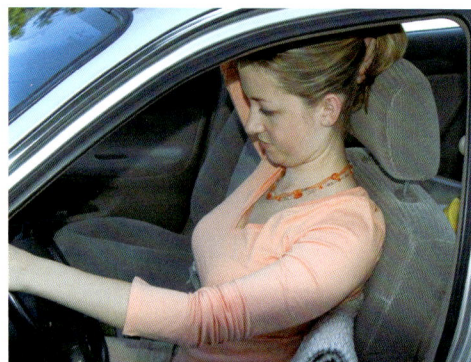

Lengthen your neck against the headrest to get gentle traction in your neck.

CHECKING YOUR POSITION

You can use the position of your rearview mirror to set a standard for your new seated height. Seat yourself as directed in these instructions and then adjust the rearview mirror to give you good rear vision. Now, whenever you drive, be sure you sit so that you can use the mirror in its established position. Don't adjust the mirror; adjust how you sit!

RECAP

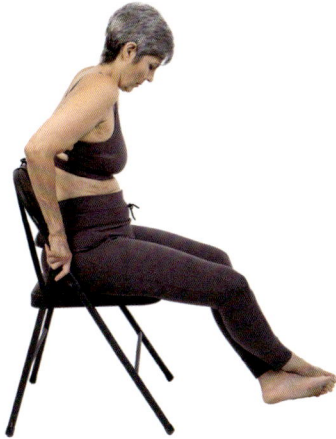

a. **Lengthen spine**

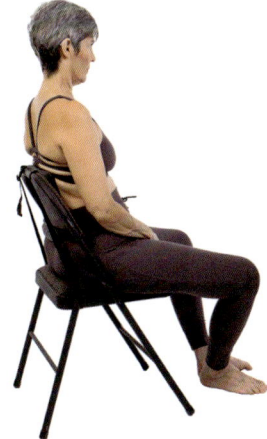

b. **Attach mid-back to chair**

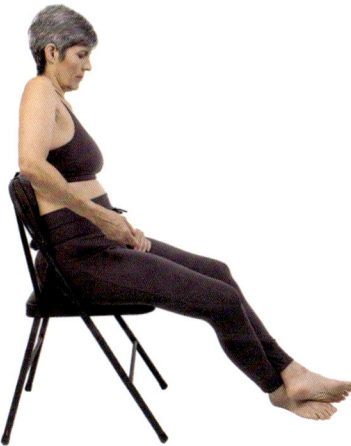

c. **Perform shoulder rolls**

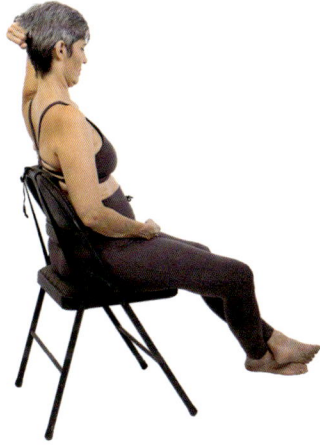

d. **Lengthen back of neck**

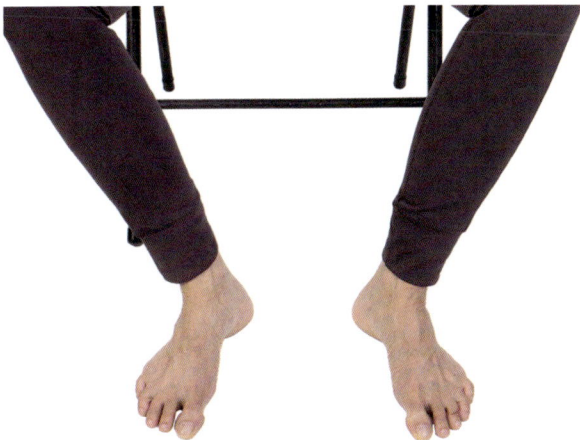

e. **Align feet in kidney bean shape**

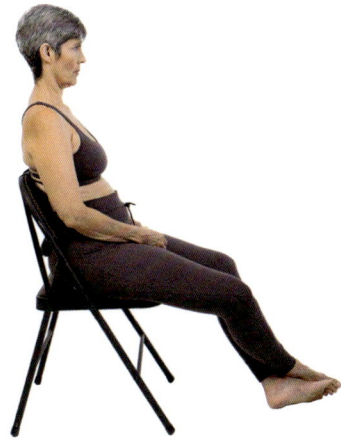

f. **Relax entire body**

2

STRETCHLYING ON YOUR BACK

Lying with a lengthened back

My youngest daughter sleeps peacefully as a baby. Notice the dome-like contour of her chest, her upper back
and neck in a straight line, her sacrum (the lowest part of her back) angled posteriorly leaving a gap between
it and the bed, and her head turned on the axis of the spine.

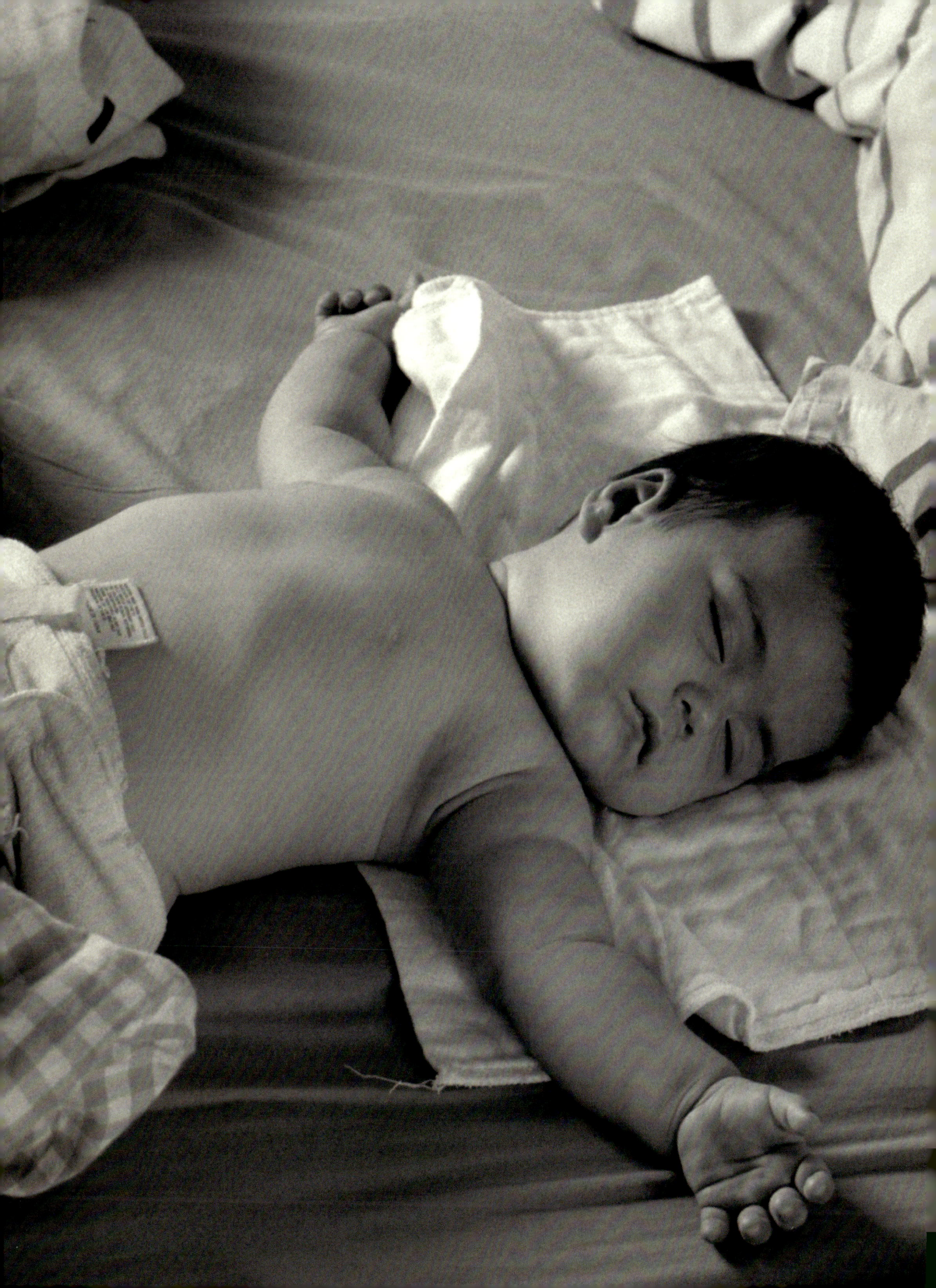

In this chapter you will learn the technique of stretchlying to elongate your spine when you lie down (fig.2-1). With this and the sitting position that you learned in the first chapter, you will gain therapeutic benefit for many hours each day—far more than that provided in any normal stretching regimen. Not only will you benefit from hours of therapeutic traction for your back, you will also enjoy improved sleep.

fig.2-2

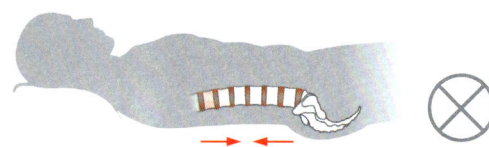

a. Lying compressed

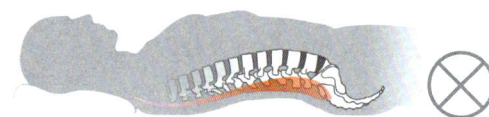

b. Lying swayed

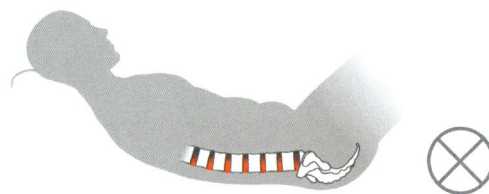

c. Lying rounded

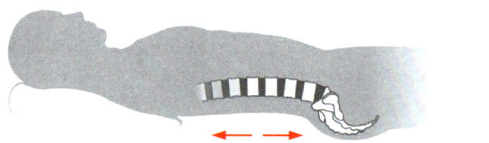

d. Lying stretched

Compromised (a,b,c) and ideal (d) ways to lie on your back.

fig.2-1

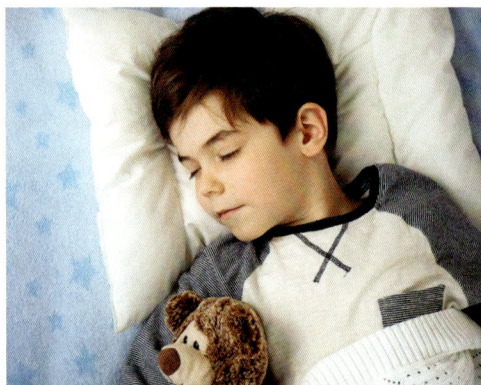

Stretchlying is a comfortable and healthy way to sleep.

A good night's sleep is nature's way of restoring and resetting the body, yet many people experience the night hours as a time of discomfort, restlessness, and even pain. Most of us understand the connection between emotions and sleep; fewer people understand the role of our sleep position.

A poor sleep position (fig.2-2a,b,c) threatens various body structures, which in turn signal the brain to change position. Tossing and turning is an attempt to find a healthy position in which your muscles can relax. If you don't succeed, and remain in an unhealthy position, you may well wake up with aches and pains because your muscles did not relax during the night (fig.2-3).

If you start the night with your body in a relaxed, comfortable position (fig.2-2d), you won't have to toss and turn to find one. You may be surprised by how long you remain in one position, and by how refreshed and comfortable you feel upon waking. Indeed, many people report waking in the same position after a whole night's sleep once they have learned stretchlying. When you have mastered the technique, it will only require a few seconds each night to get into an optimal position and enjoy improved sleep.

fig.2-3

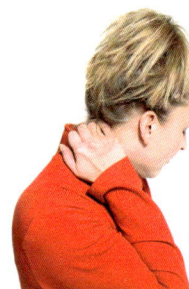

Poor sleep positions often result in aches and pains.

If you do not usually sleep on your back, you may question the value of this technique, but I encourage you to learn stretchlying for several reasons:

• You may surprise yourself by falling asleep in the stretchlying position.

- Even if you do not fall asleep, you will benefit from starting out the night with lengthened back muscles. They will retain some of the length even after you move out of this position.
- It is useful to cultivate more than one comfortable and healthy sleeping position to accommodate special circumstances, such as an injury.
- Many common exercises are performed lying on your back; stretchlying makes the exercises safer.
- Massage and other bodywork techniques usually require lying on the back. Again, stretchlying makes bodywork safer, more comfortable, and more effective.

When you first try a new sleep position, it may feel contrived, cumbersome, and not conducive to sleep. Begin each night by stretchlying for five minutes, then move to whatever position helps you fall asleep. Over time, you will probably surprise yourself by drifting off while stretchlying.

BENEFITS

- Improves quality of sleep

- Decompresses spinal discs

- Decompresses spinal nerves

- Improves circulation around the spine

- Resets the resting length of back muscles

- Improves breathing pattern

I had a severe back pain that used to especially interfere with my workouts. Since [learning] how to stretchlie on my back, I did it every night before falling asleep and now, three weeks later, I am completely pain free and back to my full workouts with no problem.

Marius Stalionis, Chicago, IL

The pain was so severe that my entire body was tense trying to fight it. There was no relief at night. No position would alleviate the throbbing. I would wake up as tense and weary as when I went to bed. People noticed the limp and the dragging of my left leg. Walking the dog was torture. Trying to mask the pain became impossible. Thoughts of surgery filled me with dread.

One of my friends suggested Esther Gokhale, who had helped her boss resolve recurring pain. I shall admit that I was skeptical. After my first session I walked out feeling better, but I believed that the relief would be short lived. That whole week was a week with minimal pain. I am still going to Esther. I have had a total of six visits. Learning is challenging. I have had no pain for four weeks. The work is not always easy, but the payoff is probably as close to a miracle as I'll ever get.

Smokey Chapman,
Palo Alto, CA

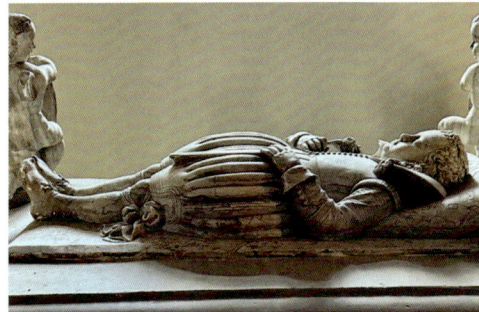

© Julie Johnson

(Germany)

57

EQUIPMENT

You will need the following:
- *Pillows: one or two for under your head and at least one for under your knees (See Further Information on page 65 for guidance on pillow thickness)*
- *A bed, a sofa, or a mat on the floor*

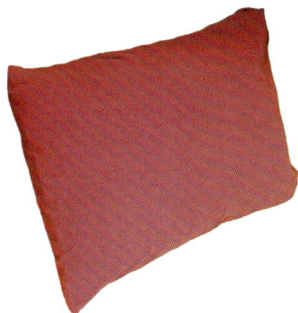

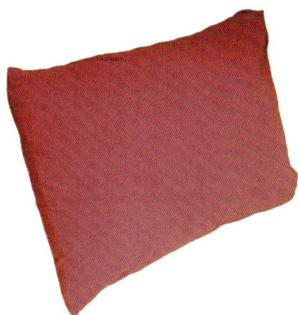

1 SIT WITH YOUR KNEES BENT AND YOUR FEET FLAT ON THE BED

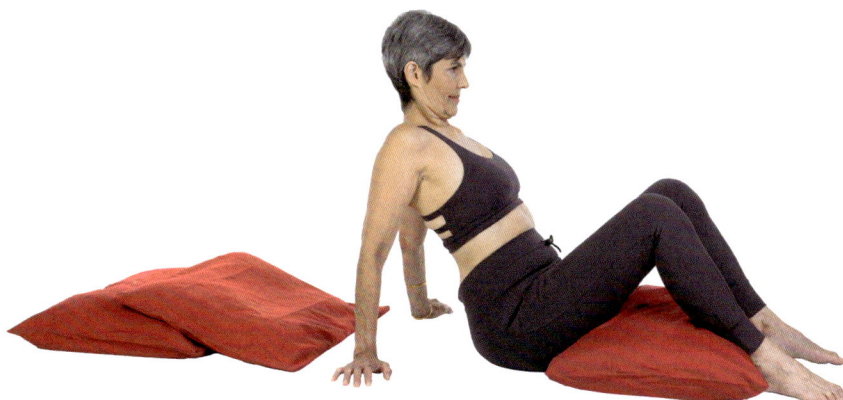

Your legs should be over (not resting on) a pillow, and your knees should point slightly out.

2 POSITION YOUR PILLOWS

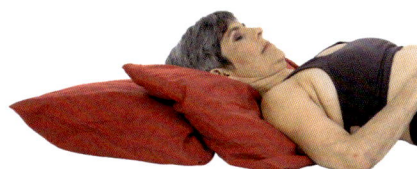

Position one or two pillows so that when you lie down, your head, neck, and 2–3 inches of your upper back will be on the pillow(s).

This pivots your rib cage, flattening your lower back.

3 PROP YOURSELF ON YOUR ELBOWS SUCH THAT YOUR UPPER ARMS FORM A 90° ANGLE WITH THE BED

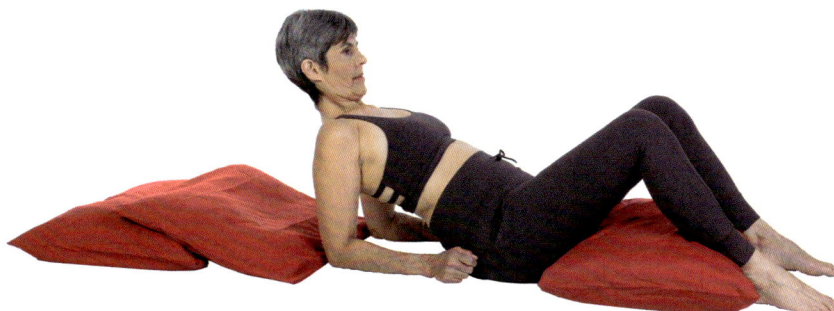

4 SLOWLY LOWER YOUR BACK ONTO THE BED WHILE LENGTHENING YOUR SPINE

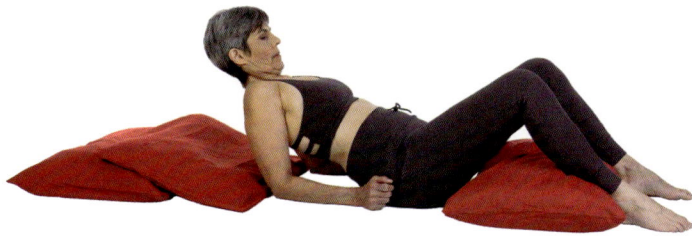

Press your elbows into the bed and down toward your feet, creating traction to gently introduce a comfortable amount of additional length into your lower back. Focus on lowering your back onto the bed segment by segment, positioning each segment further from the previous one than usual.

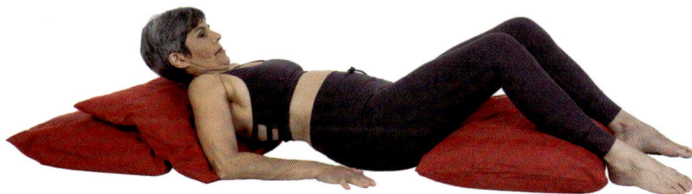

Slide your elbows out to the sides to allow the next segment to reach the bed.

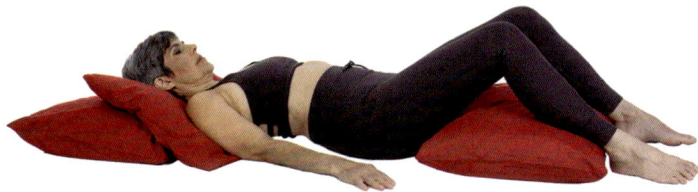

When your elbows no longer provide leverage, lower yourself the rest of the way, placing your upper shoulders and then head onto the pillow(s).

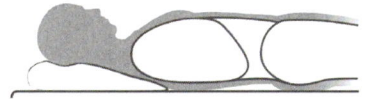

A common mistake is to arch the back as you lower it onto the bed. This shortens the back instead of lengthening it, undermining the main purpose of stretchlying. It may be helpful to think of your torso as a hammock and not as a bridge.

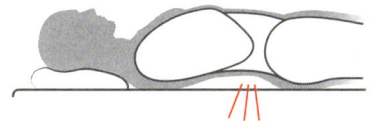

A nearly universal tendency is to tuck the pelvis during Step 4. With the discs decompressed by stretchlying, this will likely do no harm. However, if you feel any discomfort, use the maneuver in Step 10.

A PILLOW UNDER THE SHOULDERS FACILITATES HEALTHY STRETCHLYING

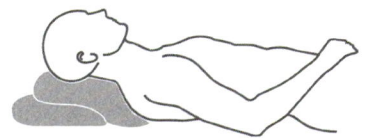

A pillow under the shoulders rotates the rib cage and decompresses the lower back.

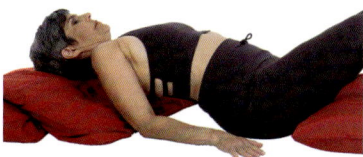

No pillow under the shoulders can result in a swayed and compressed lower back.

ACCOMMODATING A ROUNDED UPPER BACK

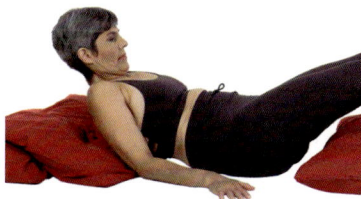

Significant kyphosis (rounding in the upper back) can be accommodated by placing an additional pillow under the head in a staircase fashion.

IDEAL AND COMPROMISED NECK POSITIONS

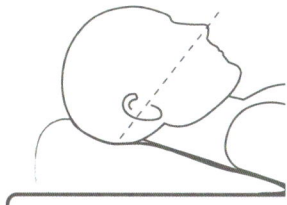

A pillow under the shoulders reduces curvature in the neck.

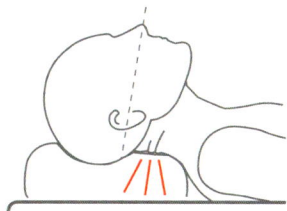

No pillow under the shoulders can result in a compressed neck.

EXAMPLES OF HEALTHY NECK POSITION

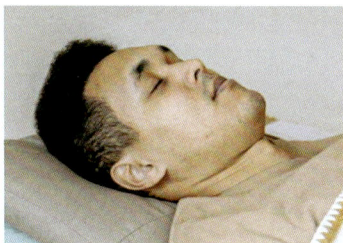

(Poland)

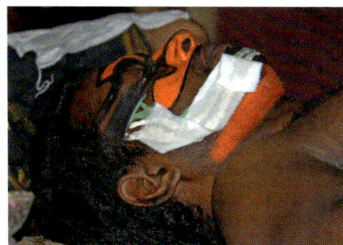

Kathakali dancer having makeup applied (India)

5 CHECK THE POSITION OF YOUR PILLOW

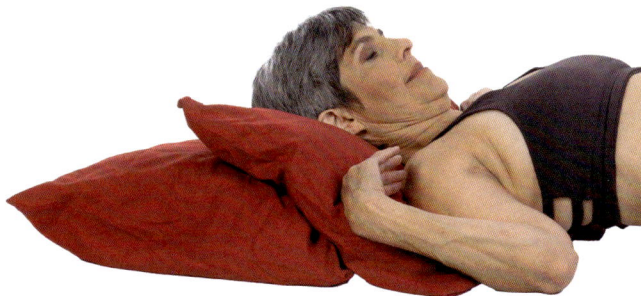

Your shoulders, neck, and head should be slightly raised on the edge of the pillow. You may have to adjust the position of the pillow if, after elongating your spine, you are too high or low on the pillow.

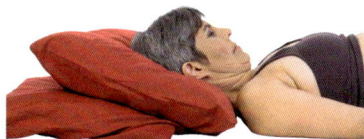

If you are too low on the pillow, it can cause your neck to curve forward.

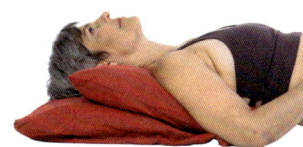

If you are too high on the pillow, it can cause your neck to sway.

6 GENTLY ELONGATE YOUR NECK

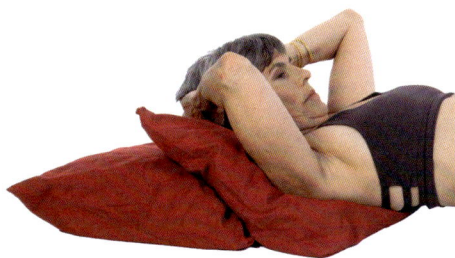

Keeping your head and neck relaxed, use your hands to lengthen the back of your neck. It is important to do this gently.

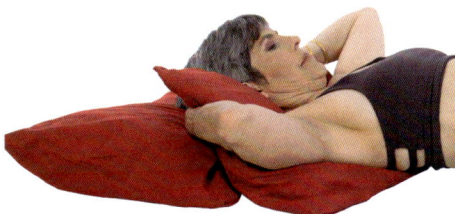

Scrunch the pillow towards your shoulders to fill any gap so your neck is fully supported.

7 SLIDE YOUR SHOULDER BLADES DOWN ALONG YOUR SPINE

HEALTHY ARM POSITIONS

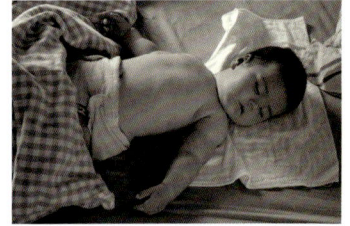

(USA)

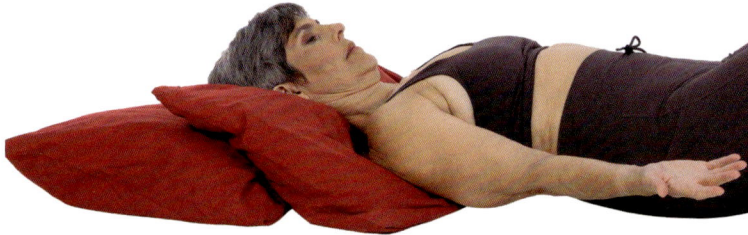

Earlier, you used your elbows to position your back, so now your shoulders may be hiked up towards your ears. Because you cannot complete a full shoulder roll with the pillow behind your shoulders, instead turn your palms up and slide your shoulders down and slightly away from your body. If the stretch in the *trapezius muscles* feels uncomfortable, back off a little.

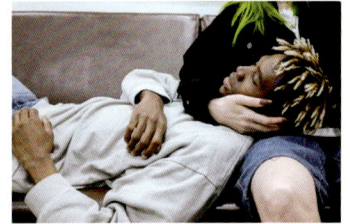

(Russia)

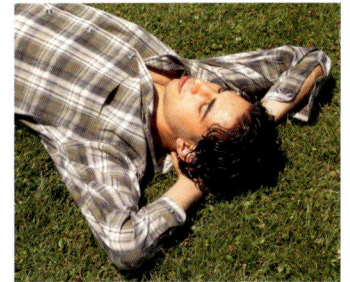

(USA)

8 POSITION YOUR ARMS COMFORTABLY AT YOUR SIDES

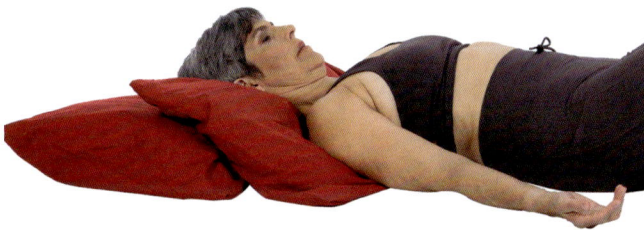

Lying with your palms up orients your arms and shoulders well.

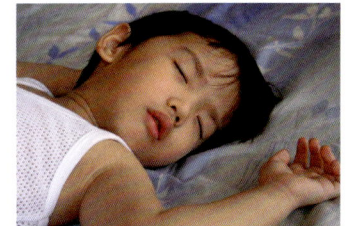

(USA)

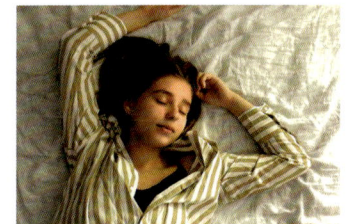

(Russia)

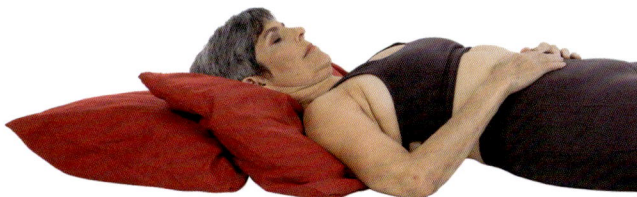

Some people find it comfortable to bend their arms softly at the elbow, resting their hands on their abdomen. Others prefer to rest their arms under or above the head.

COMPENSATING FOR TIGHT PSOAS MUSCLES

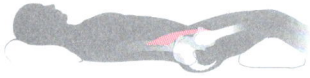

Placing a pillow under the knees compensates for tight psoas muscles, which originate at the front of the lumbar spine and end at the top of the femurs.

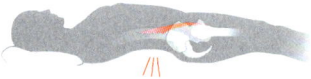

Lying with outstretched legs can cause a sway if the psoas muscles are tight.

Many people who have tight psoas muscles instinctively bend their knees to facilitate better alignment and greater comfort in the lower back (USA).

For an exercise to stretch the psoas muscles, see Appendix 1, page 220.

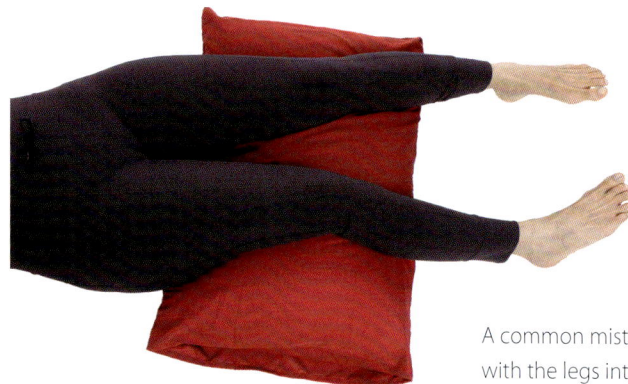

9 STRAIGHTEN AND RELAX YOUR LEGS ONTO THE PILLOW

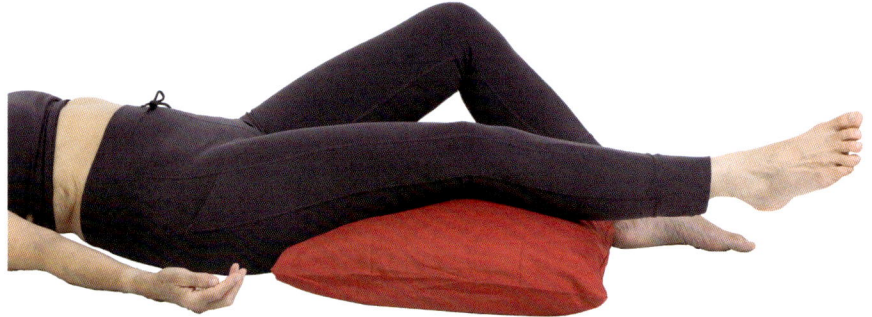

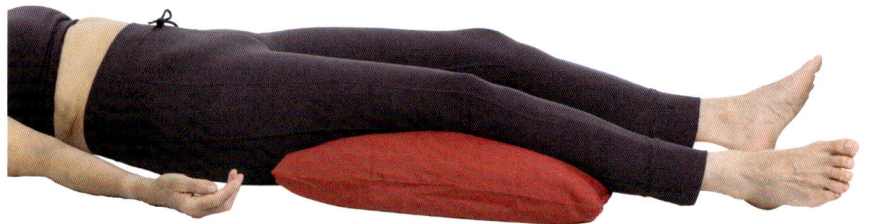

Gently rotate your legs and knees outward from the hip joint. The pillow beneath your knees supports them in a slightly bent position, relieving stress on your lower back.

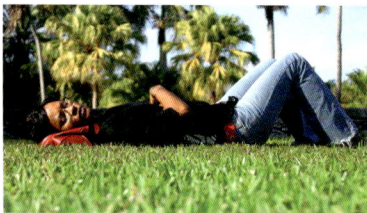

A common mistake is to lie with the legs internally rotated.

10 IF YOUR PELVIS IS TUCKED, REPEAT THE STEPS IN THIS CHAPTER, STEADYING YOUR PELVIS WITH YOUR HANDS

HEALTHY STRETCHLYING CAN HAPPEN AT MANY ANGLES

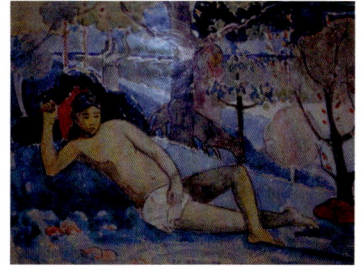

(USA)

When lengthening your spine, it is easy to unwittingly tuck your pelvis. Think about your pubic bone facing more towards your knees than towards the ceiling. If you find your pelvis still tucks during Step 4, use your hands to steady it, with the fingers facing toward your feet and the thumb hooked behind the rim of your pelvis (the *iliac crest*).

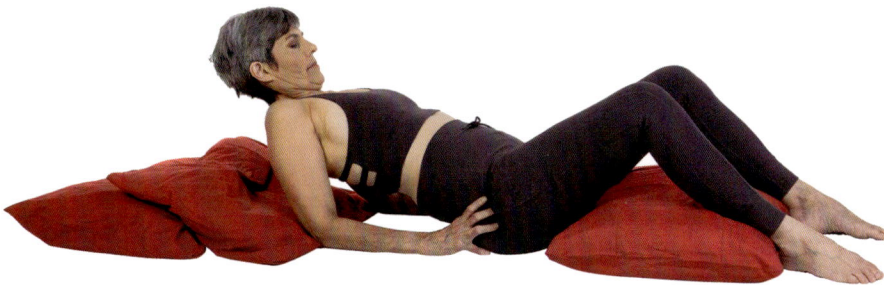

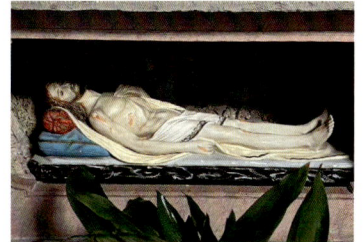

(Italy)

If you are lying on a firm surface, you should feel a small gap between your lower back and the surface you are lying on, just above your bottom. This is a good sign that your pelvis is not tucked, and you have achieved a J-spine. If there is no gap, your pelvis is probably tucked. Note that if you are lying on a mattress, it will likely conform to your body contours, so you won't feel the gap.

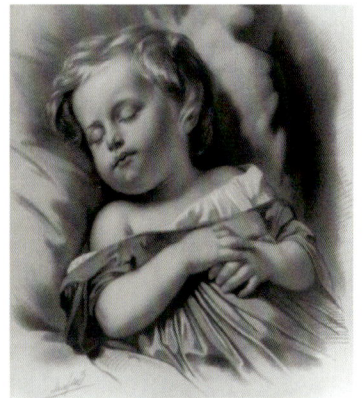

(USA)

11 RELAX YOUR WHOLE BODY

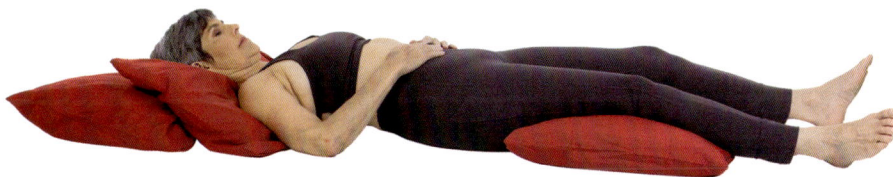

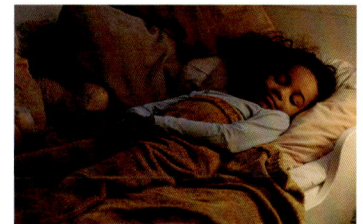

(USA)

Try to locate any tension in your body and release it. Lie in this position for five minutes, letting your muscles completely relax. If it feels comfortable, you can stay here all night if you wish.

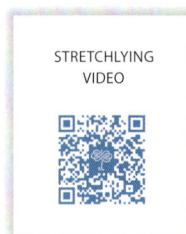

STRETCHLYING VIDEO

63

INDICATIONS OF IMPROVEMENT

When you spend an appreciable amount of time stretchlying, you will notice the same improvements as with stretchsitting: the resting length of your back muscles will increase, you'll experience less stiffness and resistance to stretch in your back, your height will be measurably taller, and you will be more comfortable even when not in traction. You will toss and turn less and experience better sleep.

Over time, your lengthened back muscles will contribute to improved circulation (which hastens healing of damaged areas), and will help to decompress discs and nerves. Normalizing this area should improve your general well-being.

As with stretchsitting, you will also notice changes in your breathing pattern. To track this, pay attention to which parts of your body move as you breathe (fig.2-4). Place one hand on your chest and one hand on your abdomen to check their relative movement. You should notice more movement in your chest and less in your abdomen, because your stretched abdominal muscles now offer some resistance to belly breathing. Meanwhile, the improved alignment of the head, neck, and upper torso facilitate easier movement in your chest. Over time, this increase in chest breathing will expand your lung capacity and support healthy architecture in your rib cage.

fig.2-4

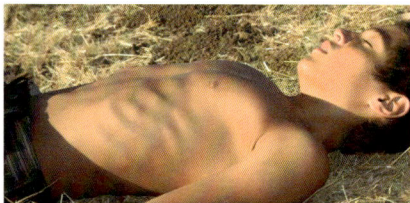

Inhalation

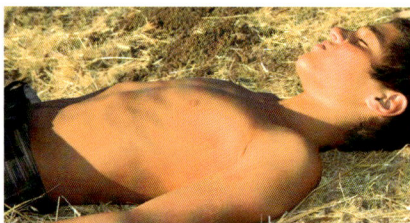

Exhalation
A healthy baseline breathing pattern expands the chest more than the abdomen.

TROUBLESHOOTING

FEELING PAIN OR DISCOMFORT IN THE LOWER BACK

• You may have very tight *psoas muscles* that are pulling your back into a sway, despite the pillow under your knees. Place more pillows under your knees until you feel no difference between Step 8 (knees bent) and Step 9 (legs on the pillow(s)) (fig.2-5).

fig.2-5

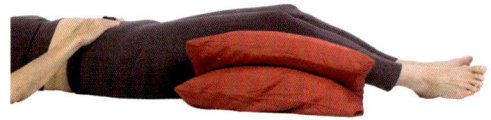

Placing extra pillows under the knees compensates for tight psoas muscles.

• You may have tucked your pelvis as you lowered your back onto the bed. If this has occurred, repeat Steps 3–9, this time placing your hands firmly on your pelvic rim to hold it stable as you elongate your back (see Step 10).

FEELING PAIN OR DISCOMFORT IN THE NECK

• You may have excessive neck curvature. Adjust the pillow(s) to a height that is appropriate to the curvature in your neck and upper *thoracic* spine. You may even have to bunch the pillow up a little to form a "cervical roll," though make sure you are not encouraging your neck to curve more than it does already (fig.2-6). You are aiming for comfortable support and the elimination of tension. This may require experimentation with pillows of different firmness and thickness.

fig.2-6

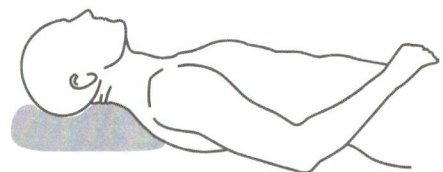

If you have excessive neck curvature, you may not be able to lengthen your neck a great deal. Support what curvature you have, and slowly work in the direction of lengthening the back of your neck.

- You may have overstretched your neck. If you feel uncomfortable, ease up a bit until you feel comfortable. Overstretching the neck muscles, especially if done abruptly, can trigger muscle spasms.

FEELING DISCOMFORT AT A POINT OF CONTACT WITH THE BED

You may have local inflammation that is causing discomfort. Sleep on your side for now (as described in Chapter 4, "Stretchlying on Your Side") and return to this technique later.

SNORING

Though good alignment can help reduce snoring even when you lie on your back, your problem may be too severe to overcome in this way. Sleep on your side rather than on your back to get a good night's sleep. If you suspect sleep apnea, consult a sleep expert.

FEELINGS OF EXPOSURE

You may feel exposed and vulnerable stretchlying on your back. Focus on the comfortable feeling in your body and you will likely soon get used to the new position.

FURTHER INFORMATION

BEDS

People often ask me for recommendations on beds. After learning to stretchlie, you will find that you tolerate a greater variety of sleep surfaces. For example, a night spent on a bed with a slight sag or on a hard surface will not cause damage or trigger protective tightening in the spinal muscles (fig.2-7). In stretchlying, your discs are decompressed, so they can tolerate distortions in the shape of the spine much better than compressed discs can.

An ideal bed is neither too firm nor too soft. It gives a little to accommodate the uneven contours of your body (especially important for wide-hipped, narrow-waisted people who sleep on their side), but does not let your heavier parts sink too deeply into the bed. The bed should not let your trunk sink too much relative to your arms, or your hips sink too much relative to your trunk. I recommend a high-quality, medium-firm mattress.

PILLOWS

The right pillow for you depends on how much rigidity and curvature you have in your *cervical* (neck) and upper *thoracic* spine. A good pillow reflects your current baseline posture but encourages your neck to move in the direction of the ideal, albeit gradually (fig.2-8). It does not perpetuate or, worse, exaggerate unhealthy curvature (fig.2-9, fig.2-10). A good pillow has enough substance to hold a baseline shape, yet enough softness to be caressing and conducive to relaxation and sleep. One solution is to use two pillows—the lower one filled with a firm substance (like buckwheat hulls or kapok) and the upper one with a soft filling (like goose down or synthetic fill).

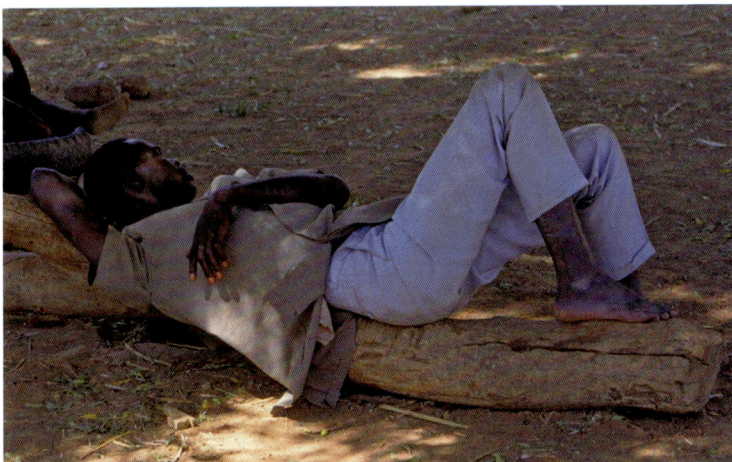

fig.2-7

If you have a decompressed spine, you will tolerate a wide range of mattress firmness. The "bed" in this photograph is "extra-extra-firm," but is not causing the sleeper any problems (Burkina Faso).

fig.2-8

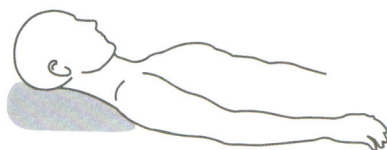

A pillow placed under your head and slightly under your shoulders serves to elongate your neck and lower back.

fig.2-9

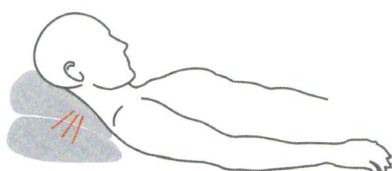

A high pillow placed only under the head and not the shoulders causes your head to jut forward, distorting your neck.

CERVICAL PILLOWS / ROLLS

Cervical pillows and rolls, like lumbar cushions, are based on misguided notions about what constitutes normal and desirable curvature in the human spine (fig.2-10). Cervical pillows and rolls are designed to support "natural" curvature in the neck or create it if it isn't there. My approach encourages you to lengthen rather than curve your cervical spine. A normal rectangular or square pillow of a thickness and firmness appropriate to the shape of your neck works best.

Only if you have significant curvature in your neck and your neck is somewhat rigid, should you use a cervical pillow (or bunch your pillow under your neck). In this case the cervical pillow is a transitional device that allows the excessively curved portion of your neck to relax against a surface rather than be unsupported. The cervical roll should never exaggerate the curvature you already have. It should have a thickness intermediate between the curvature in your neck and the ideal (little or no curvature). Over time, you will be able to reduce the thickness of the cervical roll until you don't need one any more.

fig.2-10

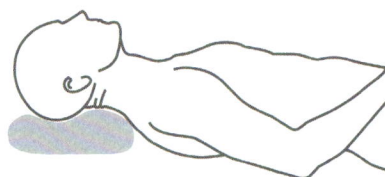

Cervical pillows may cause your neck to extend excessively. Use them only for transitional purposes.

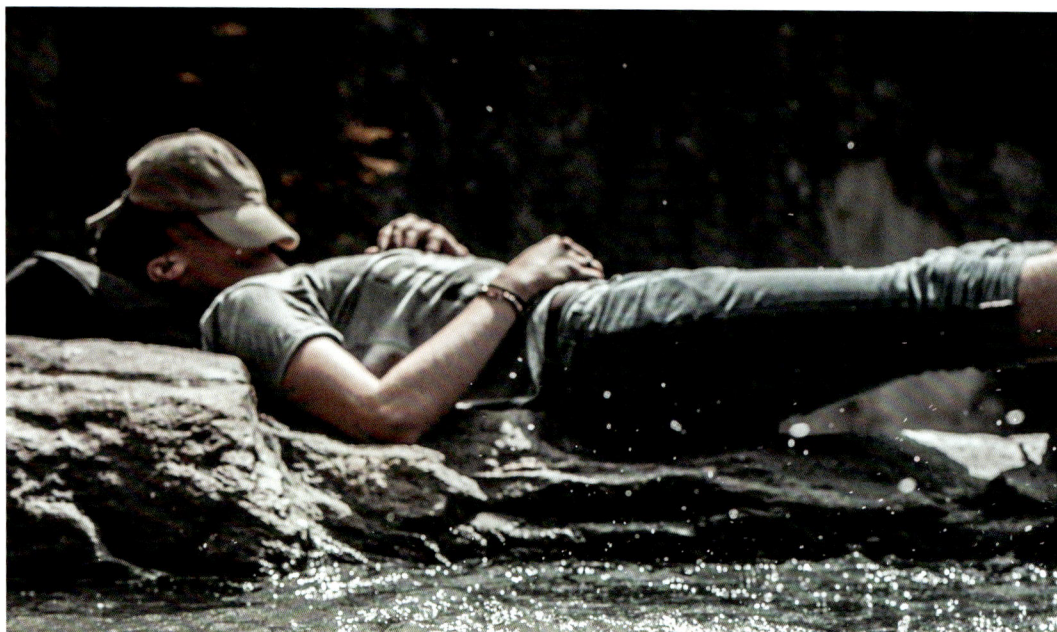

(Canada)

RECAP

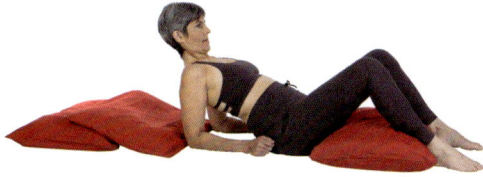

a. Prop yourself up on your elbows with knees bent

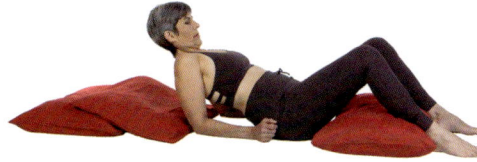

b. Push with your elbows to elongate your lower back

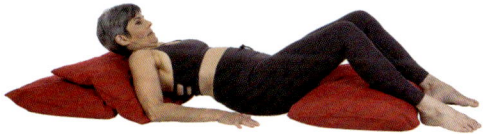

c. Unroll back onto bed, one segment at a time

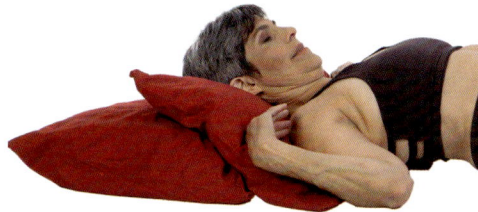

d. Make sure upper back is on pillow

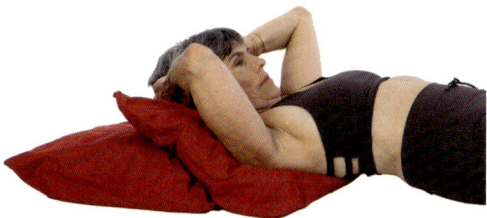

e. Lengthen back of neck

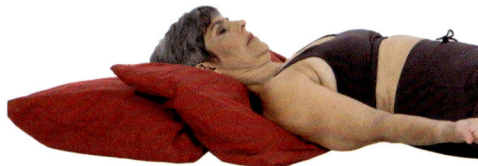

f. Slide shoulders down toward feet

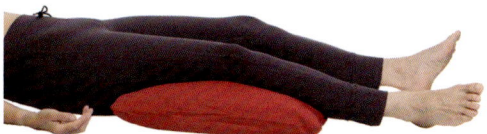

g. Straighten and relax legs onto pillow(s)

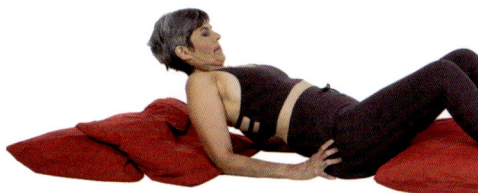

h. Check for pelvic tuck; start over if necessary

3

STACKSITTING

*Positioning your pelvis as the
foundation for your spine*

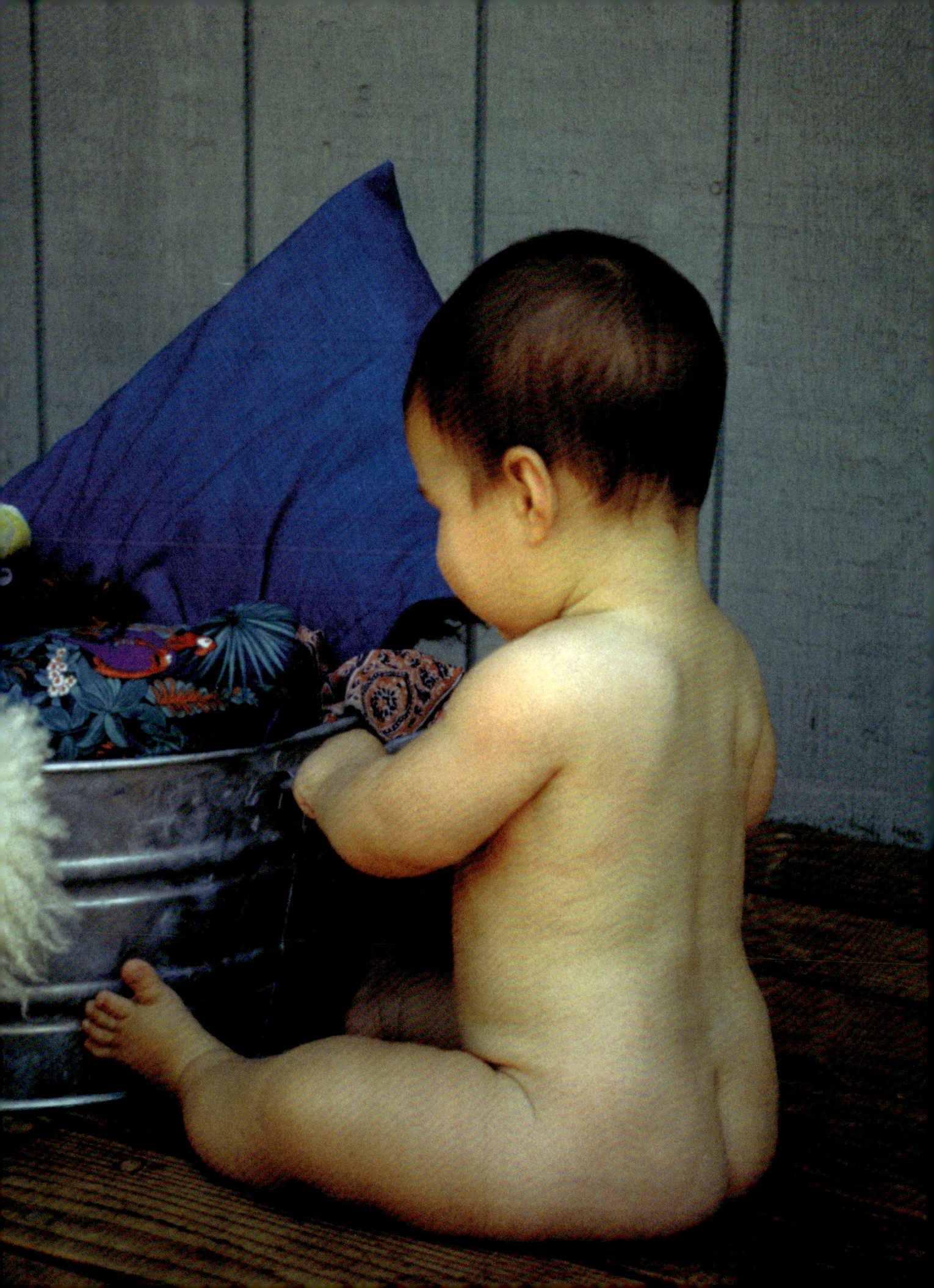

In the adjacent photographs (fig.3-1), notice that the rider on the left sits upright while the rider on the right sits with a familiar slump. How would you fix the posture of the man on the motorbike? Most people would ask him to "sit up straight," "straighten up," or pull his shoulders and neck back to be more upright. He certainly could do that, but it would require tension in his lower back muscles to maintain the position. He would then be upright but tense, with his lower back compressed and compromised. After a while, he would probably return to slumping. Many people alternate between tense muscles and a slumped back, neither of which is healthy.

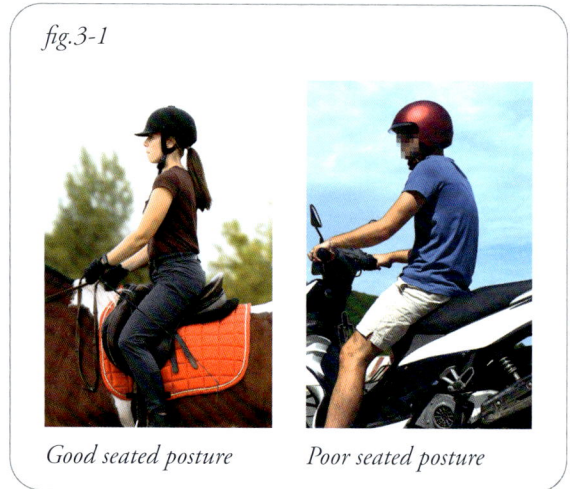

fig.3-1

Good seated posture   *Poor seated posture*

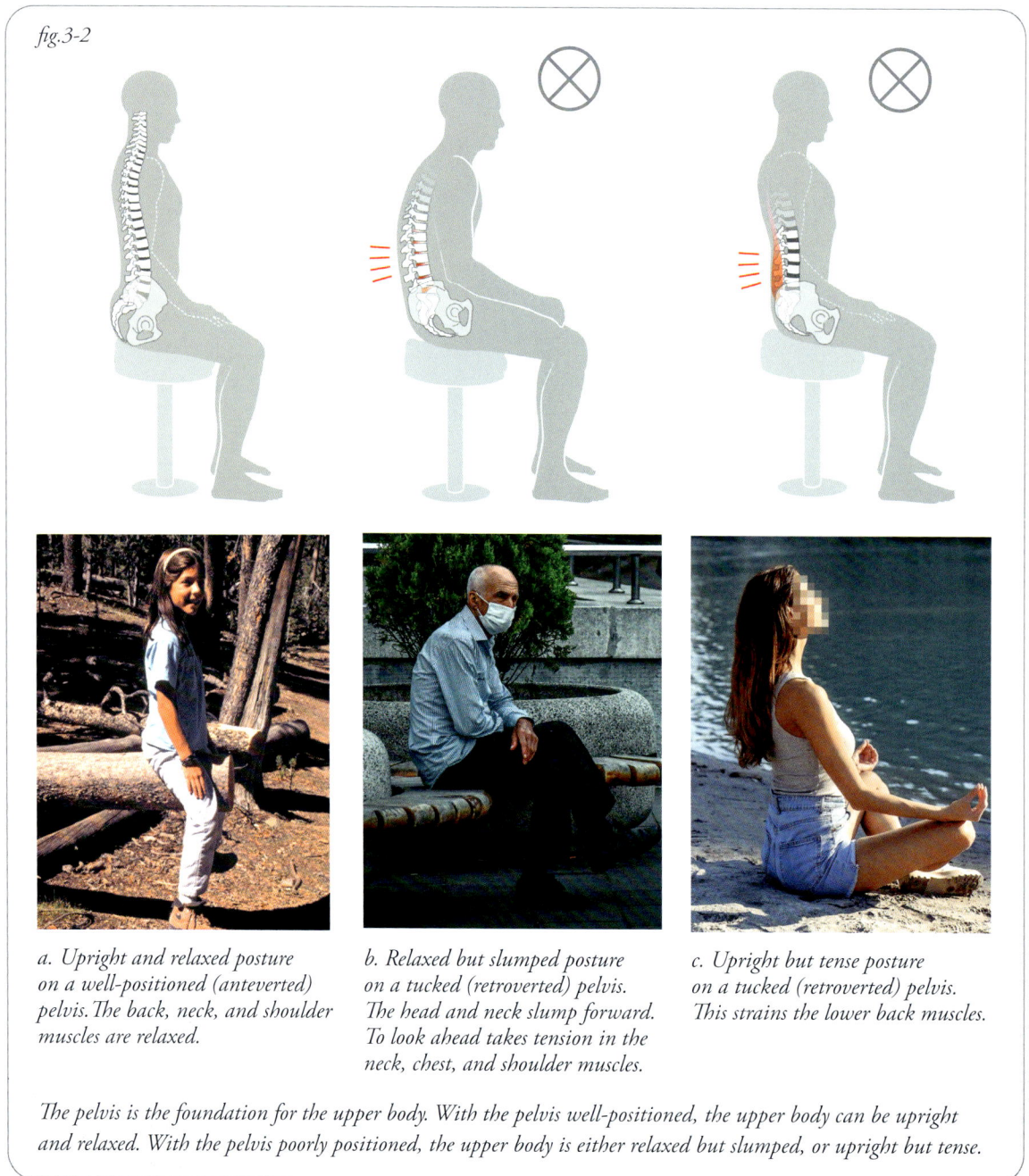

fig.3-2

a. Upright and relaxed posture on a well-positioned (anteverted) pelvis. The back, neck, and shoulder muscles are relaxed.

b. Relaxed but slumped posture on a tucked (retroverted) pelvis. The head and neck slump forward. To look ahead takes tension in the neck, chest, and shoulder muscles.

c. Upright but tense posture on a tucked (retroverted) pelvis. This strains the lower back muscles.

The pelvis is the foundation for the upper body. With the pelvis well-positioned, the upper body can be upright and relaxed. With the pelvis poorly positioned, the upper body is either relaxed but slumped, or upright but tense.

What is needed to break this cycle is a shift in the pelvis. This piece of our anatomy serves as the foundation for the spine and the rest of our structure. In our species, the pelvis is designed to be tipped forward (*anteverted*). When your pelvis is anteverted, the rest of your spine can stack well, so that you can be both upright and relaxed without requiring a lot of muscle tension to support your spine (fig.3-2a). When your pelvis is poorly positioned, you will be either relaxed but slumped (fig.3-2b) or upright but tense (fig.3-2c).

One way to gauge pelvic position is to imagine that you have a tail (fig.3-3). If you look again at the picture of the two riders in fig.3-1 and imagine they both have tails, the one sitting upright would have her tail behind her, whereas the rider who is slumping would be sitting on his tail.

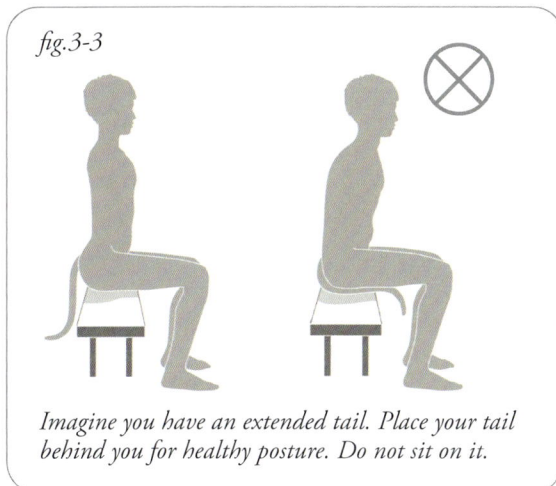

fig.3-3

Imagine you have an extended tail. Place your tail behind you for healthy posture. Do not sit on it.

In this chapter, you will learn more about the art and science of sitting. In Chapter 1, you learned how to use a backrest to place your back in therapeutic traction as you sit. But a backrest isn't always available, and sometimes, even when one is available, it is not practical to use it (for example, when you eat). In this chapter, you will learn how to sit well without a backrest.

This chapter also lets you experience a key concept of the Gokhale Method. Contrary to popular belief, good posture is not something that requires a grand effort. It is, for the most part, relaxed. What it takes is the right positioning of the bones, which enables the muscles to relax. When your pelvis is well-positioned, your vertebrae will stack easily with a minimum of muscle tension, like a tower of building blocks positioned on a stable foundation (fig.3-4). I call this "stacksitting."

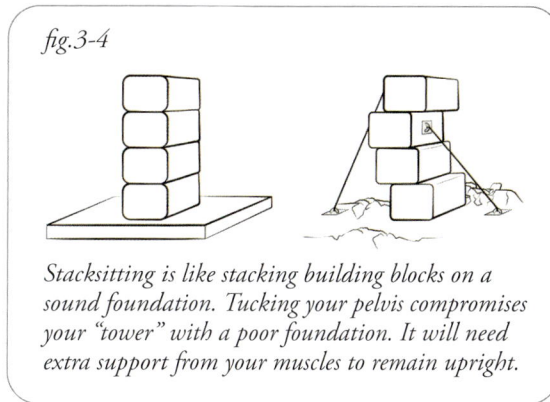

fig.3-4

Stacksitting is like stacking building blocks on a sound foundation. Tucking your pelvis compromises your "tower" with a poor foundation. It will need extra support from your muscles to remain upright.

THE WEDGE

In people who have tucked their pelvis for years, the surrounding tissues have adapted to this architecture. The muscles, tendons, fascia, and ligaments in the groin area, as well as the hamstring muscles, tend to be short and tight, while the muscles in the buttocks tend to be weak and underdeveloped. To compensate for this distorted baseline position, it is helpful to sit on a wedge (fig.3-5, fig.3-6).

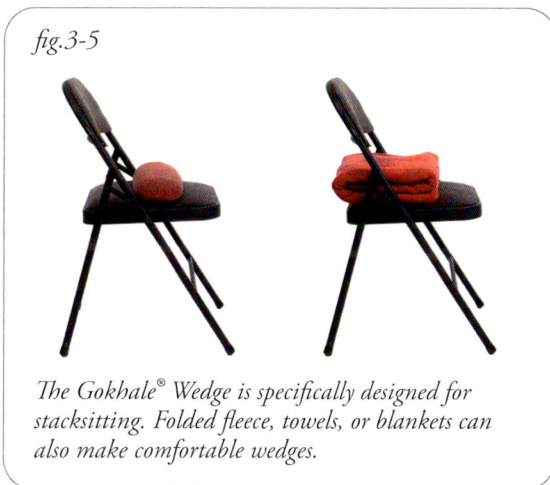

fig.3-5

The Gokhale® Wedge is specifically designed for stacksitting. Folded fleece, towels, or blankets can also make comfortable wedges.

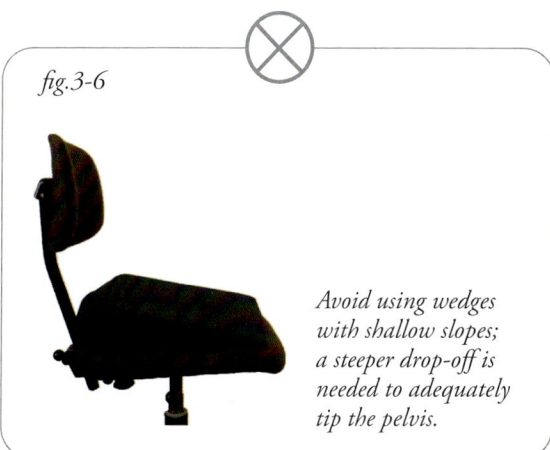

fig.3-6

Avoid using wedges with shallow slopes; a steeper drop-off is needed to adequately tip the pelvis.

Due to differences in L5-S1 angle, body shape, and muscle tone, everyone has their own unique requirement for wedge height and consistency. A good wedge facilitates tipping the pelvis forward (*anteversion*), and can transform your sitting experience quite dramatically. You may find that your spine immediately stacks effortlessly and comfortably on its base, and you can sit for hours in one position. Especially during the period of transition, as you train your body, a wedge will compensate for the compromised structures in the pelvic area. When a wedge is not available, an alternative is to perch on the very front edge of a firm chair, allowing your pelvis to tip forward (fig.3-7).

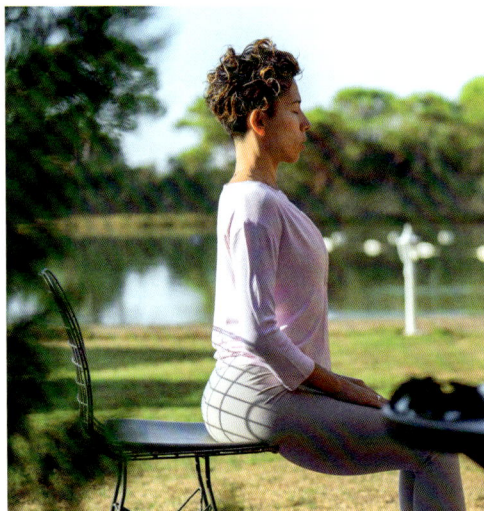

fig.3-7

If a wedge is not available, perch on the front edge of your chair, preferably with one or both thighs slanted downwards.

THE ANTEVERTED PELVIS

When your pelvis is anteverted, your back muscles relax, which has implications far beyond comfortable sitting.

One important effect is improved breathing. With relaxed back muscles, there is an elastic movement in the spine (fig.3-8a).

The new elasticity in the torso promotes good circulation, which promotes tissue health around the area of the spine, and improves overall health. Normalizing this area can have a positive effect on all of your muscles, organs, and other tissues.

This concept is so important that it bears repeating:

- The tissues around the spine remain healthy only if they have good circulation.
- Good circulation around the spine happens only if there is movement in the area.
- Nature's way of providing movement in this area is through a healthy breathing pattern.
- A healthy breathing pattern can happen only if the muscles in the area can relax appropriately.
- The muscles in the area can relax only if there is a sound stacking of the bones.
- And the bones stack well only if the pelvis is positioned well.

With relaxed chest (*pectoral*) muscles, breathing also causes an expansive movement in the chest (fig.3-8a). Over a period of years, this movement increases the size of the rib cage and the capacity of the lungs.

Incidentally, you may notice that your abdomen becomes less involved in breathing, except when you need extra oxygen for cardiovascular exercise, playing wind instruments, singing, and such.

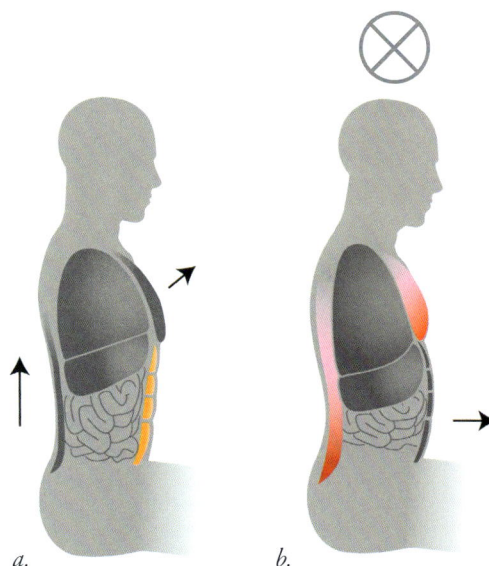

fig.3-8

a.   b.

When your back and pectoral muscles are relaxed and your abdominal muscles have good tone (a), your resting breathing action will be primarily in the back and chest. If your back and chest are tight and/or your abdominal muscles are flaccid (b), your resting breathing action will be mainly in the belly.

Another effect of pelvic anteversion is that your pelvic organs will be supported by your pubic bone and well-aligned connective tissues (fig.3-9a). With a tucked pelvis (fig.3-9b), the main supporting structure under the pelvic organs is the rather flimsy Kegel (*pubococcygeus*) muscle. In my experience with students, a tucked (*retroverted*) pelvis predisposes for organ prolapse and urinary incontinence.

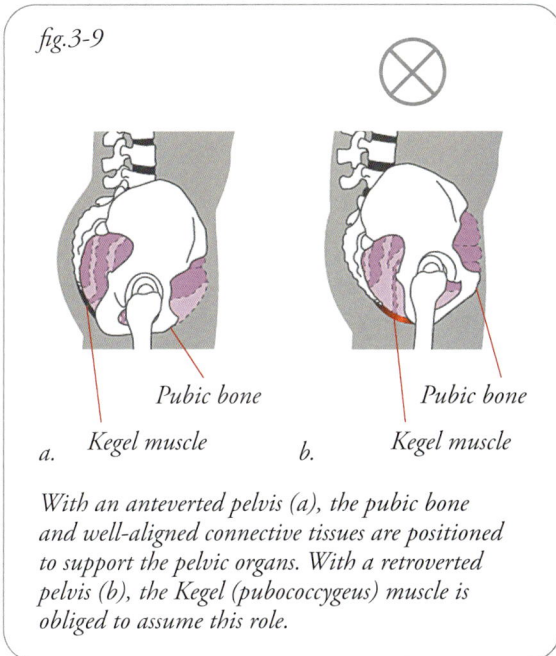

fig.3-9

Pubic bone

Pubic bone

a. *Kegel muscle*   *b.* *Kegel muscle*

With an anteverted pelvis (a), the pubic bone and well-aligned connective tissues are positioned to support the pelvic organs. With a retroverted pelvis (b), the Kegel (pubococcygeus) muscle is obliged to assume this role.

By anteverting the pelvis, you will be restoring normal architecture and function to the pelvic organs. You will also be protecting the wedge-shaped L5-S1 disc (see fig.F-26 on page 21).

PROCEED SLOWLY

If you are not used to this position, learning to antevert your pelvis may be difficult. Stacksitting and stretchlying on your side (Chapter 4) help to cultivate the habit. The wedge or the bed "hold" your pelvis in place, so you do not have to consciously maintain this position. Proceed very slowly and gently. Initially, practice a few minutes several times a day, gradually lengthening the time as the position becomes comfortable. When not sitting with a wedge, try to maximize the time spent sitting in traction as you learned to do in Chapter 1.

Caution

If you have a diagnosis, or any suspicion, of a herniated disc in the lower lumbar area (L5-S1), it is extremely important that you not antevert

your pelvis prematurely. Doing so may pinch off the herniated portion of the disc (fig.3-10). Wait to do this and the following chapter (stretchlying on your side) until you have the guidance of a qualified Gokhale Method teacher. Chapters 1, 2, and 5 teach you safe ways to lengthen your spine, which will make you more comfortable and can accelerate the healing of the herniated disc.

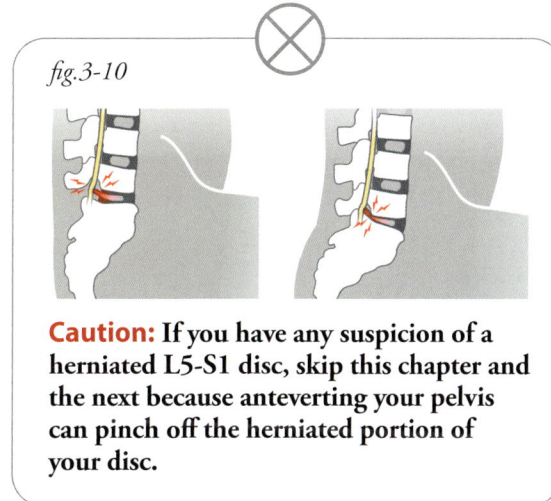

fig.3-10

Caution: **If you have any suspicion of a herniated L5-S1 disc, skip this chapter and the next because anteverting your pelvis can pinch off the herniated portion of your disc.**

BENEFITS

• Allows you to sit comfortably for hours

• Relaxes back muscles

• Facilitates elastic action of breathing

• Provides strong support for pelvic organs

• Facilitates optimal circulation throughout the back

• Allows for repair and optimal function of surrounding tissues and organs

This fine-tuned method has taught me to correct spine and rib cage positions I had not even known were causing my back and shoulder pain! Now, if I notice I'm hunching or sitting or standing in a painful way, I can correct it immediately. It feels as though a great burden is lifting off of my shoulders.

Grace Nix, San Francisco, CA

EQUIPMENT

You will need the following:
- *A full-length mirror or camera screen*
- *A stool or chair with a firm seat*
- *Comfortable form-fitting clothing that permits you to evaluate the position of your pelvis and shape of your spine. Don't wear jeans, which can distort your baseline position and make it difficult to evaluate your posture.*

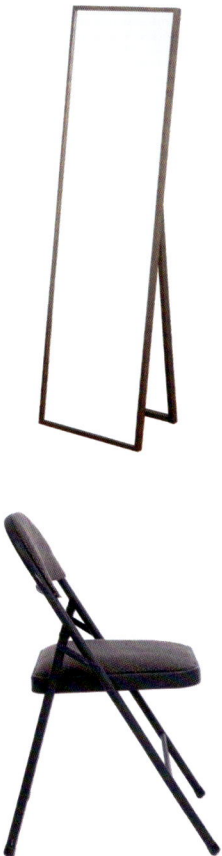

In the first part of this lesson you will analyze how you currently sit, evaluating where you need to make adjustments. In the second part, you will experiment to make those adjustments, attaining a healthy and well-aligned seated position.

EVALUATING YOUR HABITUAL POSTURE

1 PLACE A CHAIR SIDEWAYS IN FRONT OF A MIRROR, OR HAVE A FRIEND TAKE A PHOTO OF YOU SO THAT YOU CAN SEE YOUR BODY IN PROFILE

2 SIT ON THE FRONT OF THE CHAIR AWAY FROM THE BACKREST

Try to assume your habitual sitting posture rather than what you perceive to be correct. Your posture may resemble one of these images.

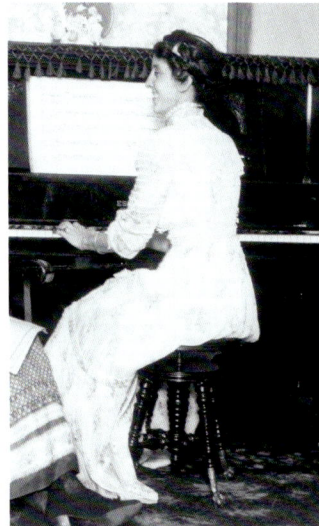

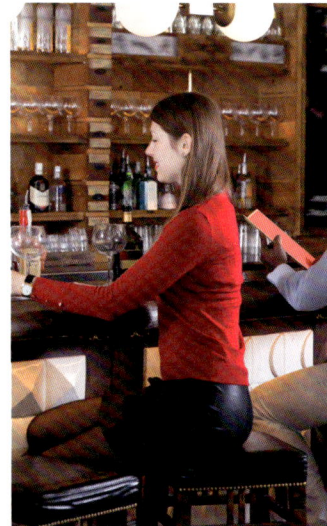

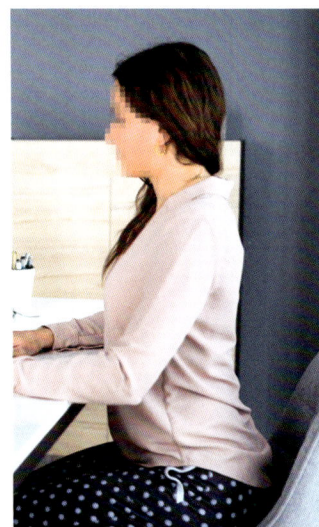

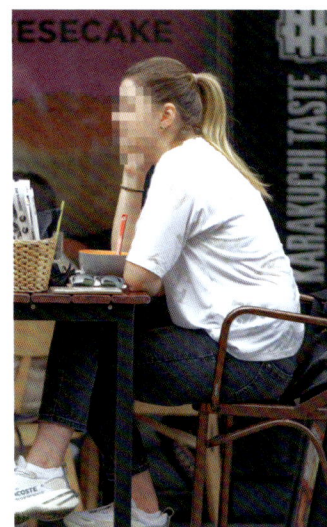

3 ASSESS THE POSITION OF YOUR PELVIS

Compare your pelvic position in the mirror or on the screen with the positions in the photos and drawings on this page.

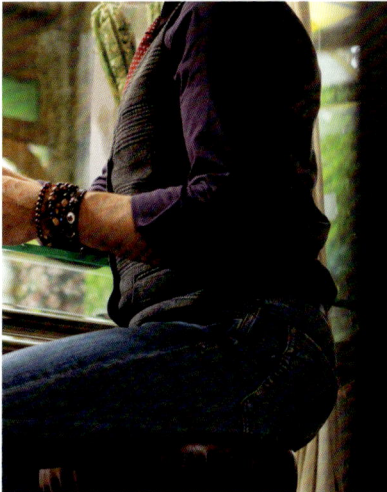

ANTEVERTED

An anteverted (tipped) pelvis is the ideal. The man on the left has his behind behind him. If he had a tail, it would be out behind him (see fig.3-1, fig.3-3).

An anteverted pelvis allows you to be both upright and relaxed.

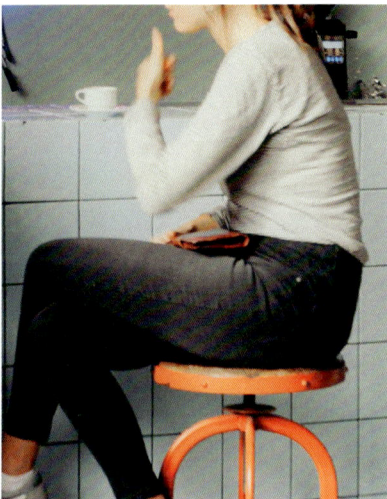

Ideal (anteverted)

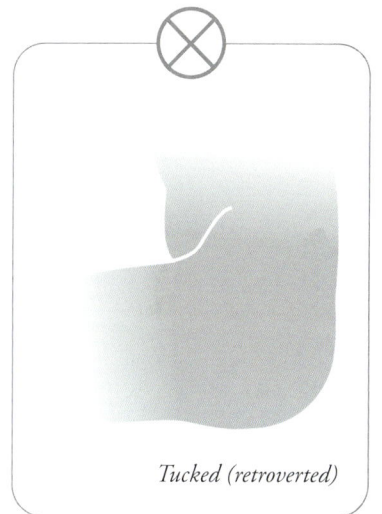

TUCKED

A tucked (*retroverted*) pelvis threatens the discs in the lumbar spine. The woman on the left and the man below both have a tucked pelvis. Their tails would be under them.

With a tucked pelvis you have two postures available to you: relaxed and slumped (woman on left) or upright and tense (man below).

a. Relaxed and slumped

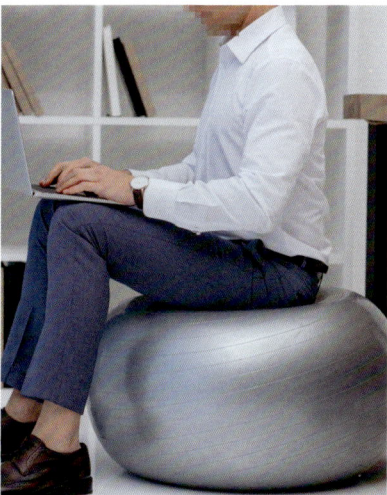

Tucked (retroverted)

b. Upright and tense

IDEAL AND
COMPROMISED
LOWER BACK SHAPES

ASSESS THE SHAPE OF YOUR
LOWER BACK

Compare your pelvic position in the mirror or on a screen
with the photos and drawings on this page.

Ideal (straight)

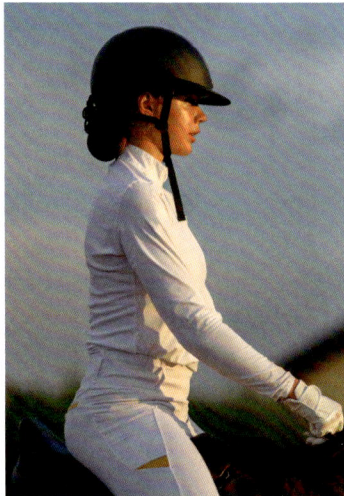

STRAIGHT

A healthy lower back is relatively
flat, has relaxed back muscles,
and decompressed discs.

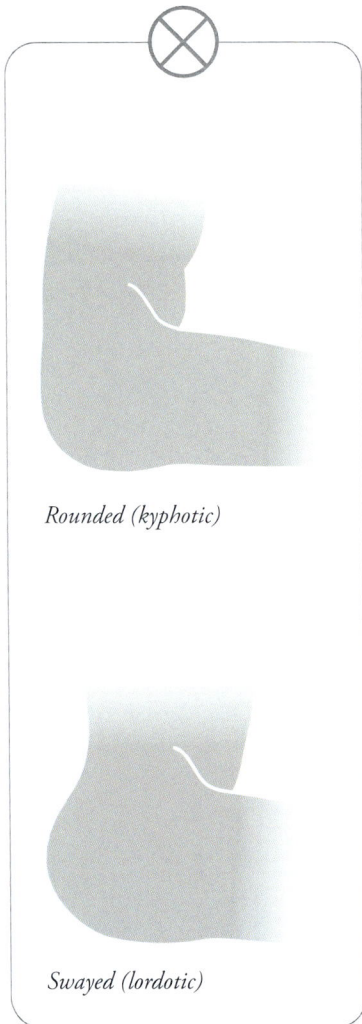

ROUNDED (KYPHOTIC)

A rounded (*kyphotic*) lower back
causes discs to bulge posteriorly,
in the direction of the spinal
nerve roots.

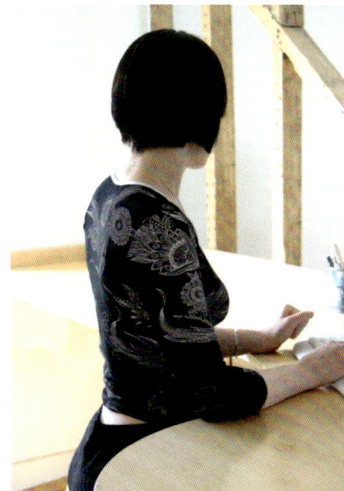

Rounded (kyphotic)

SWAYED (LORDOTIC)

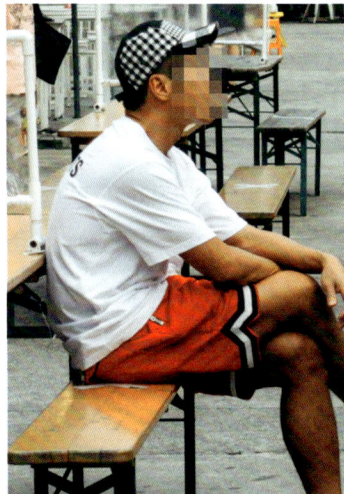

A swayed (*lordotic*) lower
back has tight back muscles,
compromised circulation, and
compressed discs.

Swayed (lordotic)

5 WITH YOUR FINGERTIPS, ASSESS THE SPINAL GROOVE IN YOUR LOWER BACK

Locate the vertical midline of the lower back. Feel the individual vertebrae lying within the groove created by the long (*erector spinae*) muscles that run vertically on either side of the spine. Is the groove deep or shallow? Are the ridges on either side like a tightly drawn bowstring or do they "give" easily when pressed on? As you run your fingertips up and down along the groove, does the depth change significantly?

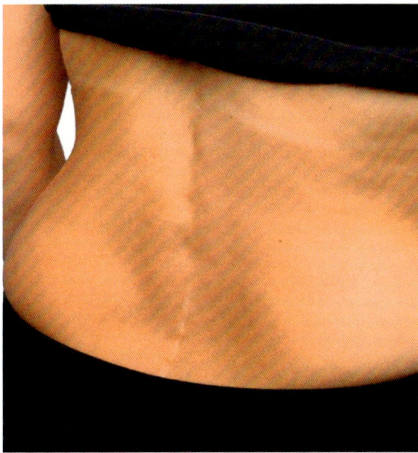

STRAIGHT

An ideal lower back has a mild groove, embedded bumps (vertebrae), and soft ridges on either side of the groove.

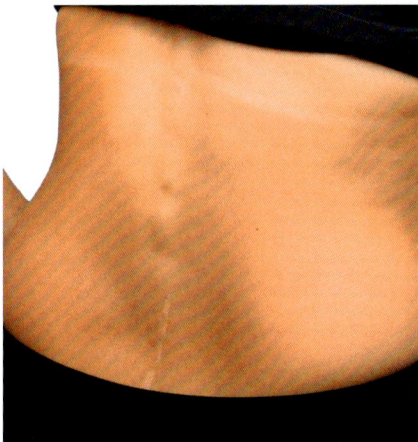

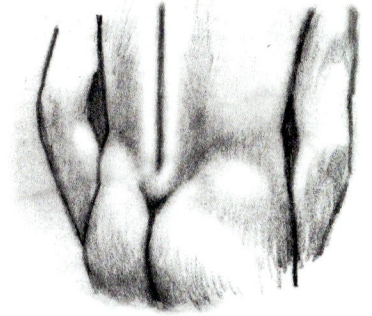

An ideal lower back with a uniformly mild spinal groove

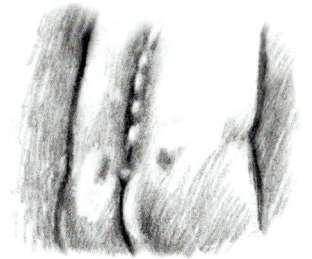

ROUNDED (KYPHOTIC)

A rounded (*kyphotic*) lower back has no groove, prominent bumps (vertebrae), and subtle or no ridges.

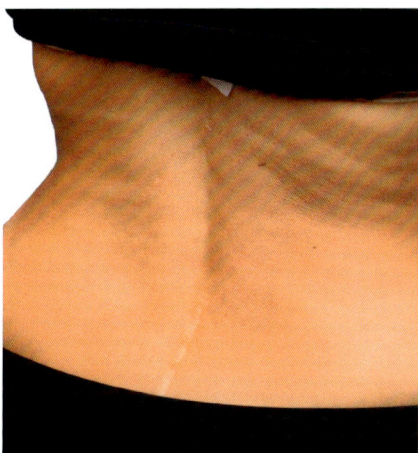

Rounded (kyphotic) lower back with no groove

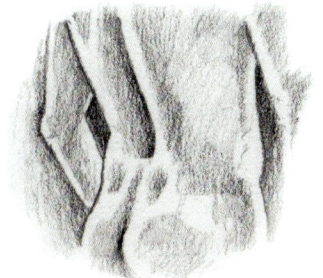

SWAYED (LORDOTIC)

A swayed (*lordotic*) lower back has a deep groove and taut muscle ridges on either side of the groove. The bumps in the midline groove are difficult to feel.

Swayed (lordotic) lower back with deep groove

If you find that your pelvis is anteverted, your lower back is straight, your midline groove is of even depth throughout the spine, and you sit comfortably, you are well on your way to the ideal sitting position.

You may not need to work through the first five steps of this section, starting on page 80. But take a look at them anyway, before tackling Step 6 on page 82.

EXAMPLES OF STACKSITTING

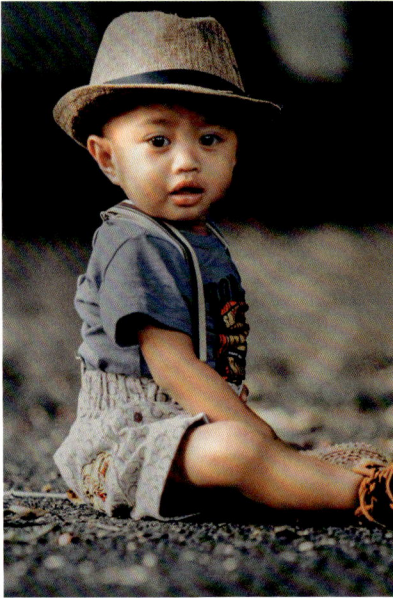

(Indonesia)

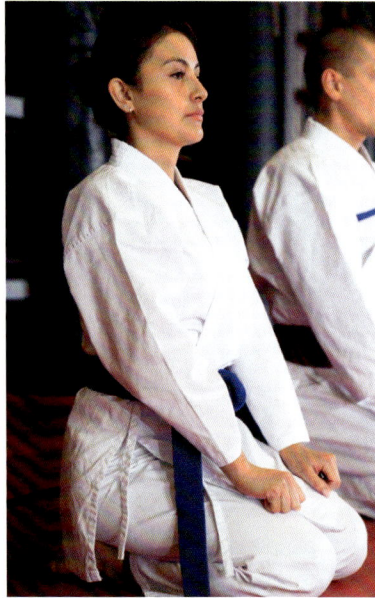

(Spain)

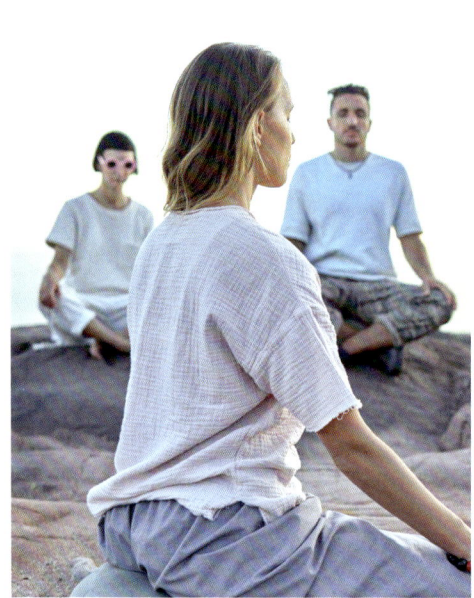

(USA)

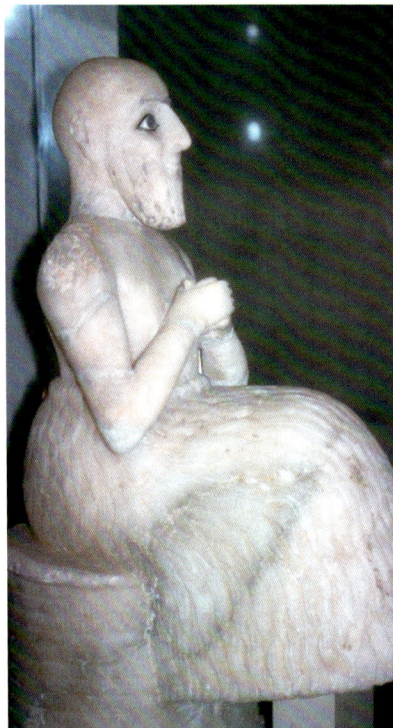

(Egypt)

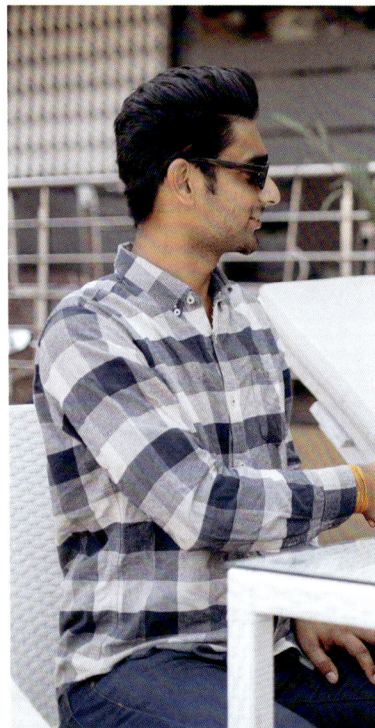

(India)

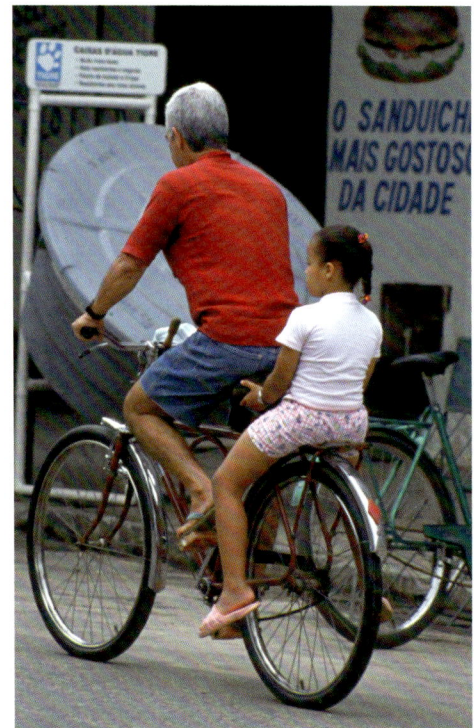

(Brazil)

EXAMPLES OF STACKSITTING

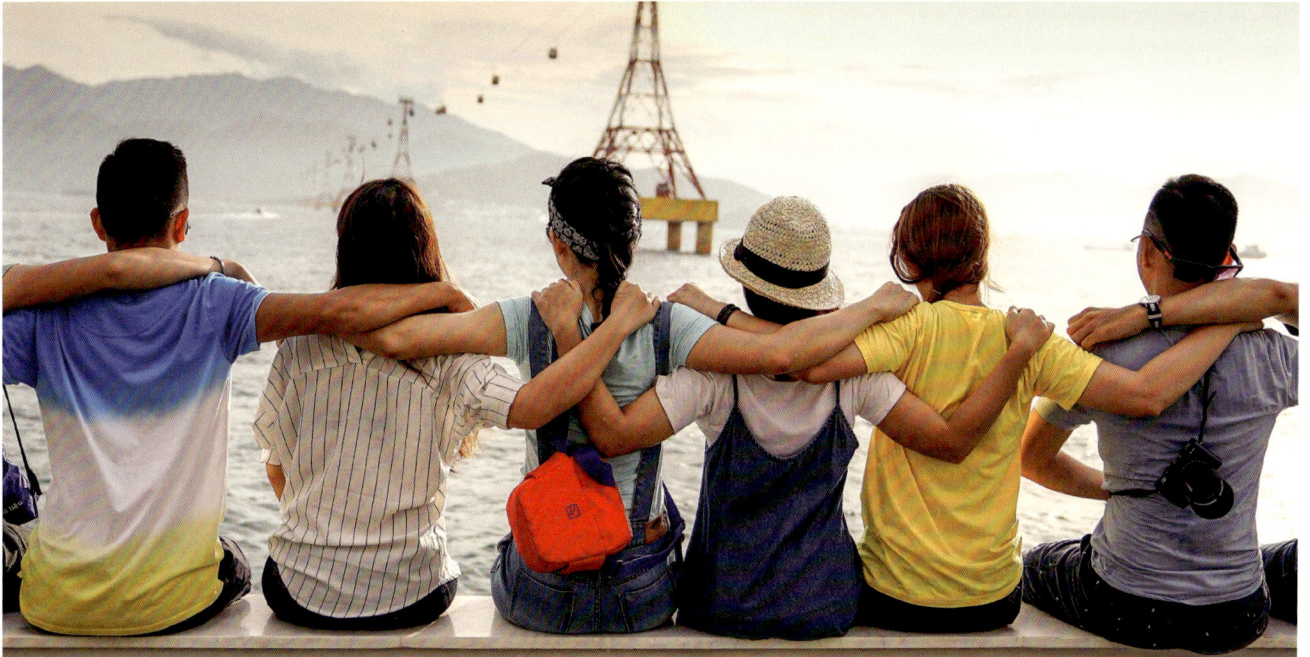

(Vietnam)

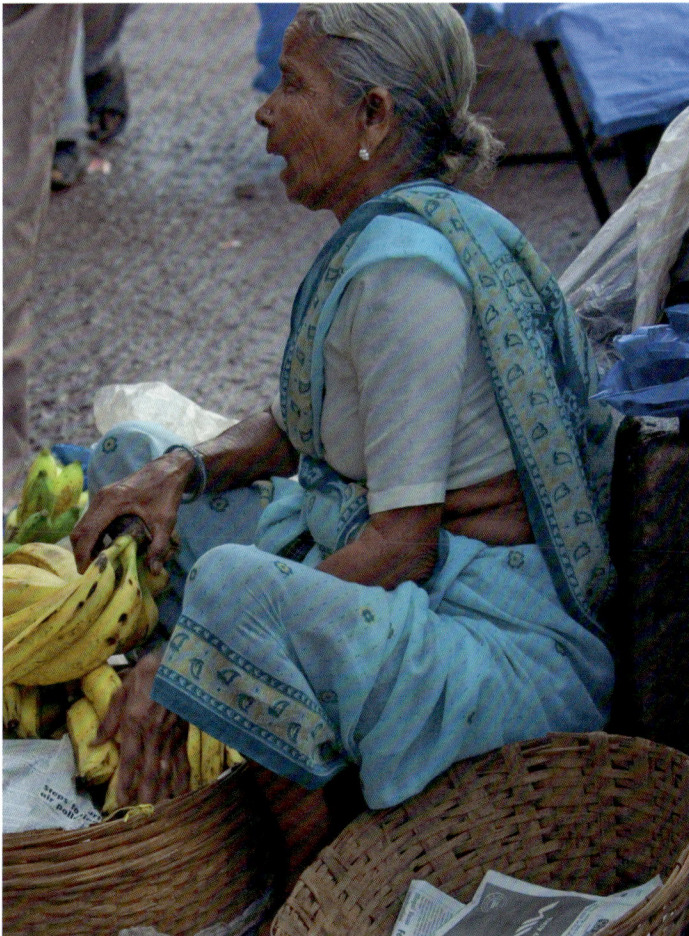

(India)

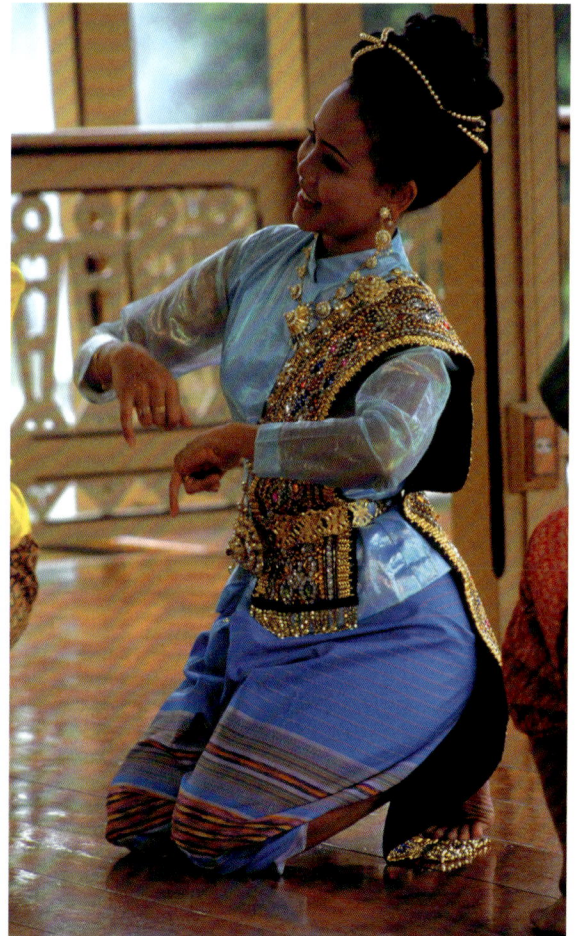

(Thailand)

EQUIPMENT

You will need the following:
* *A full-length mirror or camera screen*
* *A stool or chair with a firm seat*
* *A wedge*

The wedge should be made of a firm yet soft material: firm enough to provide support for the sitz bones (ischial tuberosities), yet soft enough to be comfortable. Most commercial wedges are too soft or too firm, and don't provide a steep enough slope. Suitable materials with which to fashion your own wedge include small wool or fleece throws, cotton batting, flannel sheets, and towels.

To make the wedge, fold the material so that it is about as wide as the chair seat but half as deep. The goal is to create a comfortable edge on which to perch your sitz bones. The drop-off at the front of the wedge helps your pelvis tip forward. Both the Gokhale Wedge and the Gokhale® Pain-Free Chair incorporate these elements (for more information visit www.gokhalemethod.com).

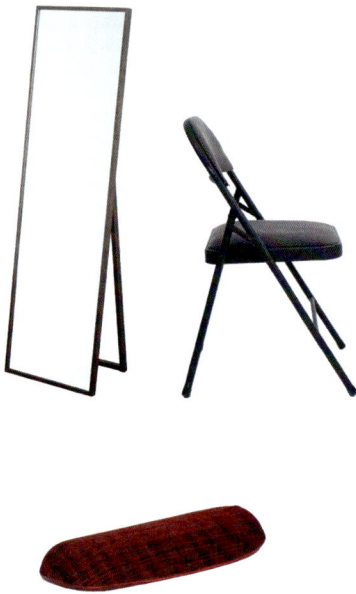

ADJUSTING YOUR SEATED POSTURE

1 PLACE A WEDGE ON THE CHAIR SO THAT YOU CAN SEE YOUR BODY IN PROFILE

Position the wedge so it helps to tip your pelvis forward when you sit.

In situations where you cannot use a wedge, you can sit on the front edge of the chair with your thighs angled downward (see fig.3-7 on page 72).

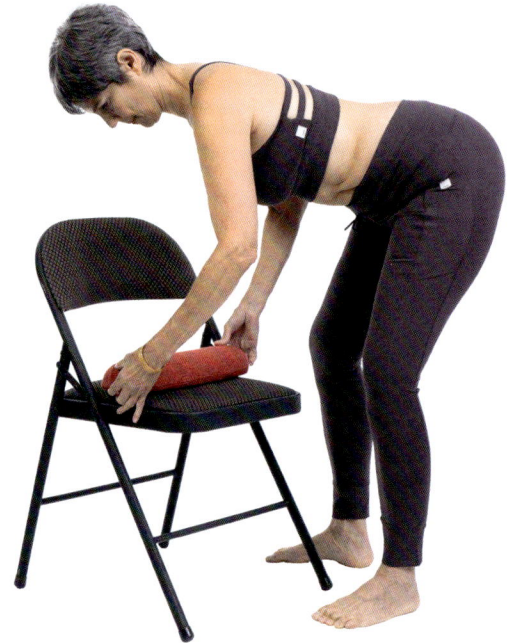

2 STAND WITH YOUR BACK TO THE CHAIR AND YOUR FEET HIP-WIDTH APART

This wide stance will help you learn to stacksit. Later, you will be able to vary your foot position and still sit well.

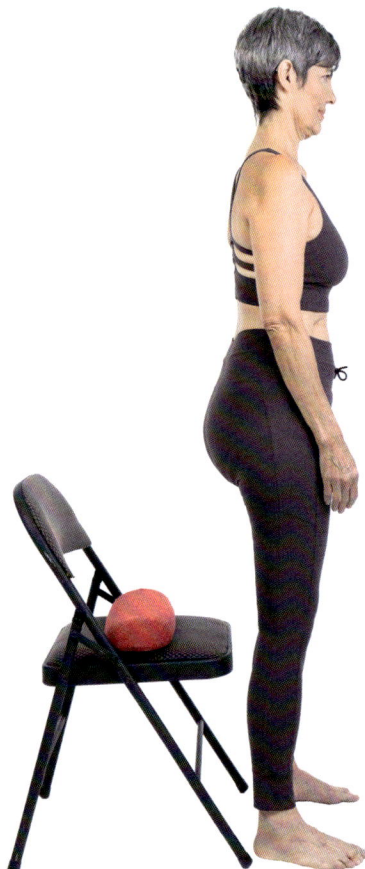

3 IF POSSIBLE, PUT YOUR FEET IN KIDNEY BEAN SHAPE

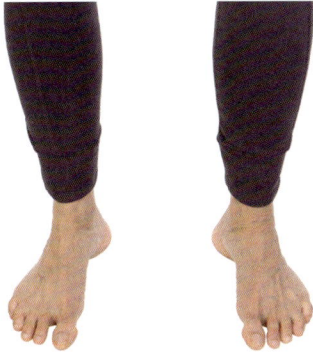

This step aligns the feet and legs optimally, but if you have trouble with it, skip it for now. You will learn more about it in a later chapter (see page 134).

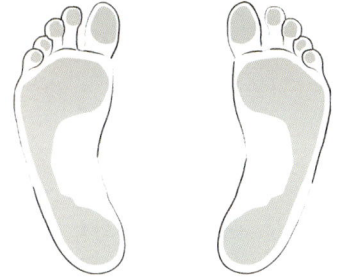

Kidney bean-shaped feet organize the bones and soft tissue of the feet, legs, and hips optimally.

4 BEND AT YOUR HIPS AND THEN AT YOUR KNEES, LOWERING YOUR SITZ BONES ONTO THE FRONT EDGE OF THE WEDGE

This tips your pelvis forward and settles your pelvis between your legs. It can be difficult to attain this position at first, yet you use it automatically whenever you seat yourself on a toilet. Try to recreate that position.

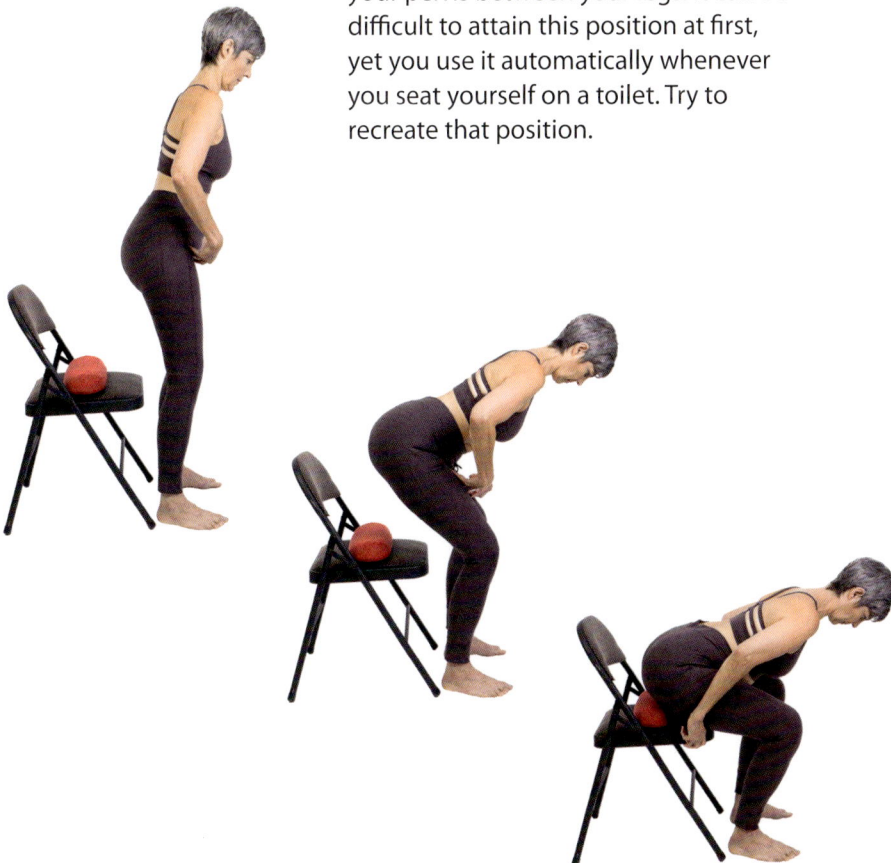

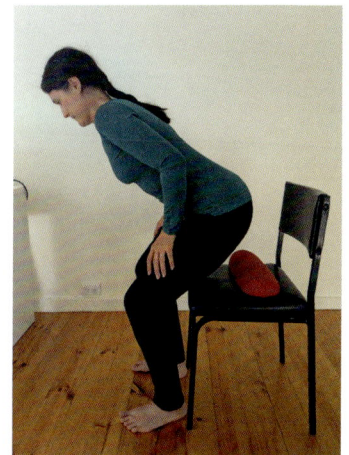

Hinging at the hip joint when beginning to sit helps position the pelvis for stacksitting (Australia).

EXAMPLES OF STACKSITTING

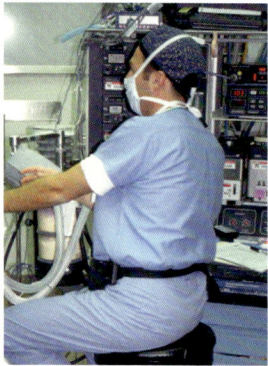

(USA)

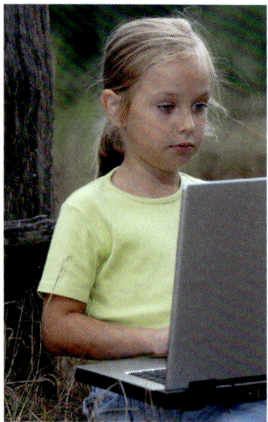

(USA)

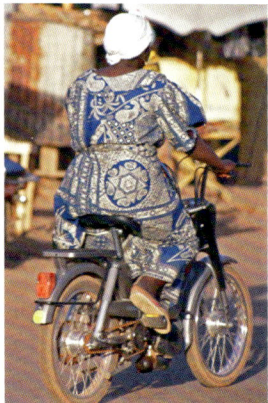

(Burkina Faso)

5 HINGE ONLY AT THE HIPS (AND NOT AT THE WAIST) TO RETURN TO AN UPRIGHT POSITION

Move your trunk as a single unit. Edit out any habit you may have of swaying your back.

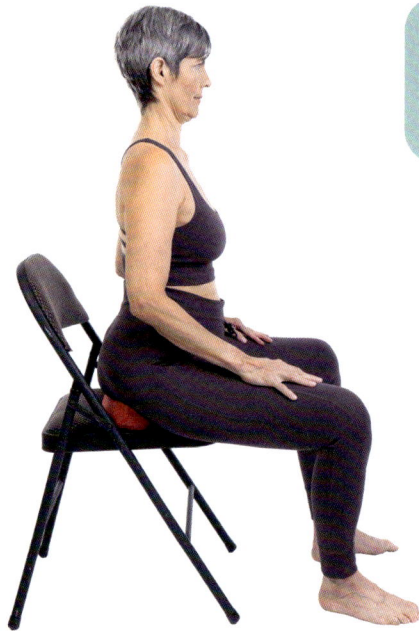

6 PERFORM A SHOULDER ROLL WITH EACH SHOULDER

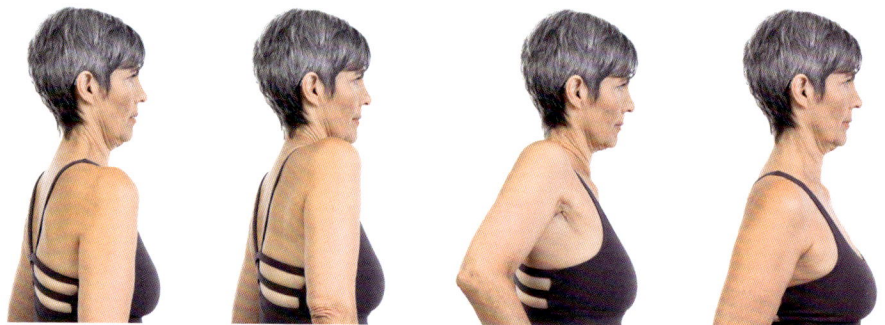

Roll the shoulder forwards, up, back, and down (see page 42). Isolate the movement to the shoulder joint, keeping your torso and head still.

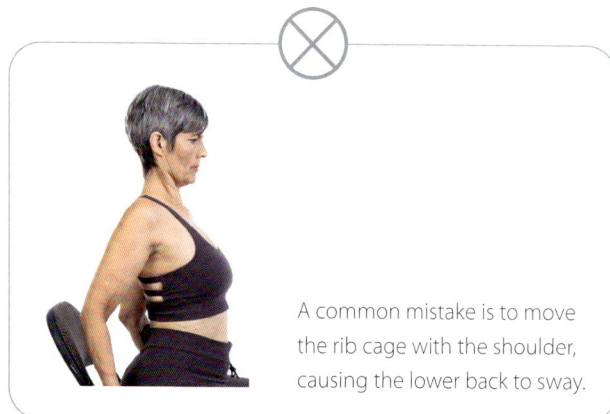

A common mistake is to move the rib cage with the shoulder, causing the lower back to sway.

7 LENGTHEN YOUR NECK

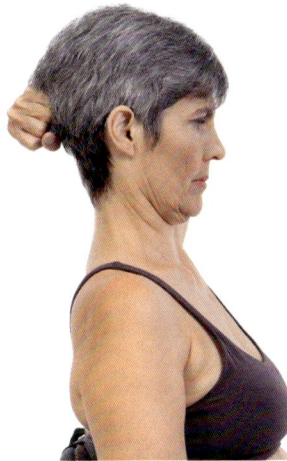

Use one of the ways you learned in Chapter 1 to lengthen the back of your neck (see page 44). Be careful not to lift your chin. Also resist any tendency to sway.

8 COMPLETELY RELAX YOUR BODY

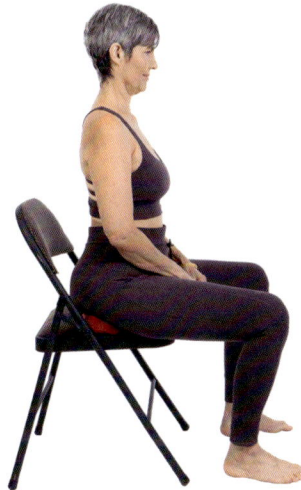

Pay particular attention to letting your upper chest relax and completely relaxing your lower back.

Checks for a good stack:

✓ Relaxed and upright: If your pelvis is positioned correctly, you will be able to become very lazy in your back muscles but remain upright. You may feel like you are slouching or leaning forward. Look in the mirror or at your screen to reassure yourself that this is not the case.

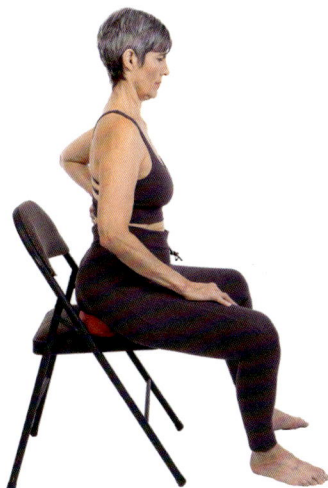

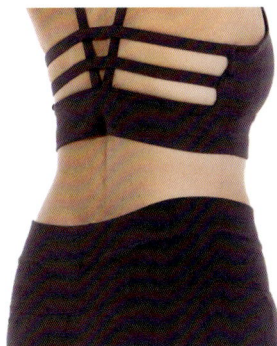

✓ Even depth of the midline lumbar groove: Feel with your fingertips for an even groove along your lumbar spine (refer to page 77).

EXAMPLES OF HEALTHY NECK ALIGNMENT

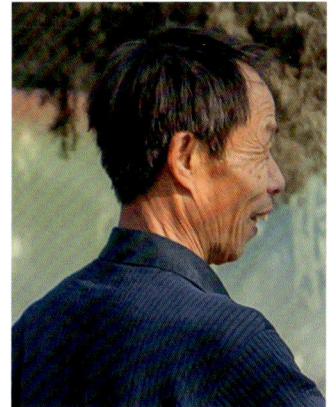

(China)

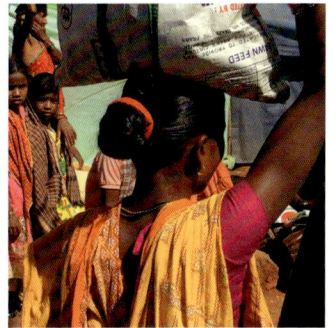

(India)

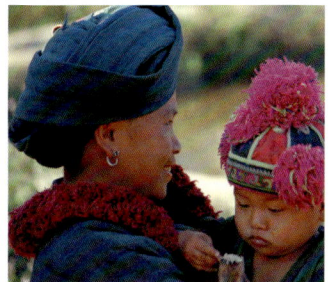

(Thailand)

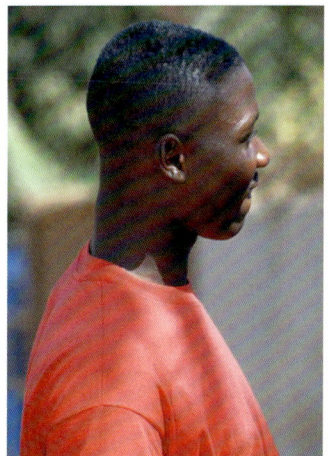

(Burkina Faso)

ART PIECES SHOWING STACKSITTING

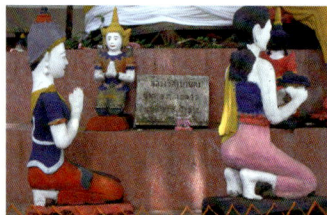

(Thailand)

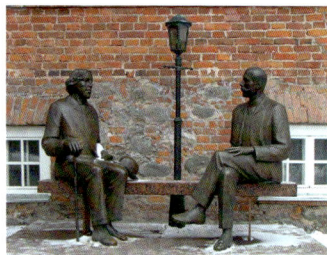

(Estonia)

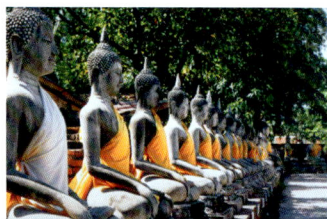

(Thailand)

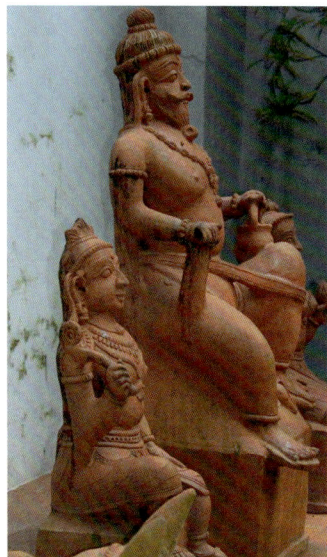

(India)

✓ A deep breath creates elongation of the spine on the inbreath and settling on the outbreath

If these three checks are in place, you have achieved a good stack.

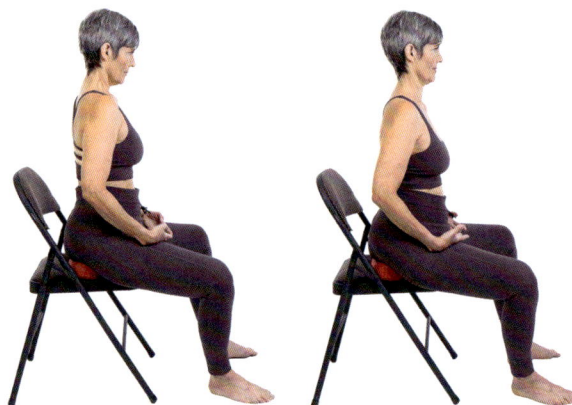

9 IF YOU FIND YOURSELF SLUMPING, TRY TIPPING YOUR PELVIS FURTHER FORWARD

There are several ways to do this. Begin with Option A and come upright to see if you still slump. If necessary, try Option B. Continue through the options until you succeed in tipping your pelvis forward enough to achieve a relaxed and upright posture.

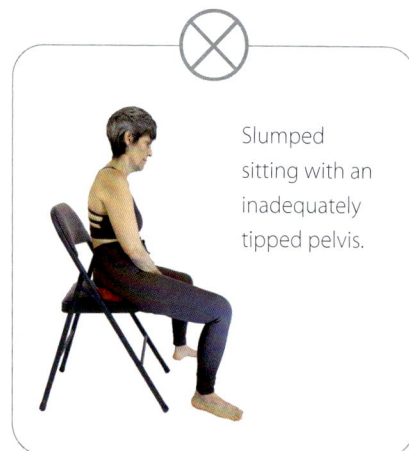

Slumped sitting with an inadequately tipped pelvis.

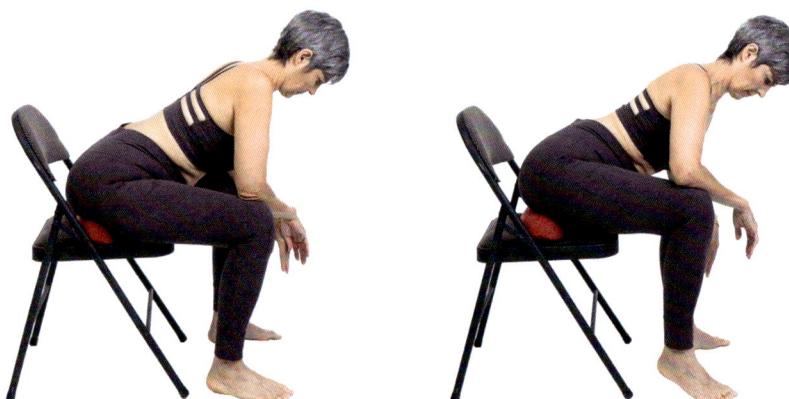

Option A
Lean forward from the hips with a straight back and rest your elbows on your thighs. Shift your weight onto your left buttock. Walk your right buttock back higher onto the wedge. Then repeat to move your left buttock higher on the wedge.

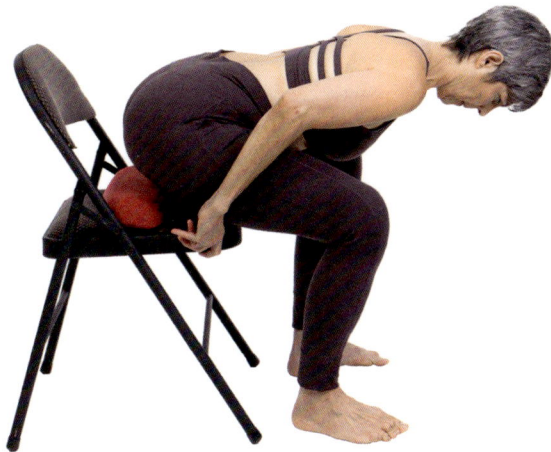

Option B
Lean forward from the hips with a straight back. Lift both buttocks a little off the chair while tipping your pelvis a little further forward. Then reposition your sitz bones on the wedge.

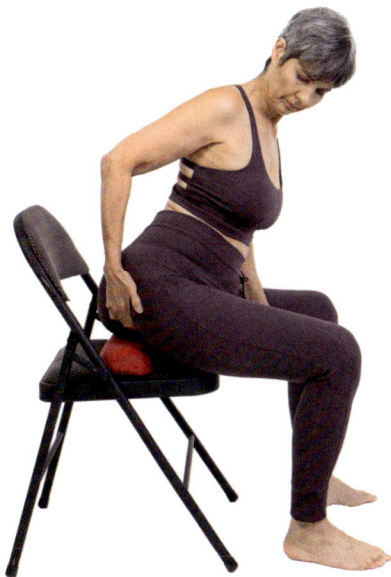

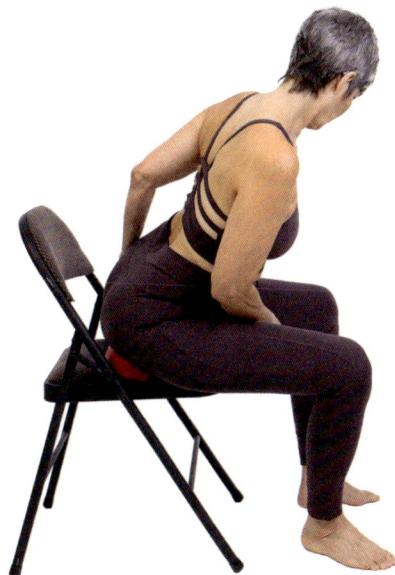

Option C
Shift your weight to your left buttock. With your right arm, reach behind and under your right buttock. Grab the flesh and pull it back as you lower the buttock onto the wedge. Repeat on the other side.

EXAMPLES OF HEALTHY PELVIC ANTEVERSION WHEN SITTING

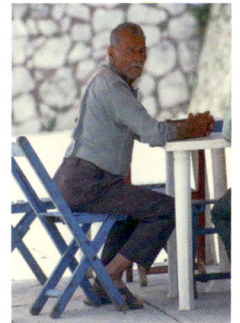

(Mexico)

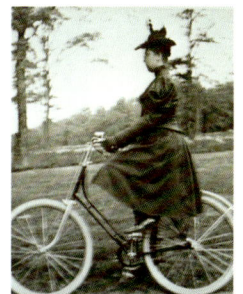

(USA)

EXAMPLES OF STACKSITTING WITH A WEDGE

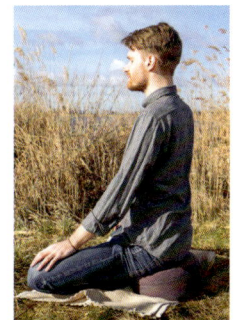

(Germany)

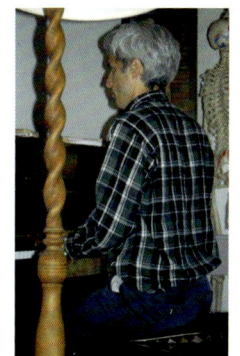

(USA)

EXAMPLES OF CHILDREN
BEING CARRIED WITH GOOD
PELVIC POSITIONING

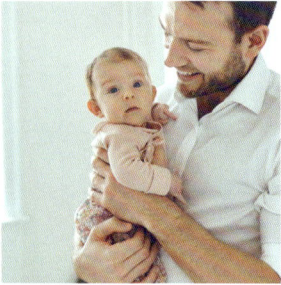

(UK)

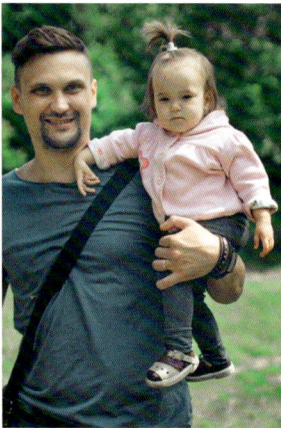

(Russia)

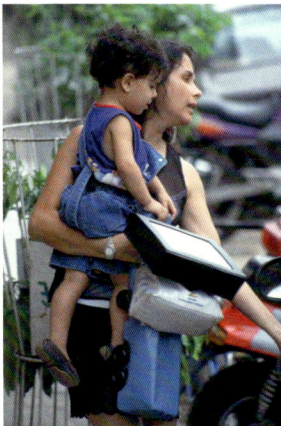

(Brazil)

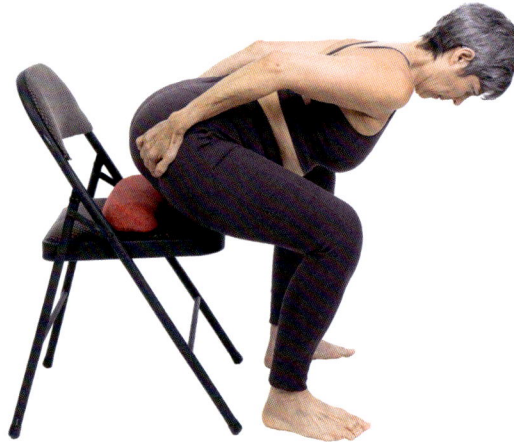

Option D
Lean forward and grab the flesh of both buttocks. Lift yourself off the chair momentarily and pull your flesh up and back. Then lower your buttocks onto the wedge.

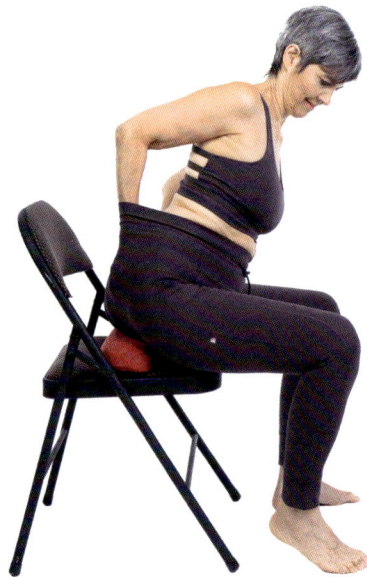

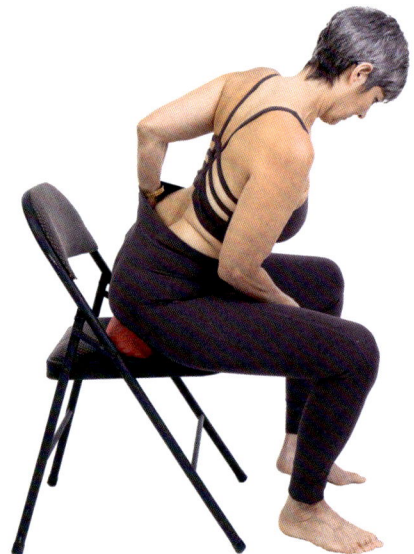

Option E
Lean forward from the hip with a straight back and rest your left elbow on your thigh. Shift your weight onto your left buttock and reach inside your pants to grasp the flesh of your right buttock. Place your right sitz bone back on the wedge. Then repeat with your left buttock. Needless to say, this move is best done in private!

10 RETURN TO AN UPRIGHT POSITION AND CHECK FOR A SLUMP OR SWAY

Roll your shoulders and lengthen your neck. Once again, completely relax your body.

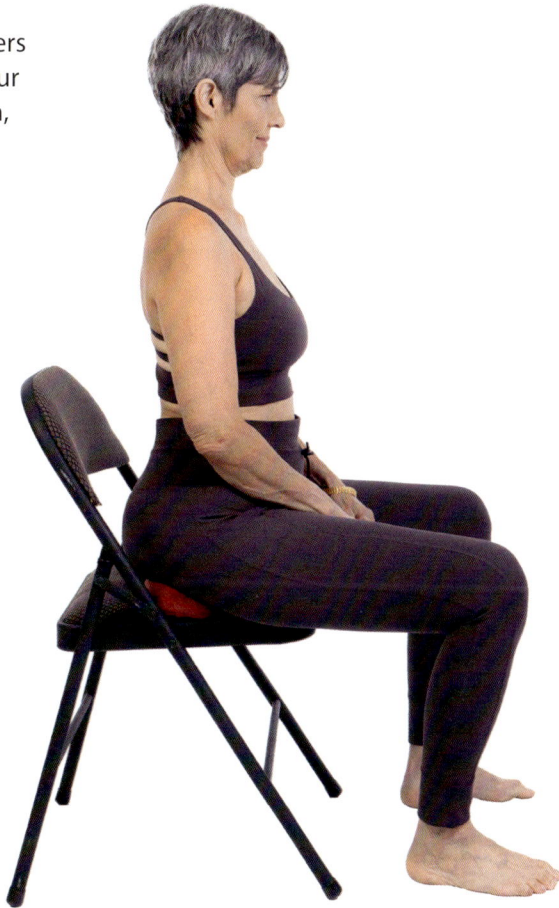

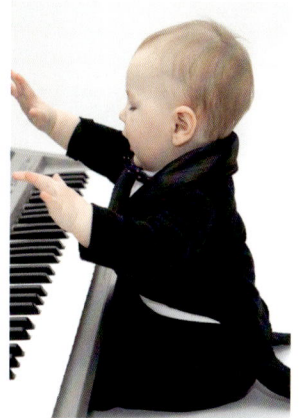

(USA)

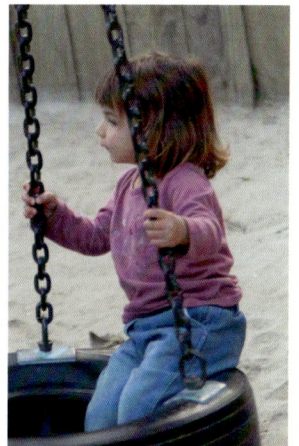

(USA)

If you still find yourself slumping, begin again from Step 1, using a higher wedge. You may need to experiment with different wedges until you find one that helps you attain the optimum sitting position.

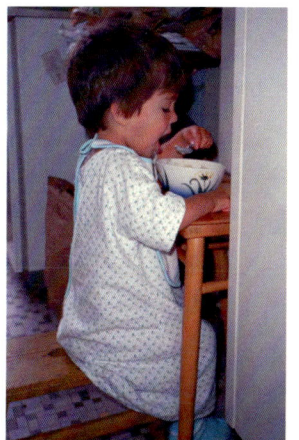

(USA)

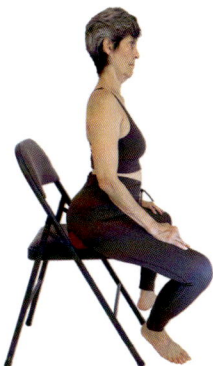

A common mistake is to end with an overtipped pelvis and a swayed (arched) lower back. You can straighten this arch by repositioning your sitz bones, one at a time, slightly further forward.

INDICATIONS OF IMPROVEMENT

As your muscles, tendons, fascia, and ligaments adjust to your new pelvic alignment, you will become more comfortable stacksitting, and will be able to sit with ease for longer periods.

When you have adopted a more upright, relaxed posture, you will notice your breathing pattern improves, increasing lung capacity and promoting good circulation.

TROUBLESHOOTING

PERSISTENT SWAY

Experiment with the height and composition of your wedge and the position of your pelvis. If your sway persists, you may be unconsciously holding on to the baseline tension your lower back is accustomed to, even though your pelvis is anteverted and stacking of the spine is available to you. See if there is any tension you can release in your lower back muscles. If necessary, use rib anchor (page 140) to actively overcome this tension for now. Over time, practice of stretchlying and stretchsitting will allow these muscles to reach a longer baseline length, allowing you to be relaxed and upright in stacksitting.

PAIN IN THE LOWER BACK

If performing any of these movements causes pain, or makes pain worse, stop immediately. Proceed to Chapter 5, where you will learn to maintain length in your spine with the inner corset technique. After mastering that, return here and apply it while you set up in stacksitting.

SORENESS IN THE LOWER BACK

If stacksitting is a significant change from your normal sitting position and feels uncomfortable, try a position that is intermediate between your old way of sitting and the ideal. Move in the direction of the ideal, but don't expect to achieve it the first time you try. You will gradually build up your ability to stacksit comfortably for longer periods. A Gokhale Method teacher can help you fine-tune your technique.

If you have misused your back in the past, your body has learned adaptive protective mechanisms, such as pain, muscle contraction, and inflammation. Pain inhibits recklessness, muscle contraction restricts mobility (preventing further damaging motions), and inflammation hastens healing. Now that you are changing the way you move, you no longer need these layers of protection, but it takes some time for your body to adapt. Continue to practice your altered, improved posture habits until your brain perceives that the area is no longer subject to repeated misuse or threat, and it will gradually adjust the instructions it sends to the lower back. Treat the area gently. Try comforting treatments, such as massage and hot baths, to coax your back into relaxation. Or consider acupuncture to "reset" the area, normalizing electrical messages between the brain and the body.

WHEN A WEDGE IS NOT AVAILABLE

You can improvise a wedge with a folded sweater or jacket, or in a pinch, the edge of a bag or shoe (fig.3-11). Or, as mentioned earlier, use the front edge of the chair as a wedge (fig.3-7). Allowing at least one thigh to slant downwards helps you achieve pelvic anteversion, which, in turn, facilitates good alignment throughout the upper body (fig.3-12). Sometimes people think they can simulate the effect of a wedge by thrusting their buttocks behind them, but if you have been tucking your pelvis for most of your life, your body architecture has adapted to this alignment. If you try to antevert your pelvis without a wedge, you will likely sway your lower back. It will take quite some time for your pelvis to settle into an ideal baseline position.

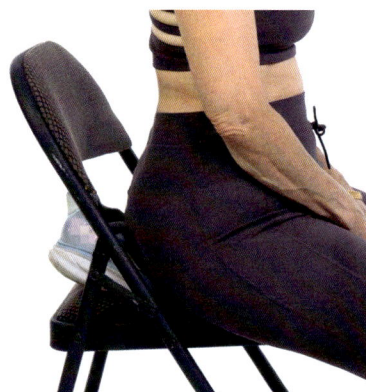

fig.3-11

Sweaters, bags, and even shoes can serve as effective wedges.

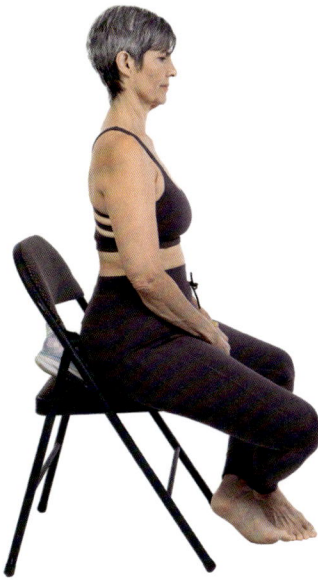

fig.3-12

Allowing one or both thighs to slant downwards facilitates pelvic anteversion by slackening the pull of the hamstrings on the sitz bones.

FURTHER INFORMATION

CONFLICTING GUIDELINES

Allowing for healthy anteversion in the pelvis is perhaps the most important and far-reaching postural measure you will learn, but I realize these guidelines may be in direct conflict with what you have been taught elsewhere. Current medical and lay thinking advocate for a "neutral" pelvis, which from a J-spine perspective is tucked. This paradigm also encourages additional tucking when stretching the lower back, "stabilizing" the lower back for lifting, and exercising the abdominal muscles, e.g. in crunches and sit-ups. This compresses the anterior portion of the wedge-shaped L5-S1 disc, compromising its integrity (fig.F-26 on page 21). It also leads to numerous other distortions throughout the musculoskeletal and organ systems (fig.3-2 on page 70). Follow my guidelines as an experiment; then evaluate how they work for you.

CHANGED LINE OF VISION

When you lengthen the back of your neck, your head naturally rotates slightly downward. This downward tilt changes your line of vision, and you may find that you gaze toward the floor. Rather than distorting your neck to look straight ahead, simply raise your eyes (fig.3-13). If you wear progressive lenses, consider using reading glasses instead to avoid needing to raise your chin.

DISTINCTION BETWEEN TIPPING THE PELVIS AND SWAYING THE BACK

Some people confuse a healthy, anteverted pelvis with an unhealthy sway in the back. There is an important distinction: swaying the back forms a curve in the upper lumbar area, while anteverting the pelvis creates a curve in the *lower* lumbar area (fig.3-14). Swaying the back is indeed unhealthy; restoring the natural arch at L5-S1 is crucial to healthy posture.

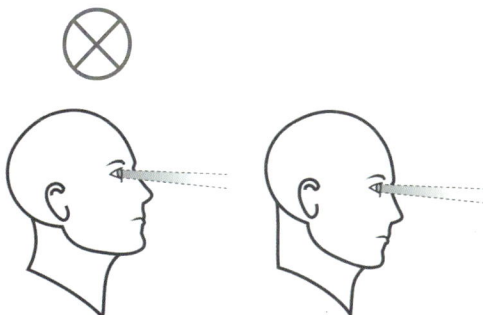

fig.3-13

After lengthening your neck, you will need to use your eye muscles to direct your eyes in a different way.

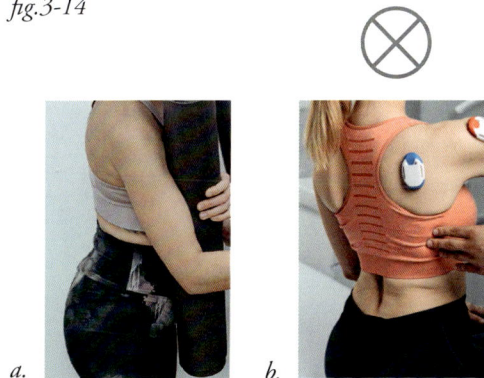

fig.3-14

a.   b.

There is an important difference between having a healthy lumbosacral arch (a), where the lower lumbar spine (L5-S1) has significant curvature and the upper lumbar spine (L1–L4) is relatively straight, and an unhealthy swayback (b), where the lumbosacral angle is small and the upper lumbar spine has significant curvature.

It is important not to combine stacksitting with stretchsitting or with placing your back against a backrest; this will result in a sway. Choose either stacksitting or stretchsitting. Many people prefer to stacksit at the dining table or when playing an instrument and stretchsit in their office chairs. We don't recommend stacksitting when driving for reasons of safety.

CHAIRS

A good chair should permit you to stretchsit or stacksit or, preferably, to switch between both. Most commercial chairs induce a pelvic tuck, upper lumbar curve, and/or hunched shoulders and are not conducive to healthy sitting (fig.3-15). A Stretchsit Cushion or Gokhale Wedge can help you adapt these chairs for healthy sitting; the Gokhale Pain-Free Chair incorporates both of these functionalities (fig.3-16). Avoid a chair with a low seat if you have tight hamstrings and/or tight external hip rotator muscles, as it will cause you to tuck your pelvis and therefore distort your alignment. Avoid a chair so high that your legs dangle above the floor, as it may distort your back (fig.3-17). If your chair does not support you well, sit on the edge, allowing your pelvis to tip forward, your thighs to angle downward, and your feet to rest on the floor (fig.3-18).

fig.3-15

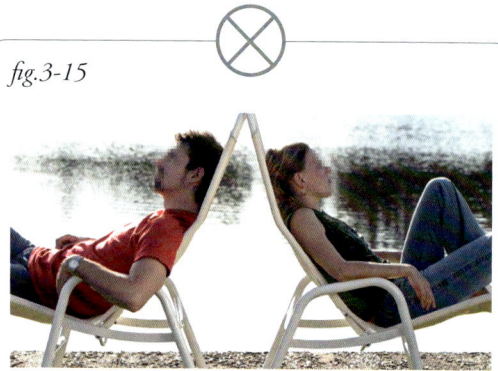

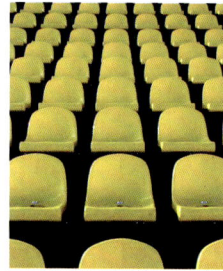

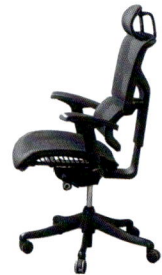

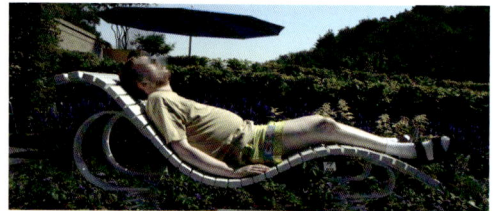

Most commercial chairs induce unhealthy spinal curvature.

fig.3-16

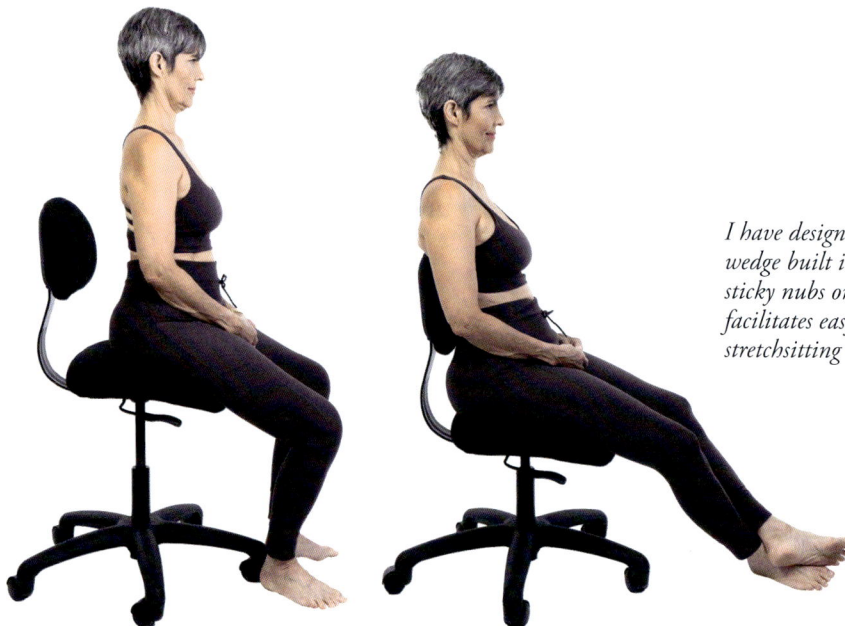

I have designed a chair with a wedge built into the seat pan and sticky nubs on the backrest; this facilitates easy transitions between stretchsitting and stacksitting.

fig.3-17

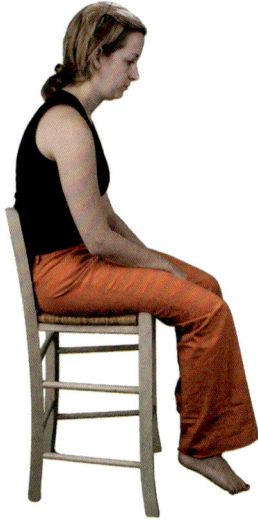

A chair that is too high may result in unhealthy seated posture.

fig.3-18

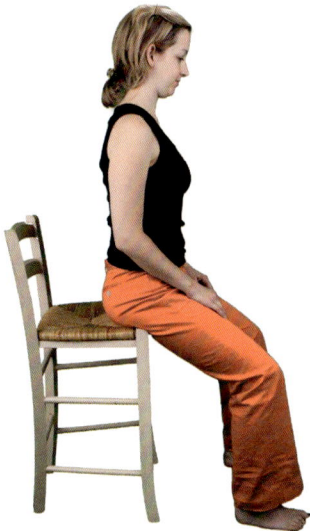

With a problematic chair, sitting on the front edge can help.

I am often asked if kneeling chairs are conducive to good posture. For people who use them well, these chairs can provide a good option for short periods of time, because the forward-tilted seat encourages pelvic anteversion. However, when not used well, the tilted seat can also contribute to a significant sway in the lower back. Settling one's weight on the knee rest for prolonged periods can also put excessive pressure on the knee and hip joints (as the thigh bone pushes into the hip socket).

FLOOR

Sitting on the floor causes most Westerners to either tuck their pelvis and round their back, or sway to be upright (fig.3-19). This is because the necessary flexibility and hip joint structure to sit well on the floor is rare in the West.

People from floor-sitting cultures have the necessary hip joint structure and hamstring and external hip rotator flexibility to be able to sit on the floor and still preserve pelvic anteversion (fig.3-20).

fig.3-19

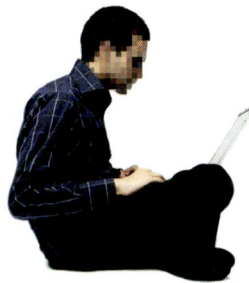

a. Tucking the pelvis and rounding the back

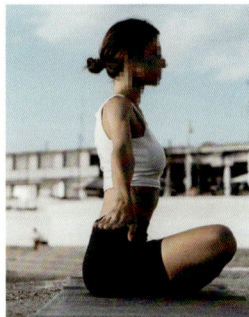

b. Swaying the back when sitting upright

Sitting cross-legged on the floor unaided is problematic for most people in modern industrialized societies.

fig.3-20

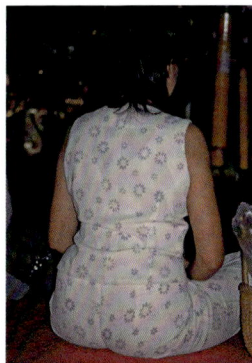

Stacksitting cross-legged on the floor unaided requires a high degree of hip flexibility and conducive hip joint structure (Thailand).

When you do sit on the floor (for example, to play with small children), it is advisable to use a sitting cushion like the traditional Japanese zafu, pillows, or a low bench (fig.3-21a). If your knees are healthy, you can sit with your buttocks resting on your heels in the Japanese "seiza" position (fig.3-21b). Another alternative is to use one or both arms to prop you up and lengthen your spine (fig.3-21c).

fig.3-21

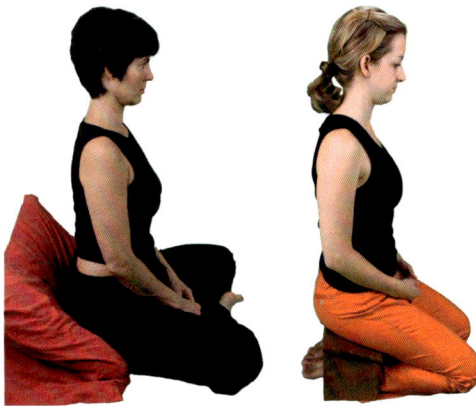

a. Using a prop facilitates stacksitting on the floor.

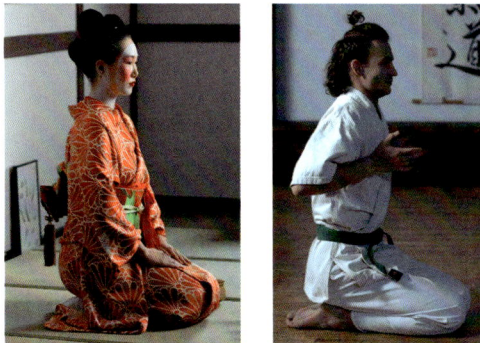

b. Sitting in the Japanese "seiza" position facilitates stacksitting but requires healthy knees and ankles.

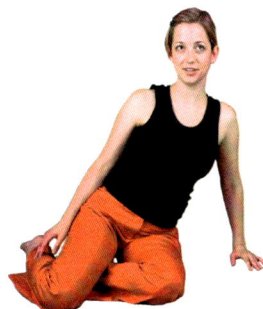

c. Using the arms to lengthen the spine facilitates sitting on the floor.

These are some healthy options for sitting on the floor.

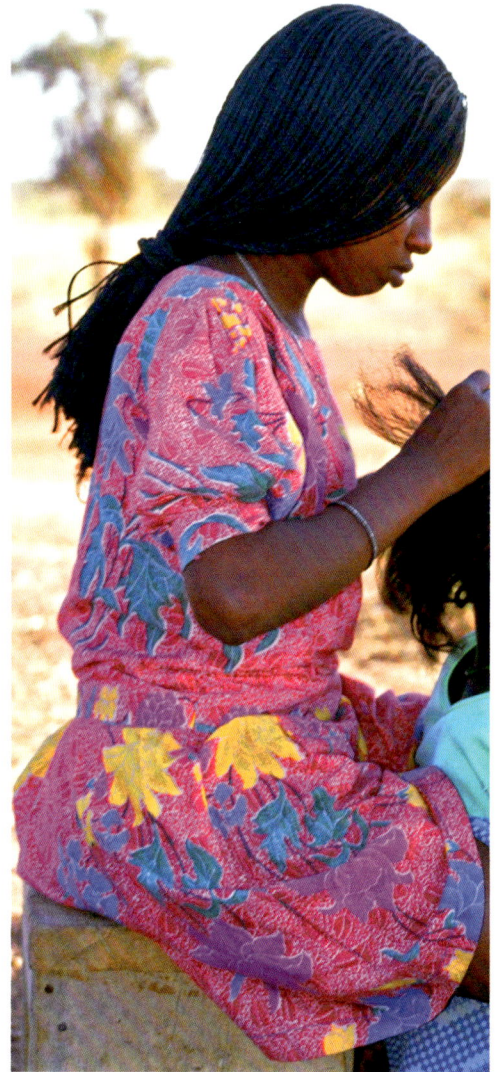

(Burkina Faso)

I couldn't sit on the floor for even a minute, because my back couldn't tolerate it. Now I can sit on the floor and play with my toddler. I still sit the way Esther taught me at concerts and lectures, and no longer come out with back pain or fatigue.

Jessica Davidson, M.D.,
Palo Alto, CA

RECAP

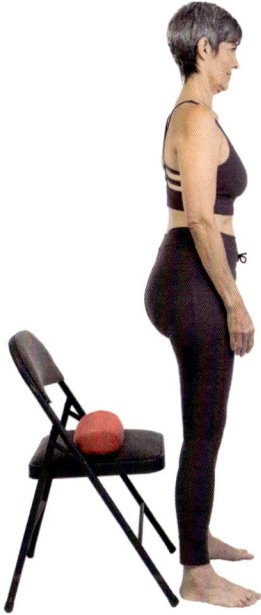

a. **Adopt a wide stance with kidney bean-shaped feet**

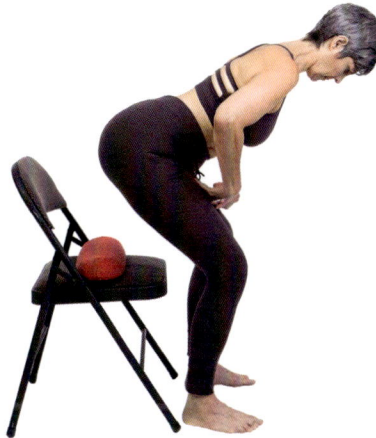

b. **Bend at your hips and then at your knees**

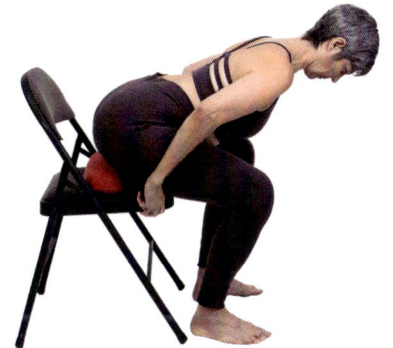

c. **Lower your sitz bones onto the front edge of the wedge**

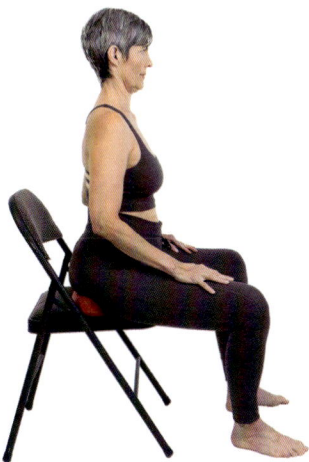

d. **Hinge only at the hips to return to upright**

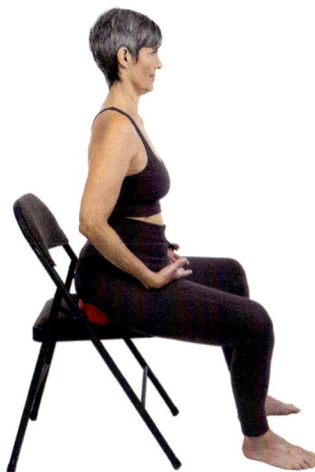

e. **Perform shoulder rolls and lengthen neck**

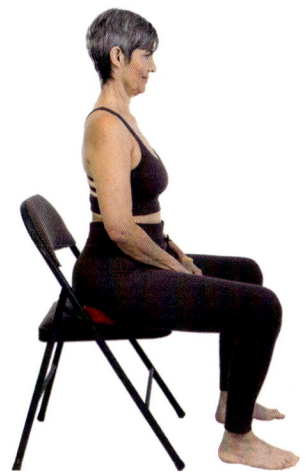

f. **Relax and check for a good stack**

4

STRETCHLYING ON YOUR SIDE

Lying with a lengthened back

This Burkinabé man is napping by his wayside stall. He has made himself very comfortable with minimal equipment. Notice that his knees are bent and his groin soft, his torso is in a straight line, his head is in alignment with his spine, and his upper shoulder is not slumped forward although he is using his upper arm as part of his pillow.

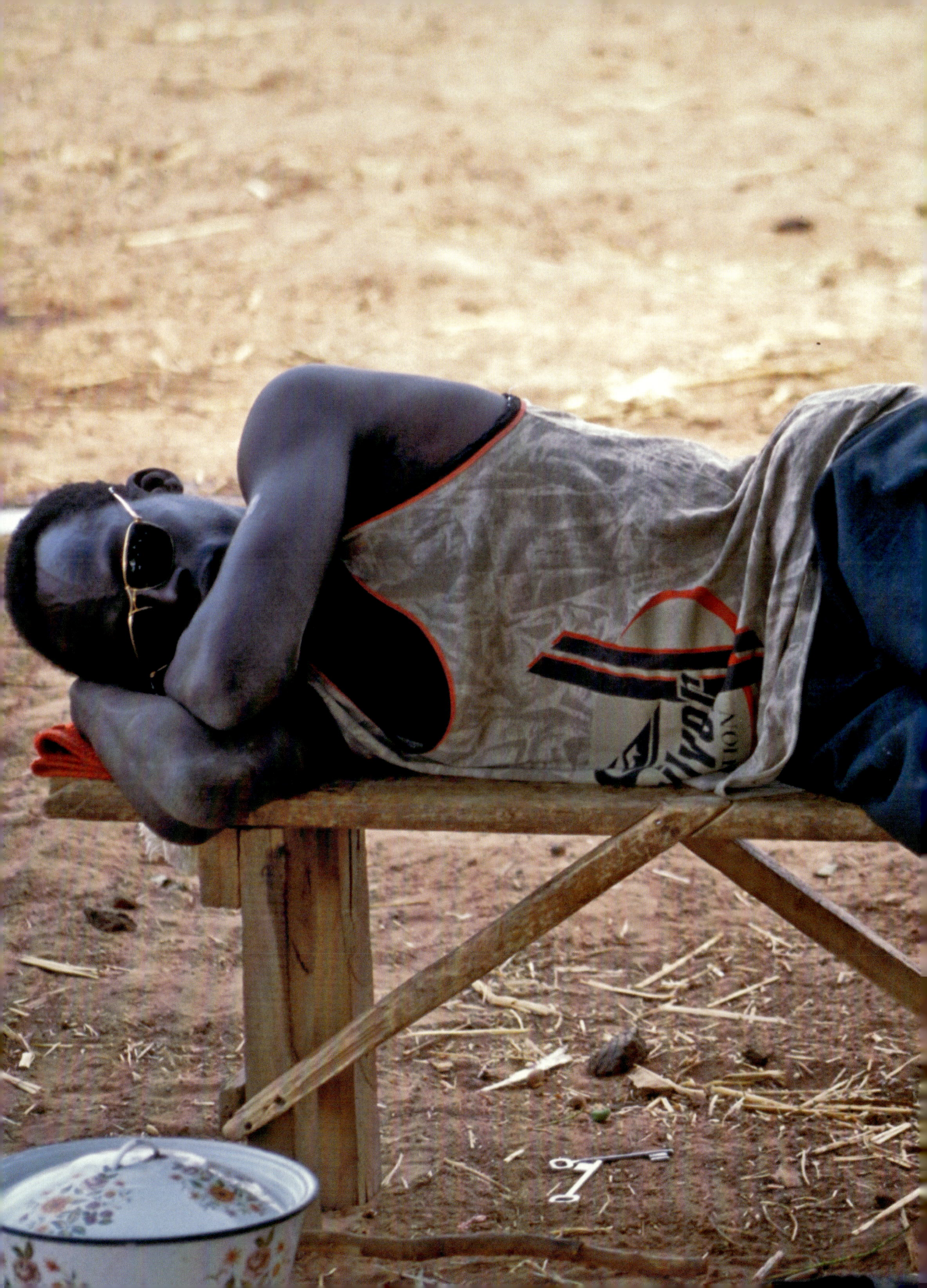

In Chapter 2, you learned a healthy way to lie on your back that also puts your spine in gentle traction. In this chapter you will learn another healthy, restful, and therapeutic sleep position: stretchlying on your side. Many people are forced to sleep on their side to reduce sleep apnea, snoring, or joint pain, and there is nothing wrong with this. Anthropological research indicates that for most of human history, it is very likely that our ancestors slept on their sides. This position allows members of a family to nest into each other for warmth, safety, and economy of ground space and cover. People living in much of the world today still tend to sleep on their sides (fig.4-1). It is certainly a natural position for us, one that we adapted to over millions of years.

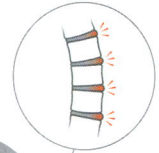

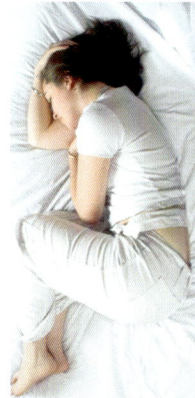
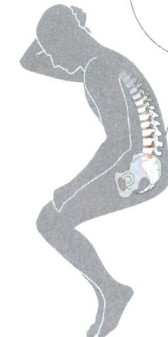

fig.4-2

a. Common "fetal" position for sleeping on the side.

b. Hunched lying position stresses discs, and even more so if the position is carried over to sitting and standing.

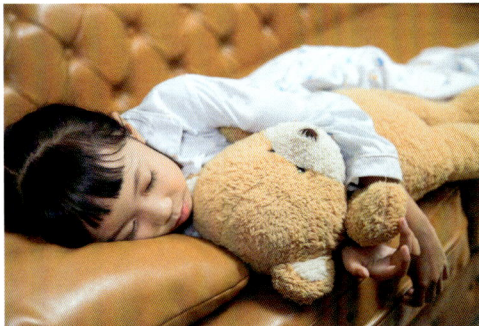

(Thailand)

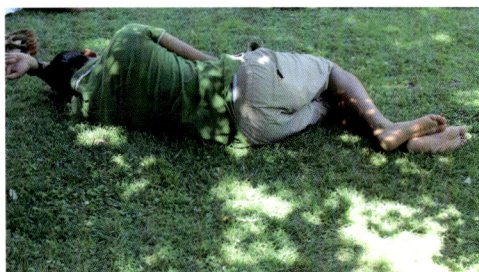

(Australia)

Lying on the side is a common sleep position throughout the world.

fig.4-3

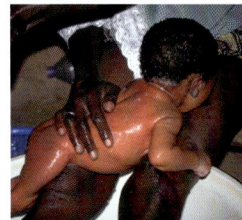

a. African newborn babies are massaged daily to stretch their spines.

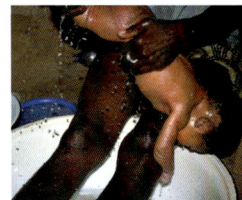

b. Part of the massage ritual involves suspending the baby upside down.

One problem is that many people who sleep on their sides assume a fetal position in which they curl their spine forward into a "C" shape (fig. 4-2a). The hunched "C" shape compresses the anterior part of the discs, forcing the contents of the discs (*nucleus pulposus*) backwards and putting pressure on the fibrous exterior (*annulus fibrosus*), causing it to fray over time (fig. 4-2b). This hunched posture, if carried over to standing or sitting, is a major contributor to disc wear and tear.

Your fetal days are over! It is time to stretch yourself out and lengthen your spine. In many African countries, newborn babies are massaged and lengthened every day by a woman specializing in this care (fig.4-3a). The massage ritual goes so far as holding the baby upside down by the ankles to lengthen it (fig. 4-3b), though I do not have enough information and experience to recommend this.

Another problem is that some people who habitually sway their lower backs carry this through into their side-sleeping position (fig. 4-4a). The *erector spinae* muscles on either side of the spine remain tense, reducing circulation in the area and compressing the spinal discs (fig. 4-4b).

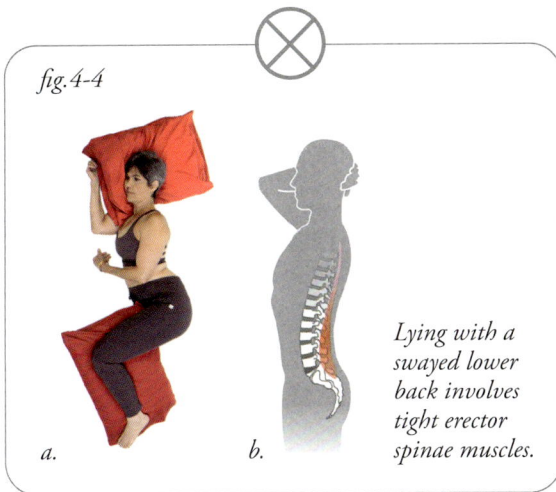

fig.4-4

Lying with a swayed lower back involves tight erector spinae muscles.

a.   b.

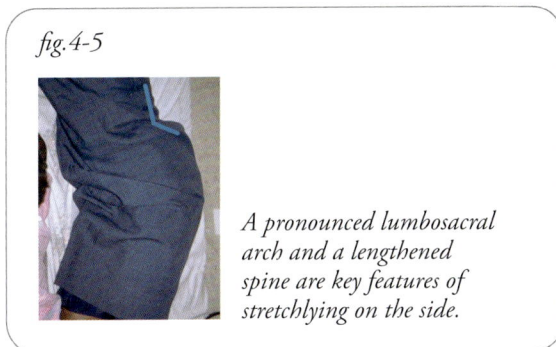

fig.4-5

A pronounced lumbosacral arch and a lengthened spine are key features of stretchlying on the side.

In this chapter you will learn to lie on your side with a pronounced lumbosacral arch and lengthened back (fig.4-5). This supports the health of your spinal discs, your nerve roots, and your other spinal tissues.

The proper position is not only comfortable; it is therapeutic. Lying with a "J" shaped spine helps the muscles in the area normalize to longer baseline lengths, improving circulation, which speeds healing. You lengthen your spine just as you do when sleeping on your back, and derive similar benefits.

Initially, the new position may seem awkward, but soon your body adapt, and you will enjoy restful sleep that is also therapeutic. Lying on your side offers a third way to put your back in gentle traction for many hours, complementing the benefits described in Chapters 1 and 2.

In addition, the position reinforces the practice of tipping the pelvis forward (anteversion). One immediate benefit from this maneuver is to soften the groin crease, improving the circulation to the legs and feet. You may notice your feet are warmer as they benefit from improved blood supply.

Even if you normally sleep on your back, we encourage you to work through this chapter. It is always useful to be able to sleep well in more than one healthy position, in case you are forced to give up your usual position because of injury, pregnancy, or some other cause.

Caution

For some people, the movements taught in this chapter constitute a major shift from their current posture. If you are one of these people, proceed very slowly and gently. Move in the direction of the ideal, but don't expect to achieve it the first time you try. **If you find that performing any of these movements exaggerates your pain, stop immediately.** Proceed to Chapter 5, which will help you maintain length in your spine. After mastering that technique, return here.

If you have a diagnosis, or any suspicion, of a herniated disc in the lower lumbar area (L5-S1), it is extremely important that you not antevert your pelvis prematurely. Doing so may pinch off the herniated portion of the disc (fig.3-10 on page 73). Wait to do this technique until you have the guidance of a qualified Gokhale Method teacher. Chapters 1, 2, and 5 teach you safe ways to lengthen your spine, which will make you more comfortable and can accelerate healing of the herniated disc.

BENEFITS

• Normalizes muscles to longer baseline lengths

• Decompresses discs and spinal nerve roots

• Promotes improved circulation and hastens healing

• Improves quality of sleep

• Creates muscle memory for an anteverted pelvis and a lengthened spine

I used to wake up with a clenched jaw and sore, tight neck and back muscles. Now with stretchlying, I wake up more relaxed, pain free and ready to move into my morning.

Nancy Shinners, Madison, WI

EQUIPMENT

You will need three or more pillows.

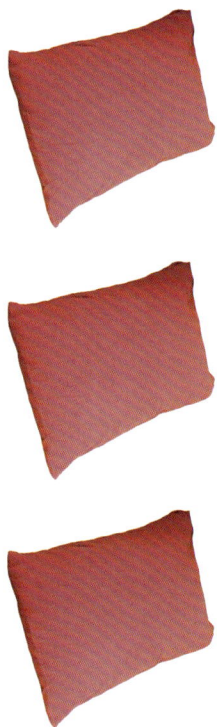

1 POSITION TWO PILLOWS UNDER YOUR HEAD

You need enough cushioning for your head and neck to be well supported while fully relaxed (one thick pillow may be sufficient). Be sure your head does not angle down, which will compromise your subsequent shoulder positioning.

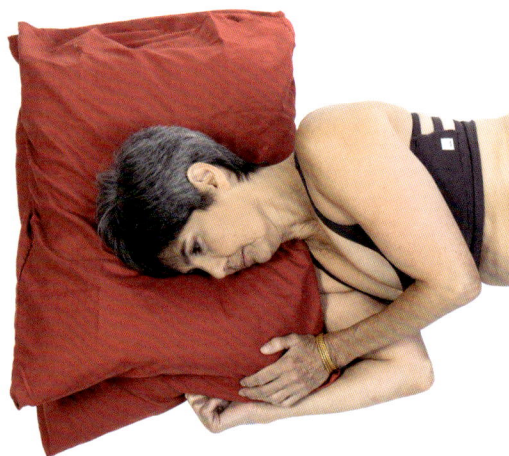

2 PLACE ONE PILLOW LENGTHWAYS BETWEEN YOUR KNEES AND ANKLES

Have your knees bent a moderate amount (see sidebar).

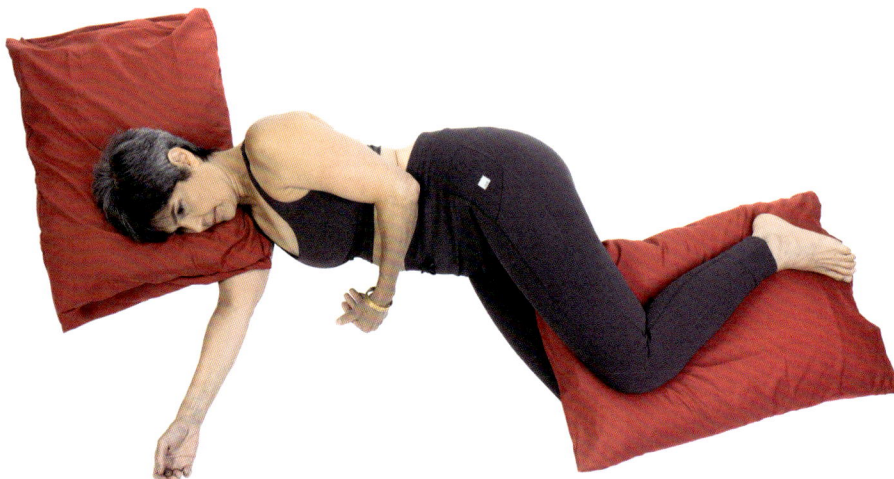

3 ELONGATE YOUR SPINE

Place your lower elbow out in front of your body, and your upper hand on the bed close to your body, with your fingers pointing in whichever direction feels most comfortable.

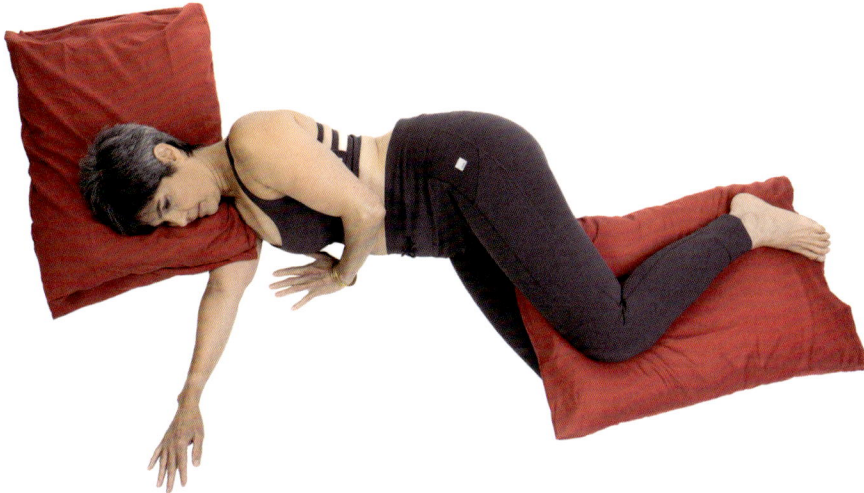

Raise your shoulder off the bed an inch or two. Push toward your feet with your lower arm and upper hand to stretch your torso away from your lower body. Relax back down onto the bed with your now-lengthened torso.

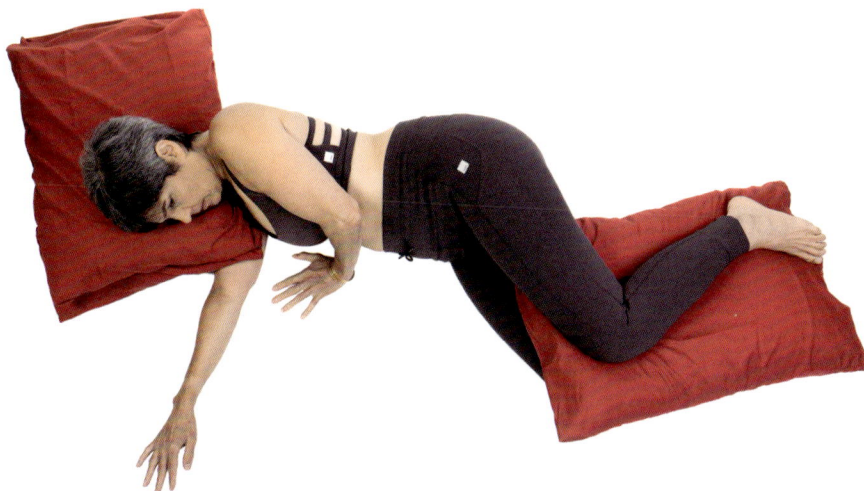

KNEES SHOULD NOT BE TOO HIGH OR TOO STRAIGHT

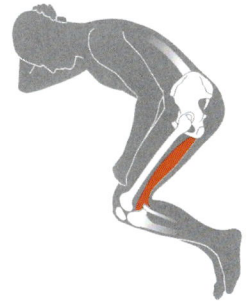

Raised knees with tight hamstrings will tuck the pelvis.

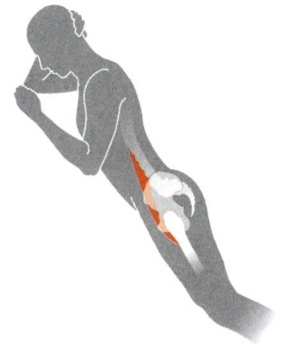

Straight legs with tight psoas muscles will sway the lower back.

ZIGZAG SHAPE

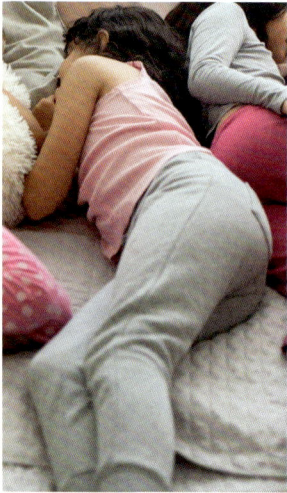

Young girl resting (Portugal)

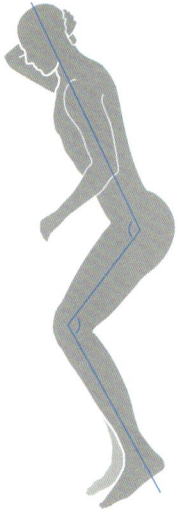

Body forms even zigzags with angles of approximately 120°

4 ANTEVERT YOUR PELVIS

Lift *only* your hips off the bed and thrust your bottom slightly exaggeratedly backwards.

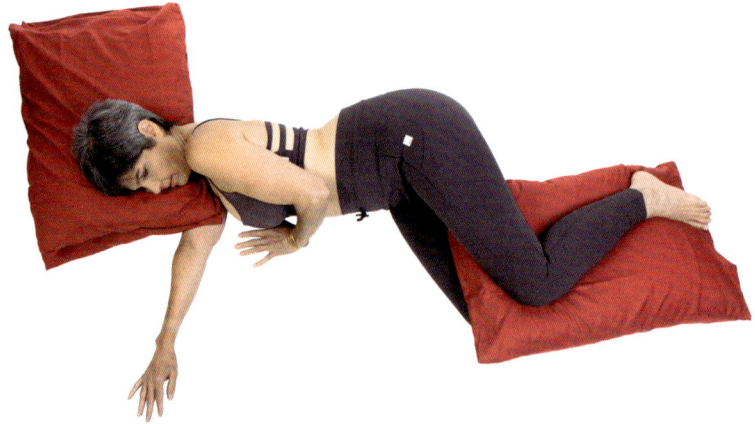

5 CHECK THE SHAPE OF YOUR LOWER BACK WITH YOUR FINGERTIPS

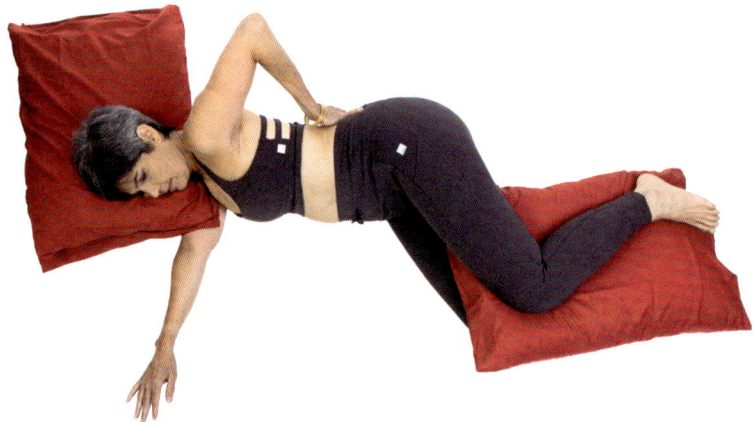

Step 4 will antevert your pelvis, but will almost always also create a sway in the lower back. To check for a sway, use your fingertips to search along your lower back midline groove for a section that is deeper than the rest of the groove (refer to page 77).

If you are concerned about swaying your back, keep in mind that you will be swayed for only a few seconds until you flatten the sway in Step 6, and that the lengthening you did in Step 3 will protect your discs from any compression caused by the sway.

A few people may have some protective stiffness in the lower back that prevents their back from swaying even when the hips have been exaggeratedly thrust back. If this is your case, you can skip Step 6 until this area becomes flexible enough that a sway could result.

6 PIVOT YOUR RIB CAGE TO STRAIGHTEN YOUR LOWER BACK

THINK OF YOUR TORSO AS A CLOCK HAND

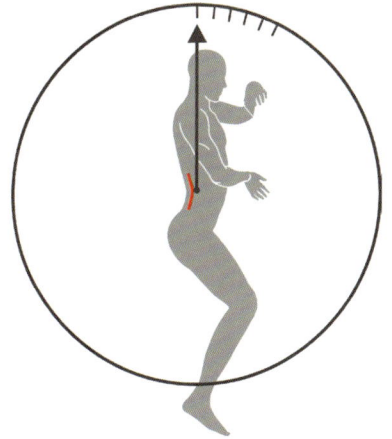

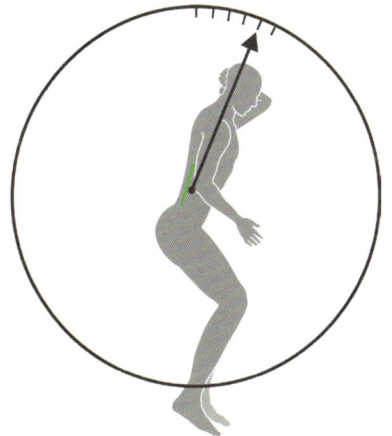

Maintaining the anteverted position of your pelvis (keep your hips exactly where they are), use your arms to lift your upper body (including your shoulder) off the bed.

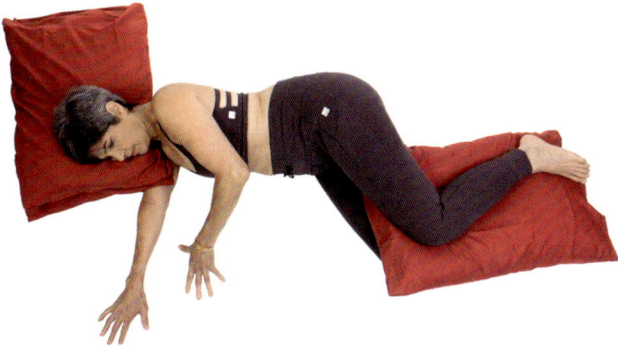

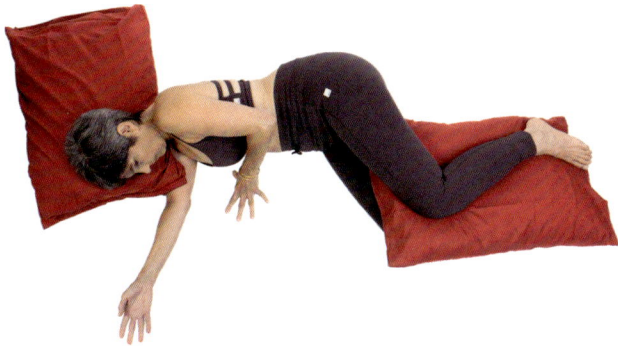

Pivot your rib cage forward a few degrees (see sidebar). Your upper rib cage will migrate forward on the bed, your lower shoulder will migrate somewhat further, and your head will migrate the furthest (bring your pillow along with you). You'll end up in a zigzag.

Lower yourself onto the bed. You should now have a "J" shaped spine.

To help you achieve the desired shape at the end of Step 6, it may be helpful to imagine your upper torso as the hand of a clock. Your upper torso pivots forward a few degrees or "minutes" until the sway in your lower back is flattened.

7 RECHECK THE SHAPE OF YOUR LOWER BACK WITH YOUR FINGERTIPS

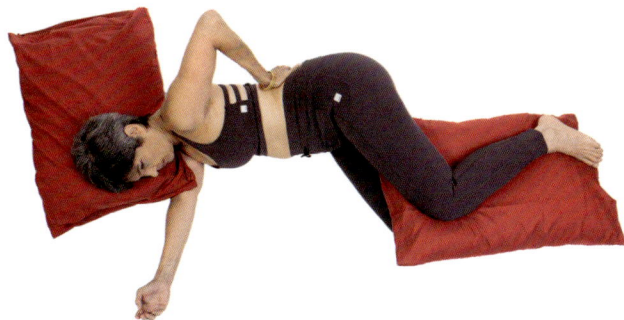

You are aiming for the midline groove running along your lumbar spine to have a uniform depth from top to bottom. Repeat Step 6 until any remaining sway in your lower back has been straightened out as much as possible.

101

AVOID SWAYING WHEN LENGTHENING THE BACK

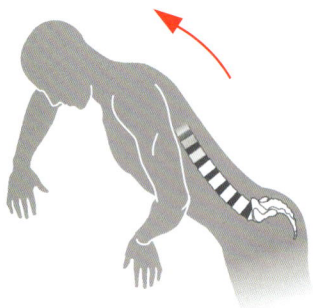

Push towards your hips with both arms to elongate the spine.

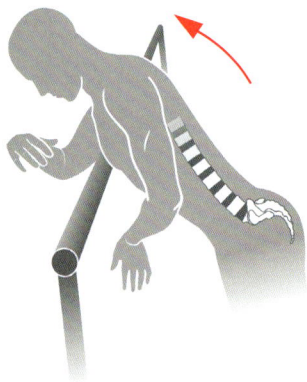

Imagine a bar that runs across the body at chest height and use it as a guide to help you push in the right direction (that is, stay close to the bar).

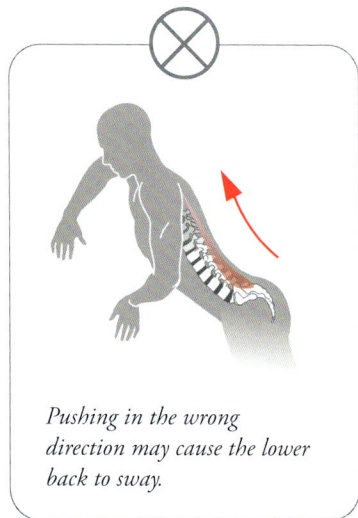

Pushing in the wrong direction may cause the lower back to sway.

8 ELONGATE YOUR J-SPINE

As you did in Step 3, raise your shoulder off the bed an inch or two. Push with your lower elbow and upper hand into the bed and down toward your hips to lengthen your spine. Take care to maintain your J shape: do not let your back arch nor your pelvis tuck.

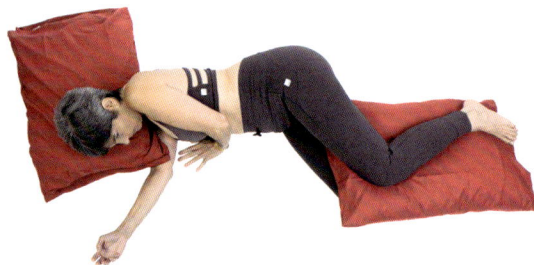

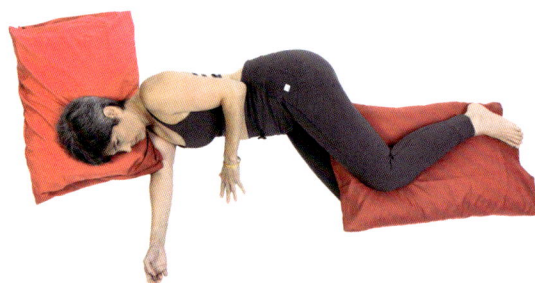

Add just half an inch (1cm) or so of extra length. Relax back down onto the bed.

You should now feel a gentle and comfortable stretch in your lower back. If the stretch is intense, back off by wriggling your rib cage down a little (be careful not to reintroduce a sway). Over time, you'll be able to stretch further with comfort.

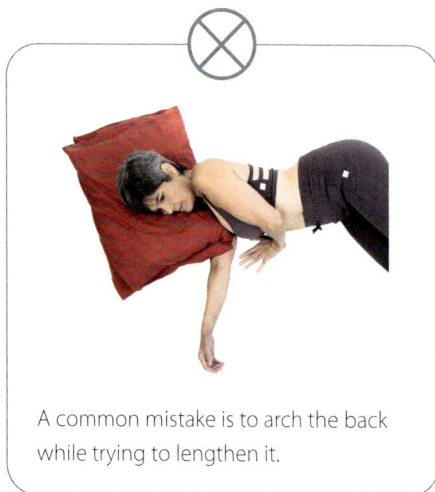

A common mistake is to arch the back while trying to lengthen it.

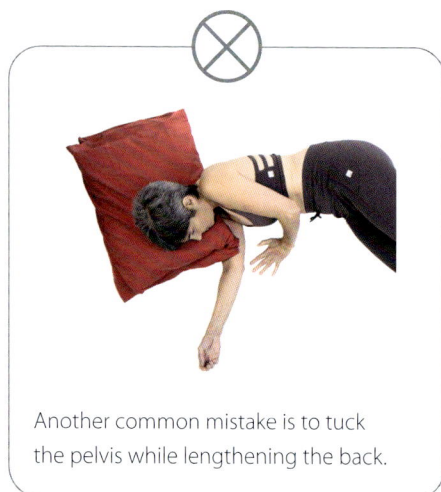

Another common mistake is to tuck the pelvis while lengthening the back.

9 LENGTHEN YOUR NECK

Raise your head slightly off the pillow and glide your head back and up to lengthen the back of your neck. It may be useful to grasp the hair at the base of your skull and then gently pull back and up. Be moderate in this action. A slight stretch is comfortable and encourages your muscles to stretch and relax; a severe or sudden stretch may cause your muscles to tighten and spasm.

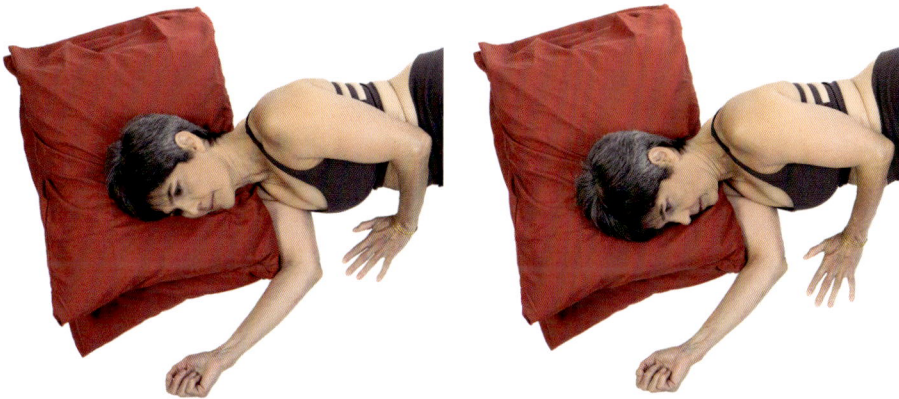

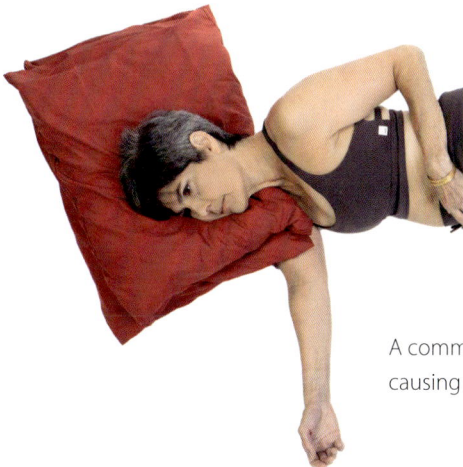

A common mistake is to raise the chin, causing compression in the neck (cervical spine).

STRETCHLYING WITH THE HEAD HIGHER THAN HORIZONTAL

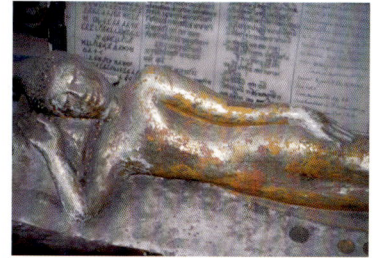

(Thailand)

All reclining Buddha images show the Buddha's head slightly elevated from the horizontal. This position is particularly comfortable as it provides ample slack in the upper trapezius, facilitating good shoulder positioning.

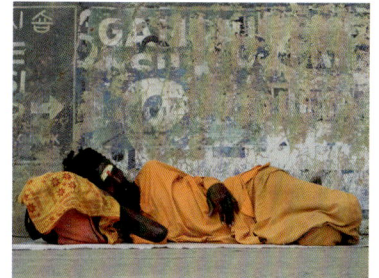

(India)

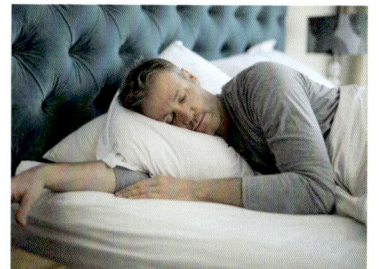

(USA)

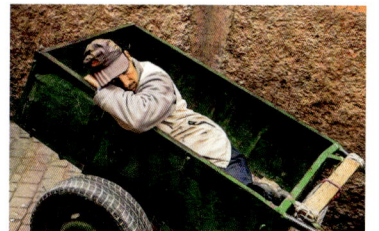

(Morocco)

THE UPPER SHOULDER DOES NOT SLUMP

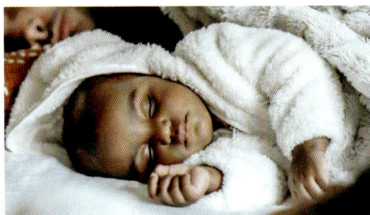

Baby sleeping (USA)

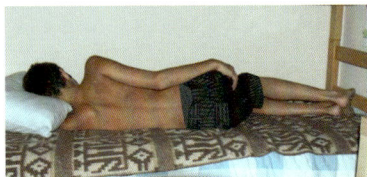

Boy lying down (USA)

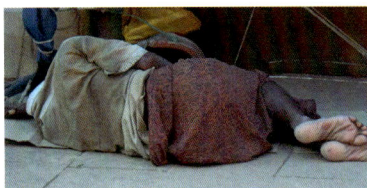

Man sleeping on street (India)

Having the shoulder rolled back allows the brachial plexus to function properly, and ensures good circulation to and from the arm. It also reduces the stress on the thoracic spine. In addition, having a good shoulder position when sleeping helps you become accustomed to healthy shoulder position during your waking hours.

10 PERFORM A SHOULDER ROLL WITH YOUR UPPER SHOULDER

Bring your upper shoulder slightly forward, then a moderate way up toward your ear, then back and down.

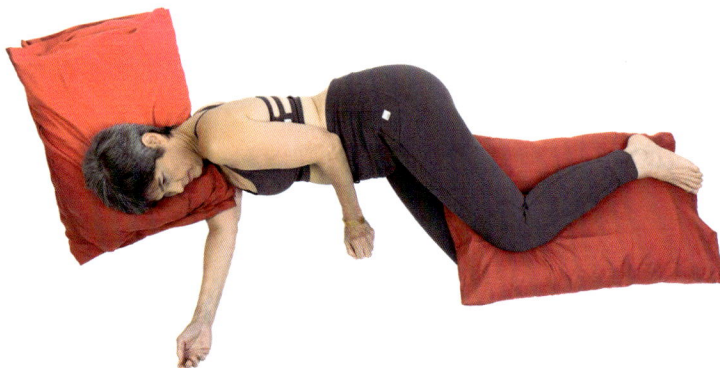

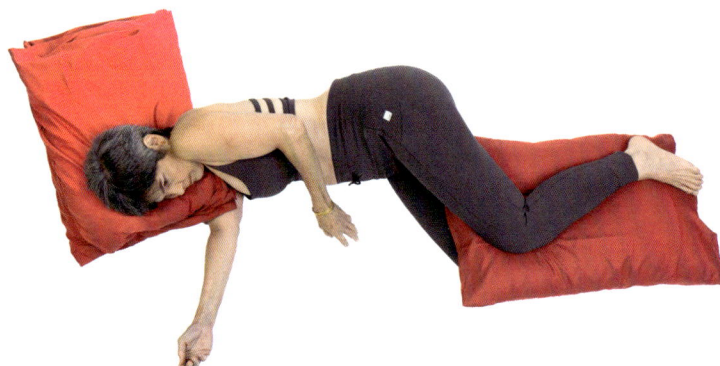

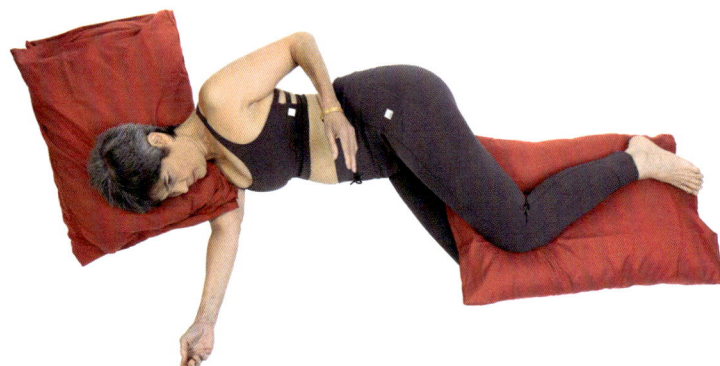

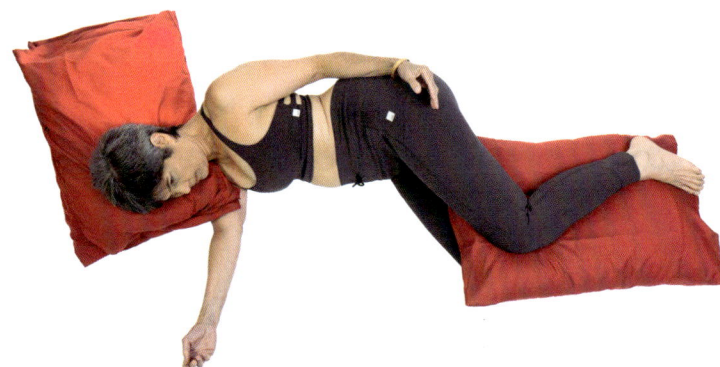

11 POSITION THE ARM THAT IS ABOVE YOUR BODY

Here are several healthy options for positioning your arm in a way that prevents your shoulder from rounding forward.

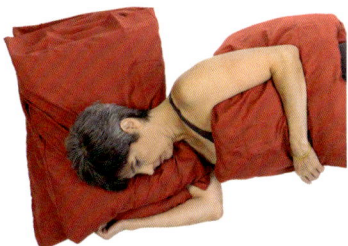

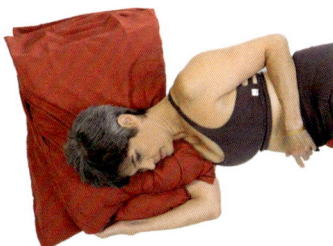

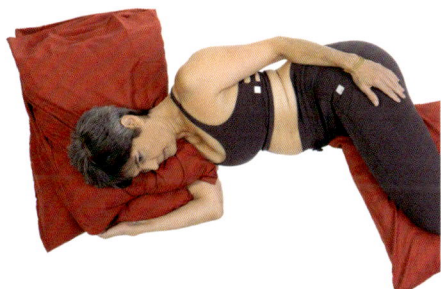

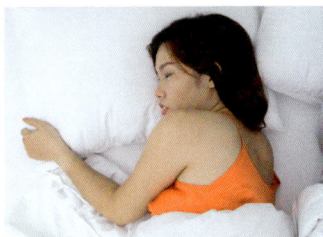

Don't allow your upper shoulder to roll forward. This stresses the upper thoracic spine and reinforces the bad habit of slumping.

12 POSITION THE ARM THAT IS BELOW YOUR BODY FOR COMFORT

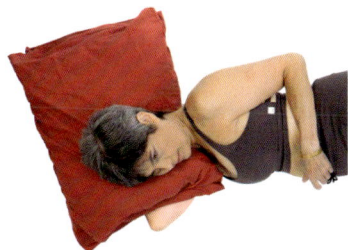

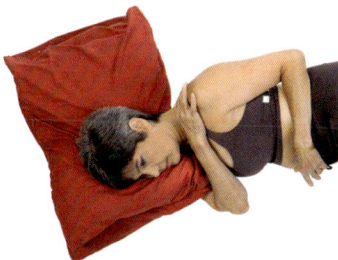

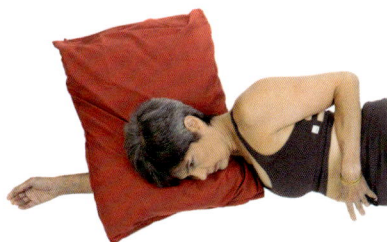

You might try placing the arm in front of your body, straight above you passing under your pillow, or under your head.

If your lower shoulder feels pinned, slide it a little forward, out from under your body. Puffing up the pillow can also help create more space for the shoulder.

THE LOWER ARM IS POSITIONED FOR CONVENIENCE

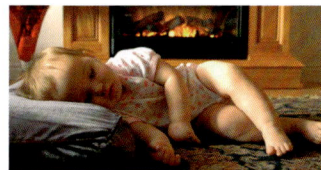

(USA)

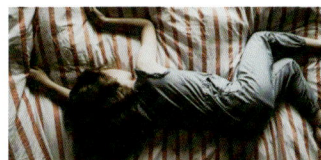

(UK)

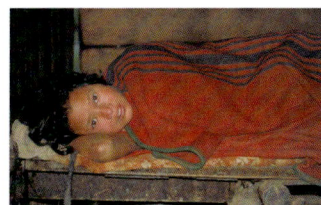

(Thailand)

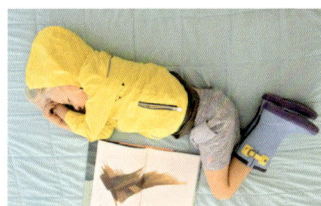

(USA)

105

INDICATIONS OF IMPROVEMENT

As with stretchlying on your back, stretchlying on your side may seem awkward at first. Soon you will find that you move into the position quickly and easily, and find it comfortable.

Stretchlying on your side provides the same benefits as stretchlying on your back: improved circulation, and decompression of discs and nerves. All these benefits contribute to increased comfort, function, and general well-being.

You will probably notice changes in your breathing pattern. The stretched abdominal muscles offer some resistance to belly breathing, resulting in more movement in your lower chest and less in your abdomen. Over time, this increase in chest breathing will expand your lung capacity and support normal architecture in your rib cage.

If you spend much of the night stretchlying, either on your back or side, the resting length of your back will increase, you will become measurably taller, and you will be more comfortable even when not in traction.

TROUBLESHOOTING

YOU CAN'T FALL ASLEEP

You may need to train your body to use this new sleeping position. Try doing some breathing meditation or perform a *body scan* (see Glossary). If some time after assuming your stretchlying position, you are still awake, revert to a more familiar position to fall asleep. As stretchlying becomes more familiar over time, one night you will probably fall asleep in this position. Eventually your body becomes so used to being comfortable and pain free that it gravitates to this and other healthy positions even during sleep.

YOUR BODY DOESN'T HOLD THE POSITION THROUGH THE NIGHT

Don't worry about this! It is normal to change positions during the night. When you start the night with your back in a lengthened position, you will derive some benefit all night long. Your back muscles will remain slightly stretched, allowing for better circulation, nerve function, and disc rehydration.

YOU ARE UNCOMFORTABLE IN THIS POSITION

Elongating your spine and anteverting your pelvis are difficult skills to learn. Go through the instructions again. Repeating the movements makes them more familiar and helps increase your mastery.

You may require a straighter spine, perhaps because of a recent back injury or a significantly narrower waist than hips. If your back is healthy and you lengthen your back as you lie down, a slight sag or twist at the waist will not cause any problem. If, however, your discs are compressed, the additional pressure from sagging or twisting may cause discomfort. Try one of these suggestions:

- Place a small pillow or towel roll between your waist and the bed (fig.4-6). This eliminates the sag in the waist that results if your hips are much wider than your waist. Use the support until your back normalizes.

- Place a pillow between your knees or thighs (fig.4-7). This eliminates the twist in your back that results from your hips being wider than your knees. Use this support until your back normalizes.

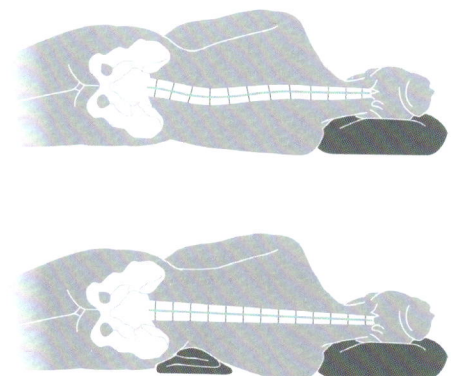

fig.4-6

The sag in the spine caused by a narrow waist and wide hips is easily remedied by putting a small towel roll under the waist.

fig.4-7

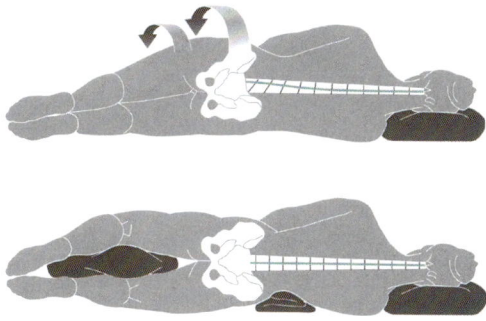

The twist in the spine caused by being narrower at the knees than at the hips when lying on the side is easily remedied with a pillow or Gokhale™ Wedge between the knees.

FURTHER INFORMATION

J OR NOT A J: THAT IS THE QUESTION

With time and practice you will become increasingly adept at recognizing a J-spine using your fingertips as in Step 7. If you are unsure, ask a friend to take pictures of you from above. Indications of a J-spine include: your bottom is behind your lower back, your back is straight, and there is a defined angle at L5-S1 where the bottom meets the back (fig.4-8a,b,c). Some people, myself included, have fleshy pads on the sides of their sacrum obscuring the juncture at L5-S1. At first glance, the contour may appear to be a sway, even if the spine itself is "J" shaped (fig.4-8d).

SLEEPING ON YOUR STOMACH

Although many people opt to sleep on their stomachs, this position can present problems. First, an ordinary pillow imposes nearly a 90° angle on the neck, which can stress or damage it. To make stomach sleeping healthier, place the head pillow so it does not force an acute neck angle. For example, place just the back half of the head on the pillow, allowing the face to angle downward (fig.4-9). Also, most people have a tendency to sway the lower back when lying face down. Placing a small pillow under the abdomen reduces the sway (fig.4-10). Before lying on your stomach, it pays to lengthen your spine by digging your elbows into the bed as you lay your torso down (fig.4-11). Young children sometimes sleep face down in a crouched position (fig.4-12).

fig.4-8

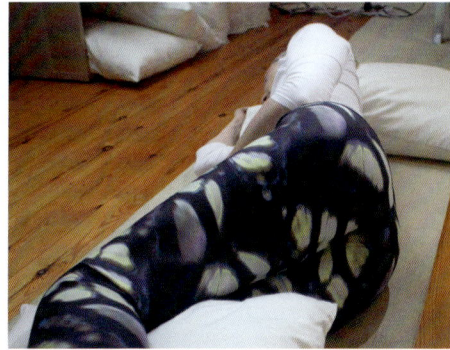

a.

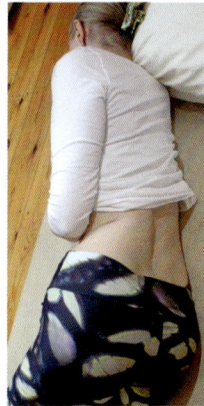

b.

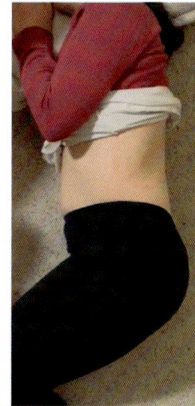

c.

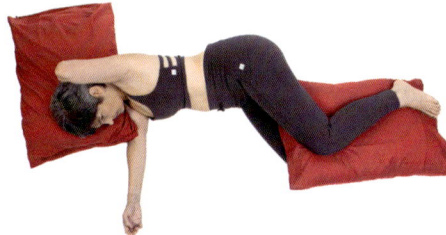

d.

Indications of a J-spine include: the "behind" is behind (a), the lumbar spine is quite straight (b), and there is a defined angle at L5-S1 (c). The curve of the hip may be incorrectly interpreted as a sway (d).

fig.4-9

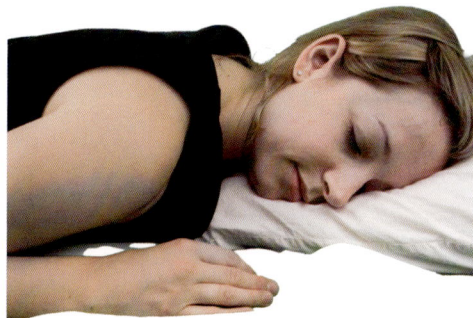

Placing a pillow to reduce strain on the neck.

107

fig.4-10

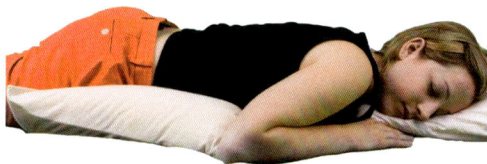

Placing a pillow to reduce a sway in the lower back.

fig.4-11

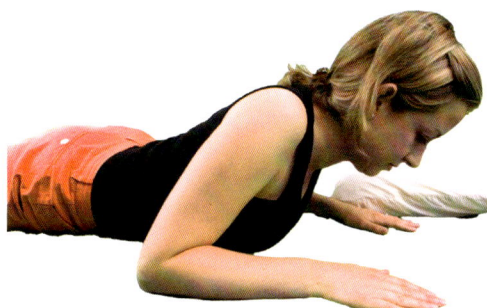

Digging in the elbows to lengthen the back.

fig.4-12

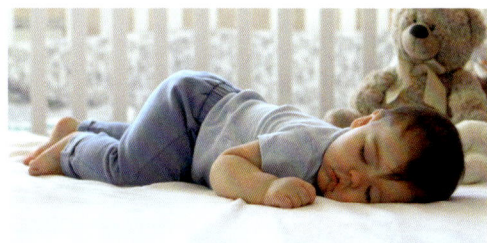

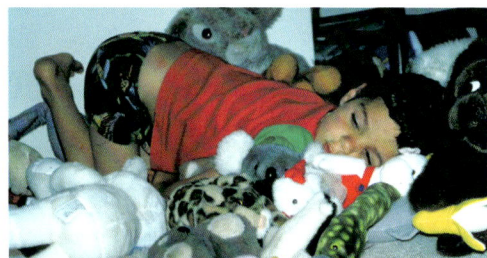

Young children have sufficient flexibility to sleep comfortably on their stomachs. They sometimes use a novel way to keep their backs well aligned.

WHAT TO DO WITH YOUR LEGS

Many people who sleep on their sides find it comfortable to straighten their lower leg, bend their upper knee, and twist their spine to place the upper knee on the bed or ground (fig.4-13). If you have compressed discs, twisting the spine can damage your discs. To reduce this risk, lengthen the spine before introducing the twist, distribute the twist throughout the spine evenly, and place a pillow beneath the bent knee (fig.4-14).

fig.4-13

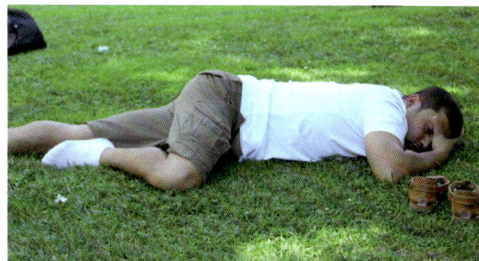

A common sleeping position that helps navigate hard sleeping surfaces and is healthy for a lengthened, well-shaped back (Australia).

fig.4-14

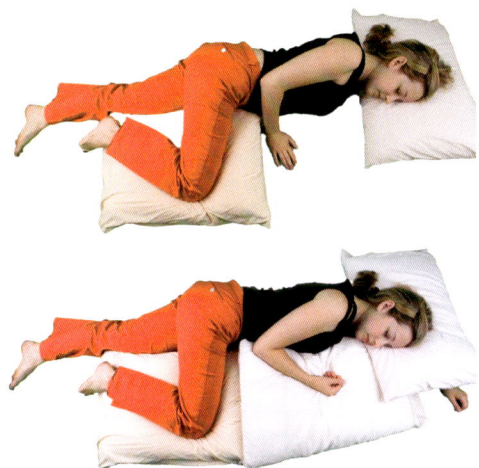

Placing pillows to reduce twisting helps protect the spine.

RECAP

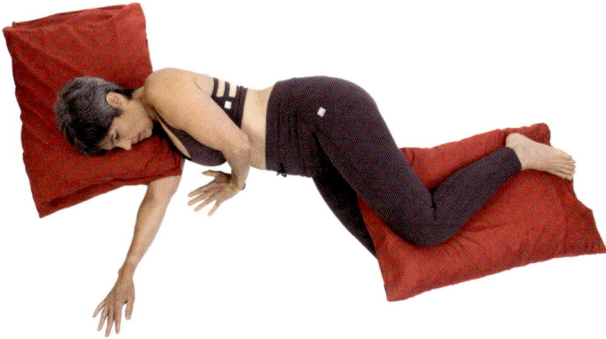

a. **Lengthen spine**

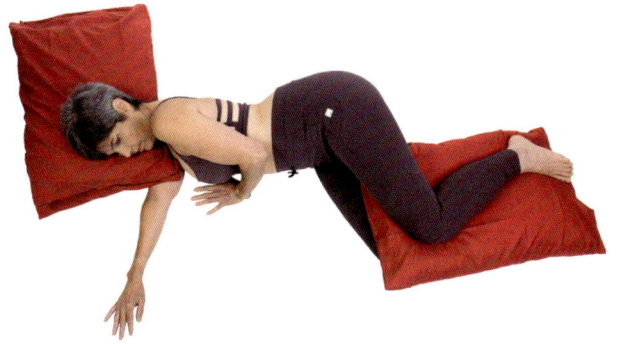

b. **Move hips backward to antevert the pelvis**

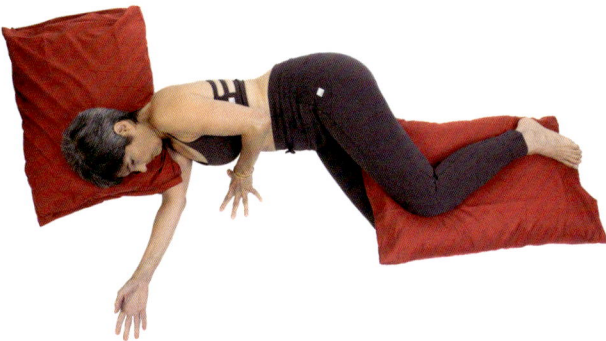

c. **Pivot rib cage forward to remove any sway**

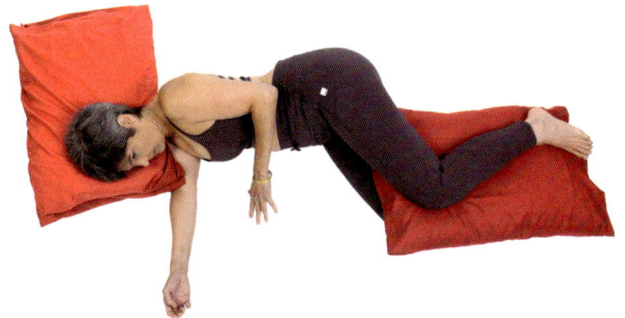

d. **Lengthen spine again**

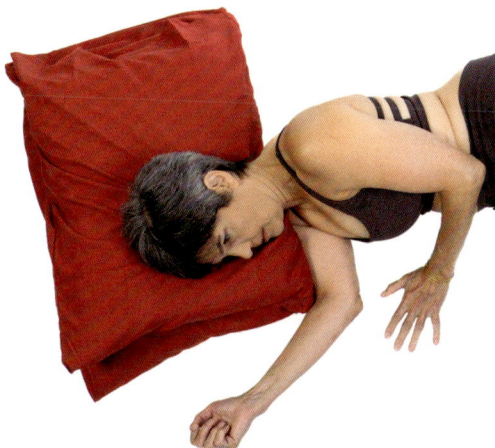

e. **Lengthen neck and rotate head forward**

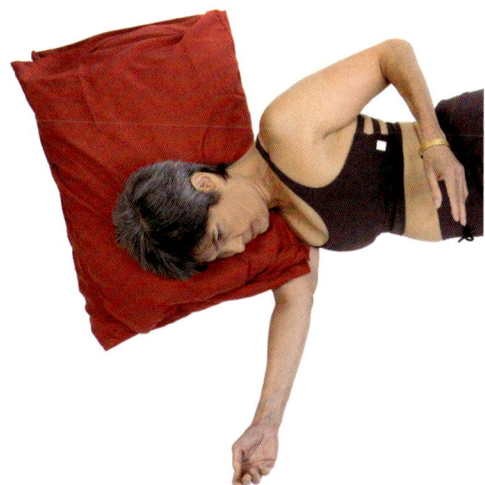

f. **Roll upper shoulder**

5

USING YOUR INNER CORSET

Using your muscles to protect and lengthen your spine

This Samburu tribesman in Kenya engages his abdominal muscles to help him elongate his torso
and protect his spine against the impact of jumping. Notice his rib cage is anchored—the front
lower border flush with the contour of his abdomen, not jutting out.

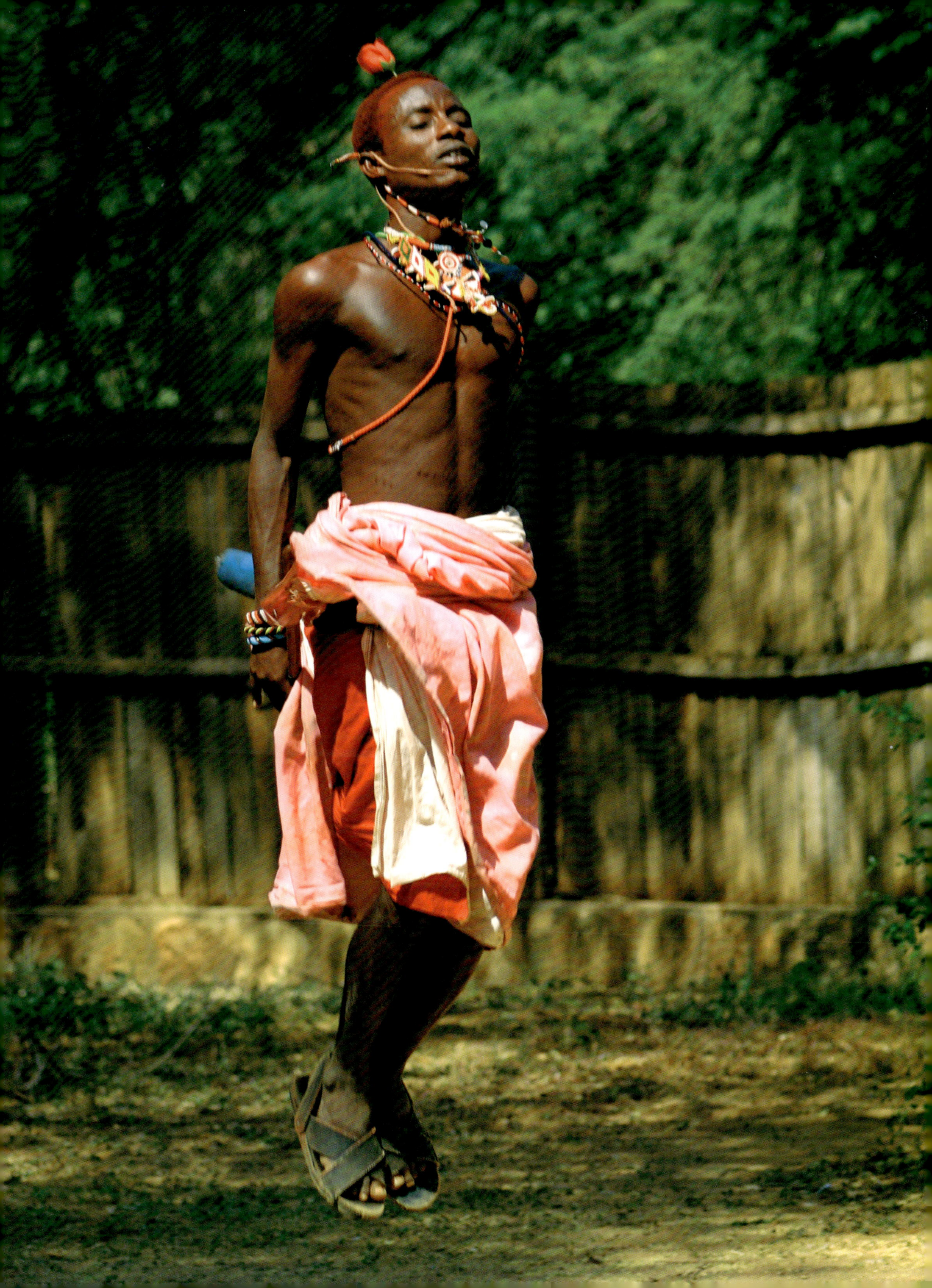

In the chapters so far, you have learned several effective ways to lengthen and protect your spine:

- Using an external object like a backrest or bed to put your spine in traction (stretchsitting, stretchlying).
- Positioning your pelvis so the vertebrae stack above it without tightening and shortening the surrounding muscles (stacksitting).
- Breathing with the muscles around the spine relaxed, to further lengthen the spine with each breath (page 72).

In this chapter you will learn a more powerful technique that gives you added length, is available to you at all times, and provides strong support to protect your elongated spine. The technique involves contracting certain muscles in your abdomen and back to make an "inner corset." This contraction causes the torso to become narrower and taller, thus lengthening the spine (fig.5-1).

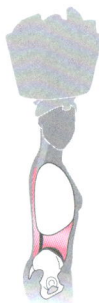

fig.5-1

The muscles of the inner corset include the intrinsic back muscles and the abdominal transversus and obliques.

The inner corset is important in situations where your discs may be challenged, such as:
- Carrying a heavy backpack, suitcase, or other object (fig.5-2a).
- Running, jogging, or engaging in other high-impact aerobic activities (fig.5-2b).
- Playing almost any sport—tennis, volleyball, basketball, or even swimming.
- Performing yoga poses that involve twists, sidebends, or backbends (fig.5-2c).
- Dancing in a way that involves impact, spinal twisting, or bending.
- Riding on a bumpy road in a vehicle with poor shock absorbers, riding a mountain bike, or sailing in rough seas (fig.5-2d).

When an African or Indian village woman carries a heavy weight on her head (fig.5-3), she is not

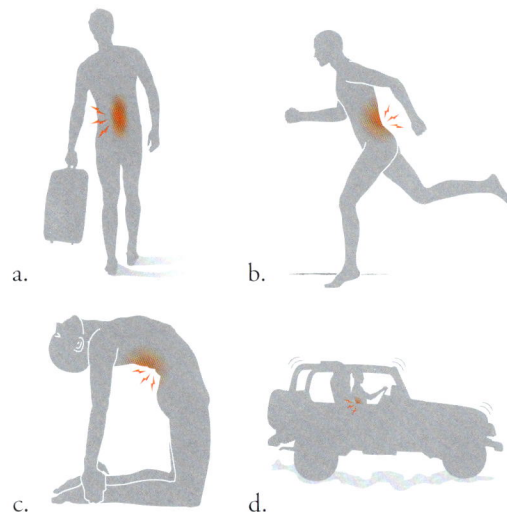

fig.5-2

a.   b.

c.   d.

Activities where not using your inner corset can result in damage.

fig.5-3

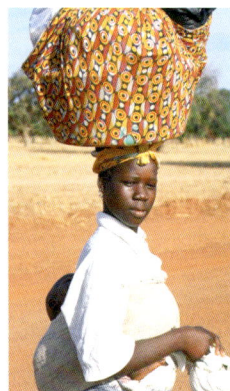
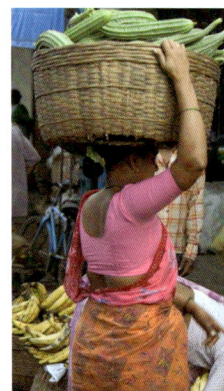

(Burkina Faso)   *(India)*

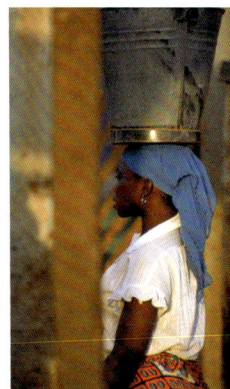
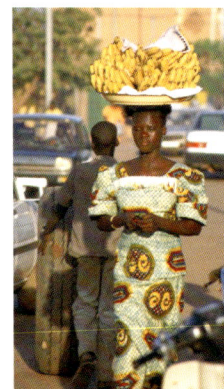

(Burkina Faso)   *(Burkina Faso)*

These women are actively using their inner corsets to elongate and protect their spines as they carry substantial weights on their heads.

passive under that weight, which would cause her discs to compress. Rather, she actively engages her inner corset; her torso becomes more slender and her spine becomes longer. In this way she protects her discs from the weight she carries. Periodically, when carrying a burden for a long time, she may lift the burden above her head with outstretched arms (fig.5-4). This action stretches her back muscles and reengages her inner corset.

Medical literature documents that in certain populations, such as the Bhil tribe of Central India, the discs of a 50-year-old look very similar

to those of a 20-year-old (fig.5-5).[48] The proper and frequent use of the inner corset muscles is perhaps why these populations experience virtually no disc degeneration as they age. In industrialized societies, on the other hand, it is considered normal to have significant disc degeneration by age 50. By using our muscles to protect our discs as the Bhils do, we can avoid the deterioration and damage that we have erroneously come to accept as normal.

In the Gokhale Method, as in conventional approaches, there is an emphasis on using and strengthening the abdominal muscles. However,

fig.5-4

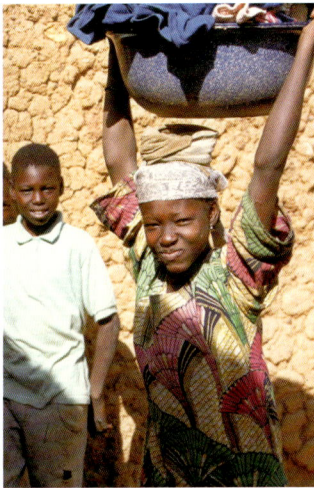

It is common among people who carry weights on their heads to stretch their back muscles and reengage their inner corsets periodically (Burkina Faso).

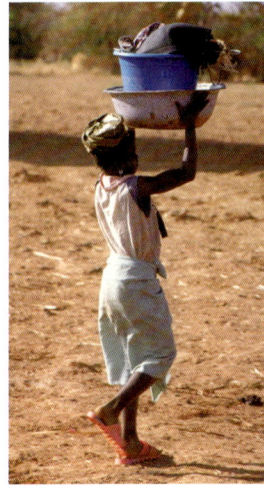

Woman placing laundry baskets on her head (Burkina Faso).

fig.5-5

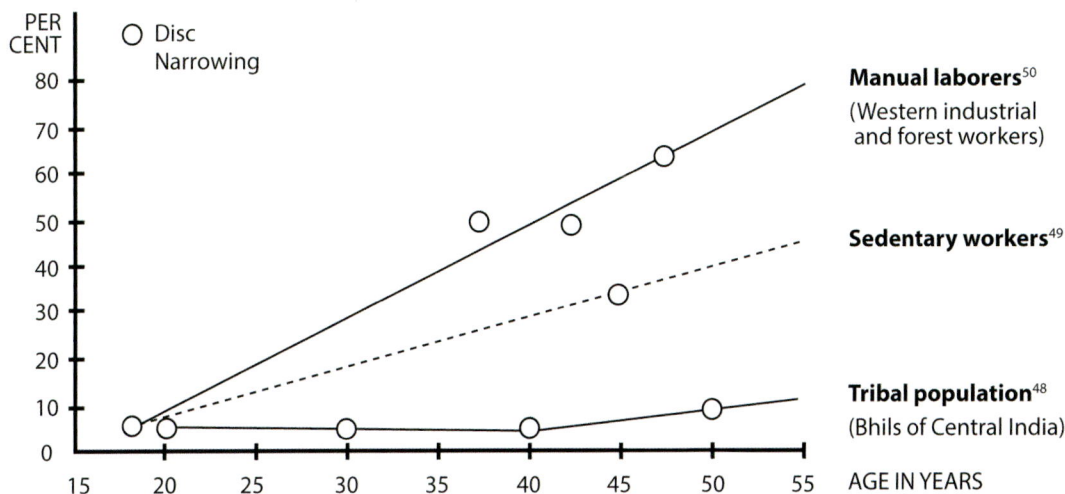

This graph [48] shows a large difference in disc narrowing with age in three different populations. There is very little disc narrowing in the Bhil tribal people of Central India,[48] more disc narrowing among Western sedentary workers,[49] and high levels of disc narrowing among Western industrial and forestry workers.[50]

113

fig.5-6

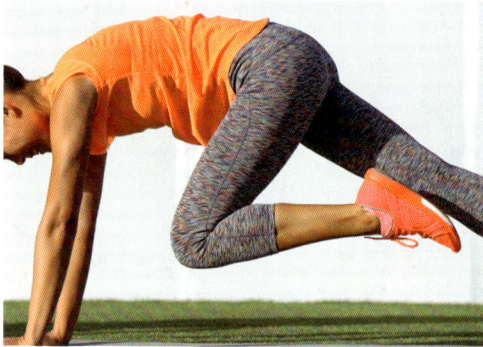

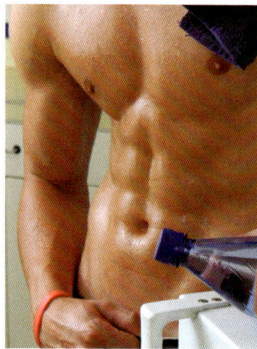

a. Many common abdominal exercises involve tucking the pelvis and rounding the back inappropriately.

b. Doing conventional abdominal exercises may result in long-term unhealthy posture changes.

fig.5-7

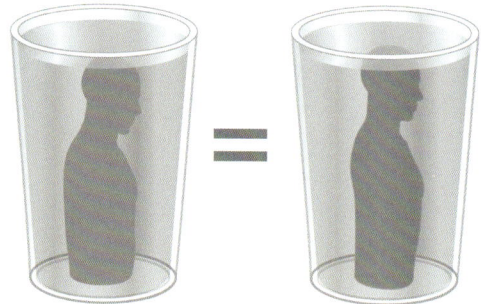

As your torso gets more slender, it must get taller because its volume stays the same.

in contrast to many conventional approaches, the Gokhale Method teaches you to isolate the abdominal *obliques* and *transversus* muscles from the *rectus abdominis* muscles so that you can lengthen and support your spine without distorting it (fig.5-6). Learning this can be challenging, especially for some highly trained athletes who must overcome firmly ingrained habits in order to isolate the different abdominal muscles.

LENGTHENING BY CONTRACTING

You might ask how you can lengthen your spine by contracting your muscles. The answer is twofold.

First, contracting the abdominal muscles causes the abdomen to become narrower. Since the abdomen has a fixed volume, it must become taller, changing its shape from a short, squat cylinder to a tall, thin cylinder (fig.5-7). This action elongates the spine, easing the vertebrae apart and decompressing the discs. The lower back feels braced, as though you were wearing the support belt commonly used by workers who carry heavy burdens. You use an inner corset made of your own muscles.

Second, certain muscles, because of their geometry, cause the spine to lengthen as they contract. For example, the *longus colli* muscles are attached to the front of the cervical spine. When these muscles contract, they force the cervical curve to straighten, thus lengthening the cervical spine (fig.5-8).

fig.5-8

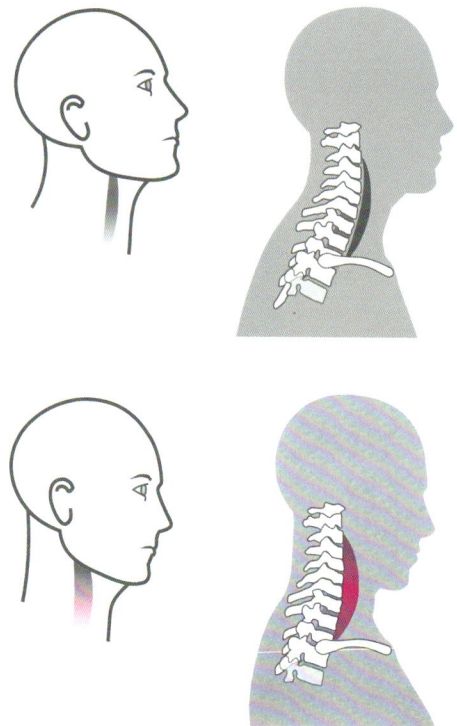

The longus colli muscles attach to the front (anterior) of the cervical vertebrae. When they contract, they cause the neck to straighten and, therefore, lengthen.

The deepest muscles of the back (*rotatores* and *multifidus*) have a more complex geometry. When contracted unilaterally (that is, on just one side of the spine), the rotatores muscles cause the spine to rotate. When contracted bilaterally, these muscles contribute to spinal elongation. It is difficult to envision how this works but we know from electromyelography studies that these muscles are involved in lengthening the spine.

The best way to strengthen and maintain the muscles of the inner corset is to use them in the course of daily activities. When you are first learning to use your abdominals in this new way, try to exercise your inner corset up to 20 times a day for a minute each time. This will help you establish the new pattern and reach a threshold level of muscle strength. It will also give the long muscles of your back (*erector spinae*) a periodic stretch and your discs a periodic decompression.

When you have integrated this new pattern into your daily life, you will find that many activities traditionally considered harmful for the back are actually healthy challenges for the muscles of your inner corset.

I now notice muscles in my abdomen that I never saw before, and I did not have to do any sit ups for them!

Mai Huong Nguyen,
Veazie, ME

I am happy to say that I am back to my normal rigorous routine in our backyard. Utilizing the technique of hip-hinging and engaging my inner corset, I feel that I am not only preventing injury but also strengthening muscles in my abdomen, along my spine, and in my thighs. The Gokhale Method has allowed me to resume gardening, and has actually enhanced my gardening experience.

Dana Seyfried,
Seaford, DE

BENEFITS

- Protects your spine in actions that involve compression, impact, or distortion

- Stretches your spine more reliably and with a stronger action than any other technique

- Stabilizes your spine in case of injury

- Provides a stable platform enhancing the power of arm and leg actions

- Improves the tone and appearance of your torso

Until I met Esther Gokhale, I had lost hope in finding relief for my constant pain caused by a severe, multilevel back injury. I had spent years working with numerous physicians and physical therapists, received a number of cortisone injections, tried virtually every available prescription anti-inflammatory medication, and endured painful diagnostic and therapeutic procedures to curb significant pain and avoid surgery. I was convinced I had explored every treatment option, but I hadn't. Upon receiving independent endorsements of Esther's technique from trusted friends, I decided to see her for pain relief.

Initially I resented her advice to revisit the way I positioned and moved my body. I felt betrayed because I had faithfully followed my prescribed physical therapy and home exercise regime. Nevertheless, I was taught and slowly relearned how to sit, stand, walk, and even lie down.

I found and strengthened areas I didn't even know needed attention. With Esther's guidance, I worked out in new ways. Friends started telling me I looked great. Thank you, Esther, for relief from pain and a new awareness of my body.

Patti Fry
Menlo Park, CA

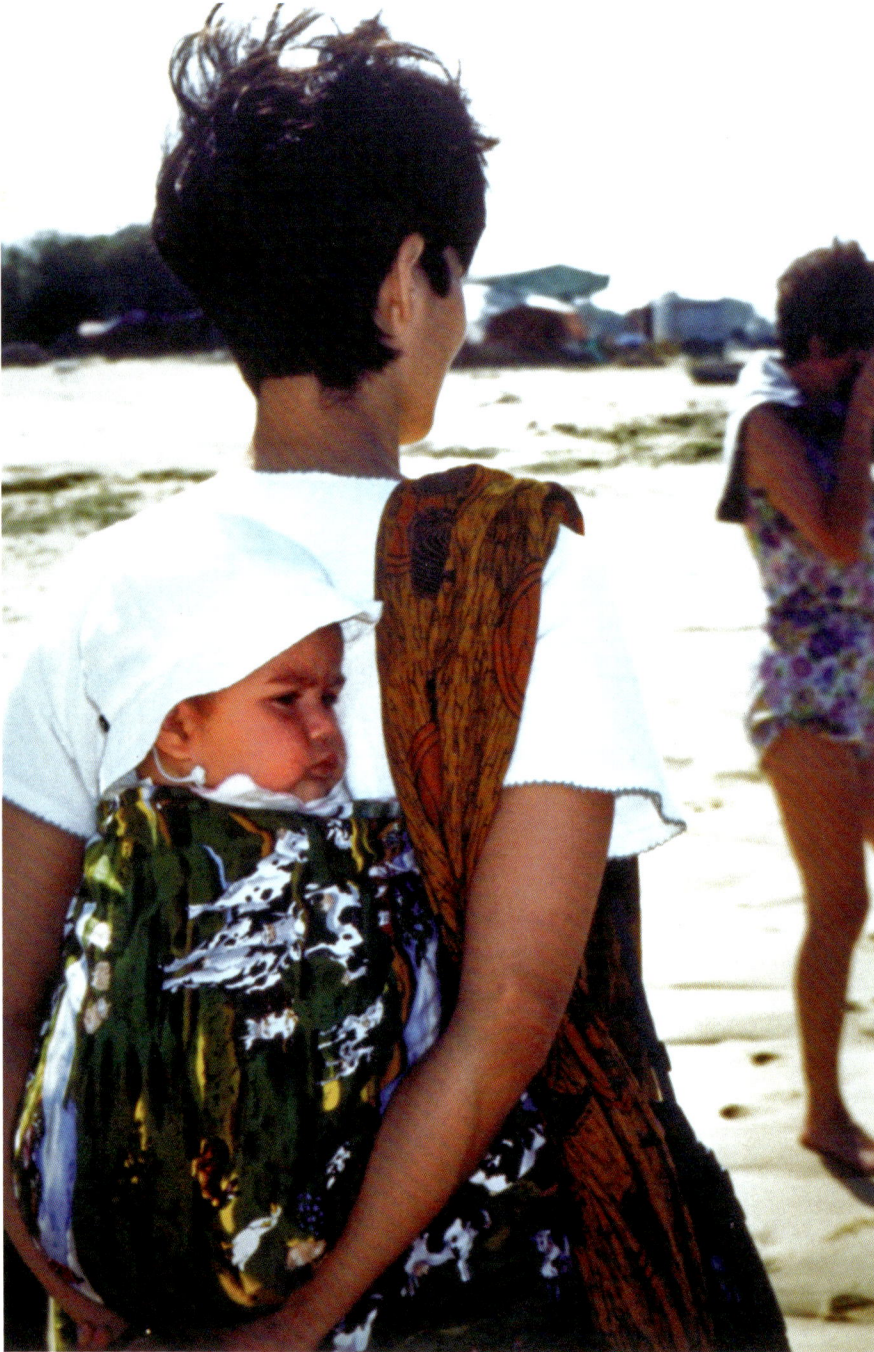

Carrying my baby on my back

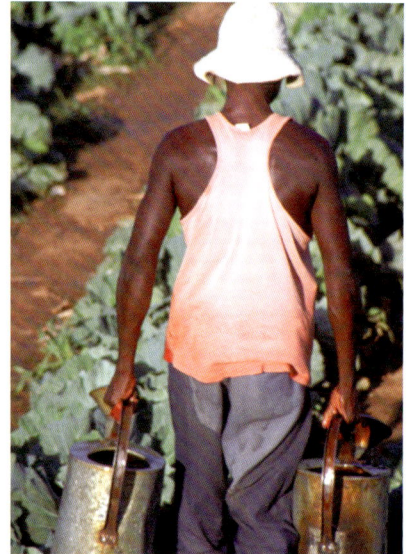

Watering crops (Burkina Faso)

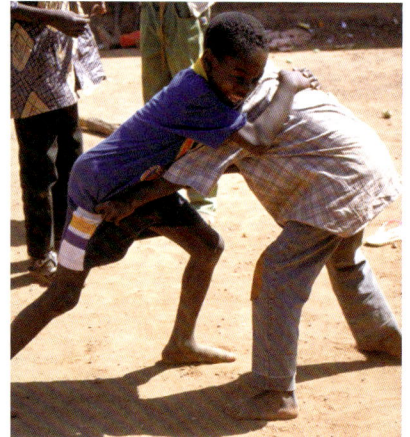

Wrestling game (Burkina Faso)

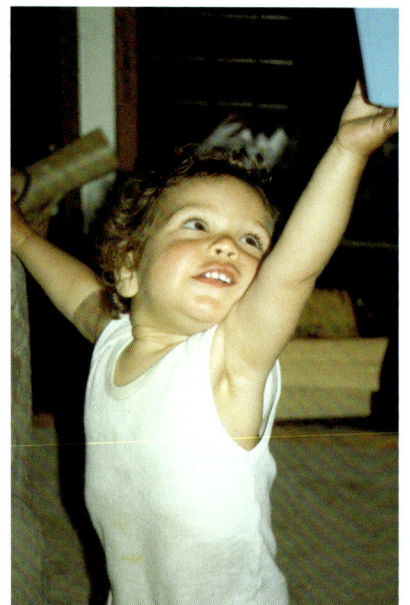

My son reaching up for a toy (USA)

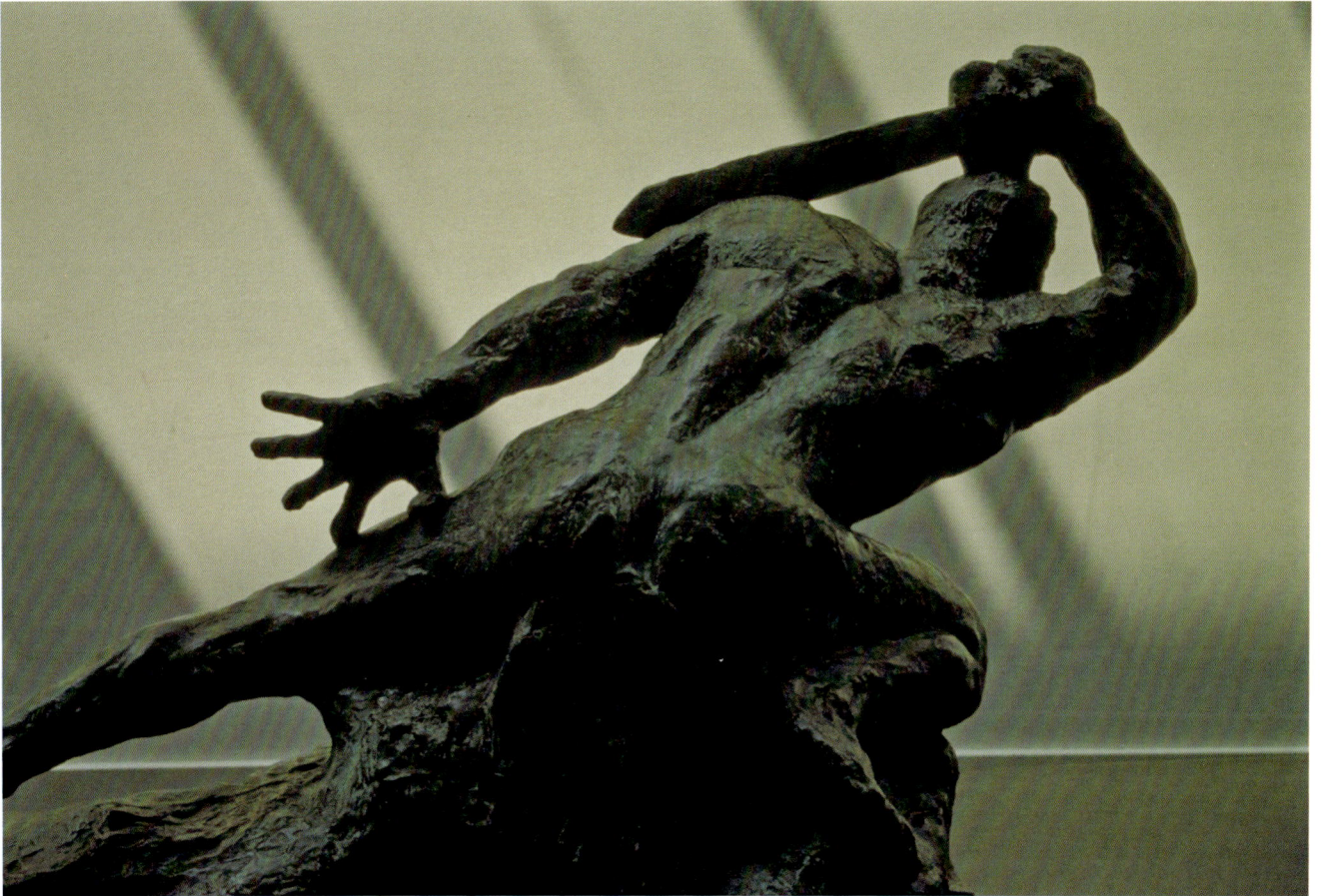

Gladiator sculpture (19th century, France)

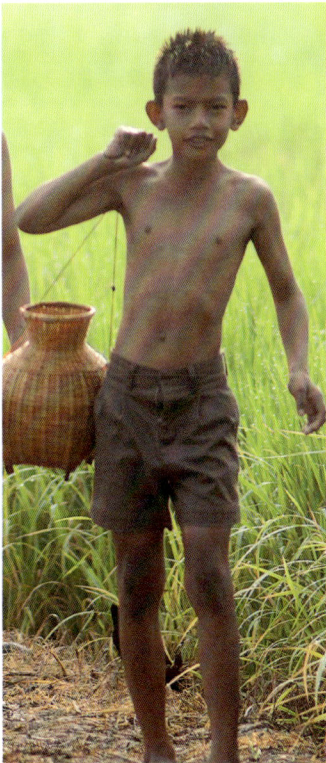

Carrying a fish trap (Thailand)

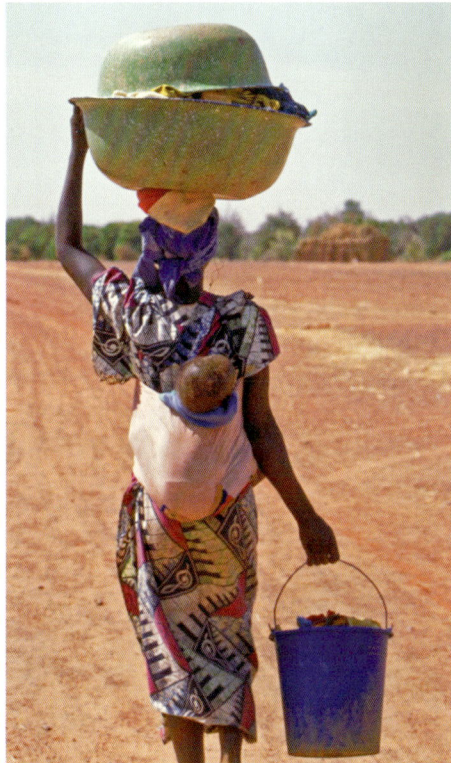

Carrying baby, bucket, and tub (Burkina Faso)

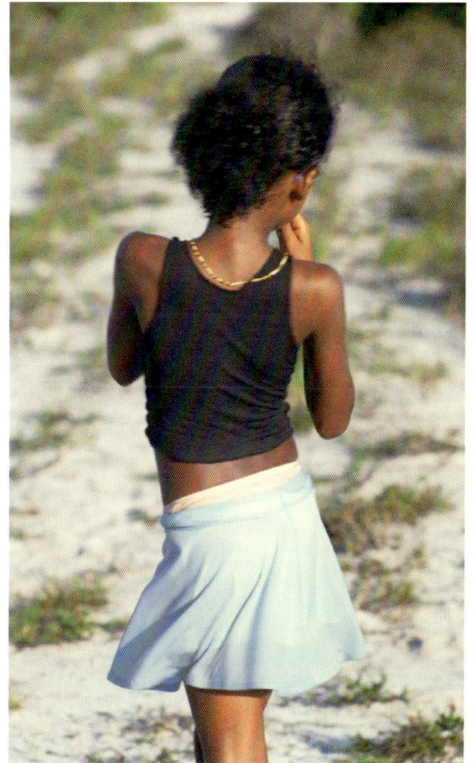

Engaging in play (Brazil)

EQUIPMENT

You will need a full-length mirror.

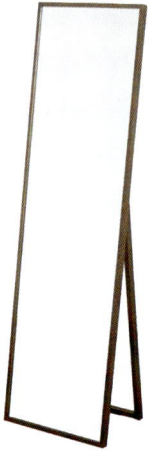

RIB ANCHOR

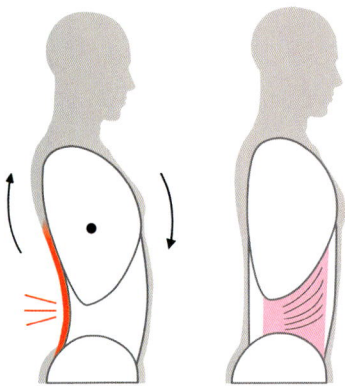

The rib anchor technique involves pivoting around an axis running from side to side roughly through the middle of the rib cage.

1 SET UP IN A "READY POSITION," WITH SOFT KNEES AND KIDNEY BEAN-SHAPED FEET

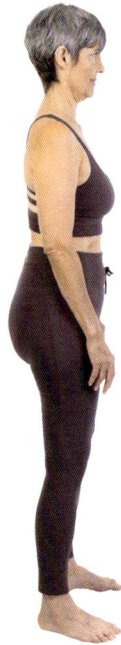

It is important to start with a healthy standing position before engaging your inner corset.

2 ANCHOR YOUR RIBS

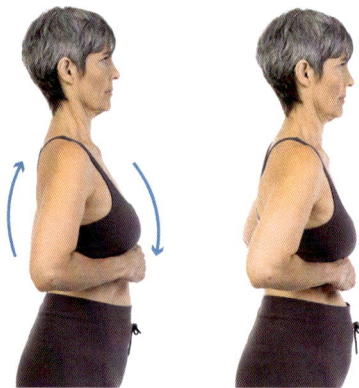

Pivot your rib cage so that the front moves down and the back moves up, pulling the lumbar spine straighter (see fig.F-27 on page 21, and page 140).

3 PLACE THE FINGERTIPS OF ONE HAND SO THAT THEY CAN MONITOR YOUR SPINAL GROOVE

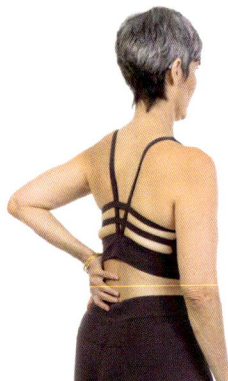

Use a light touch to check the entire lower back. Ideally, the midline groove will be a uniform depth from top to bottom (see page 77).

4 CHOOSE ONE OF THE FOLLOWING WAYS TO RECRUIT YOUR INNER CORSET MUSCLES

A. Reaching Up

With one hand, reach upward and a little forward, as though you were reaching for the top of a high cabinet. Find the direction of stretch that gives you length in your back rather than your front. Use your fingertips to check your lower back does not arch.

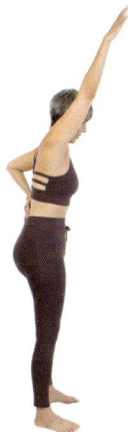

Imagine reaching up and over a bar at chest height to help engage the inner corset muscles correctly.

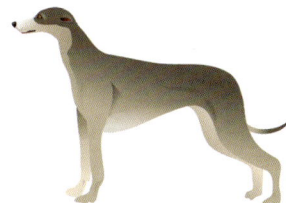

Now reach up with your other hand, too. Stretch upward as far as you comfortably can.

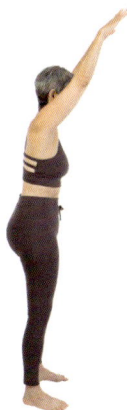

The lean abdominal area of a greyhound provides a useful image to help you engage your inner corset.

B. Pushing Yourself Tall

Push down on the rim of your pelvis with your hands to lengthen your spine. Envisage yourself going up and over an imaginary bar at chest height (see sidebar).

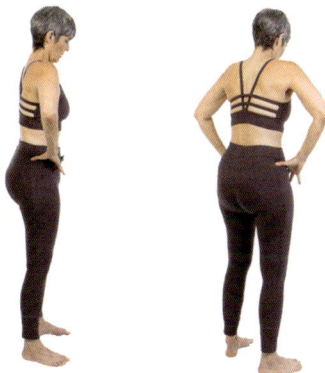

EXAMPLE OF ENGAGING THE INNER CORSET WHILE REACHING UP

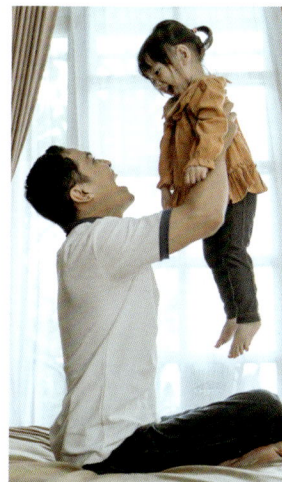

C. Imagining Entering Cold Water

Imagine walking into a cold lake or ocean. As the water level rises around your middle, you pull your torso up and away from the icy water. Take care not to sway.

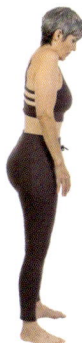

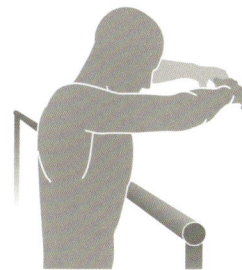

(Indonesia)

USING THE INNER CORSET TO PROTECT SPINAL STRUCTURES

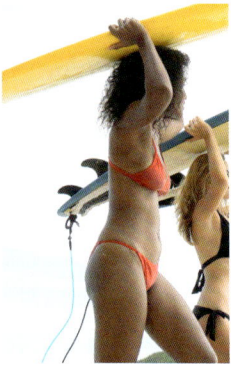

Carrying a surfboard (Brazil)

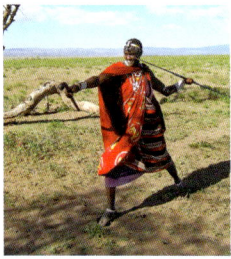

Hunting with a spear (Tanzania)

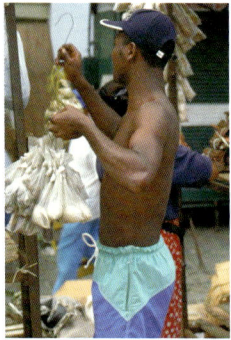

Hanging wares in stall (Brazil)

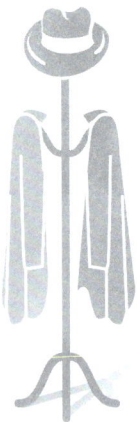

A coat rack provides a useful image to help you maintain a stable torso while relaxing your shoulders and arms.

5 BECOME AWARE OF THE MUSCLES IN YOUR ABDOMEN. ENGAGE THEM STRONGLY SO THAT YOUR ABDOMEN FEELS SLEEKER THAN USUAL

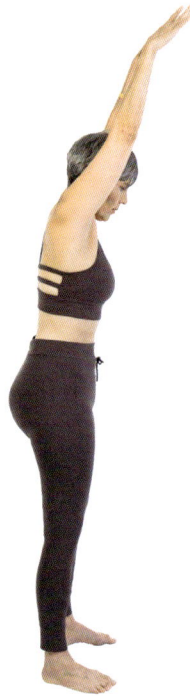

6 RELAX THE REST OF YOUR BODY, INCLUDING YOUR SHOULDERS

The goal is to restore your arms and shoulders to a relaxed position while maintaining all the abdominal support and extra length in the torso that you established in Steps 4 and 5.

It is difficult to isolate the deeper abdominal muscles. You may find, as many beginners do, that when you relax your arms and shoulders, your abdominal muscles relax too. If so, start again and proceed with care. Imagine that you are a coat rack: The spine is the sturdy, tall central support and the shoulder girdle is a coat hanging from it.

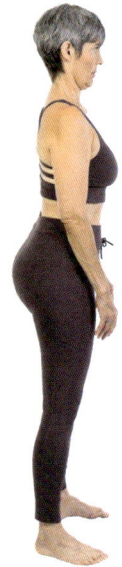

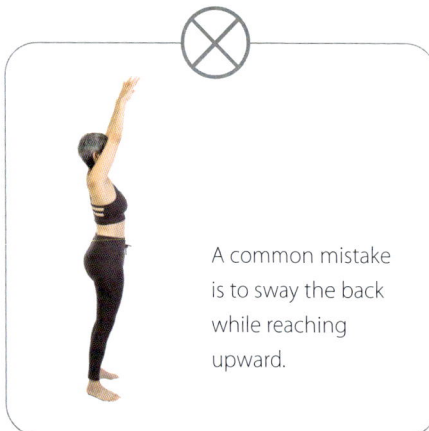

A common mistake is to sway the back while reaching upward.

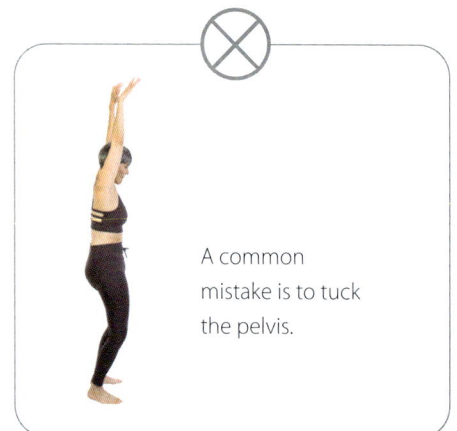

A common mistake is to tuck the pelvis.

120

7 PRACTICE MAINTAINING YOUR INNER CORSET AS YOU MOVE

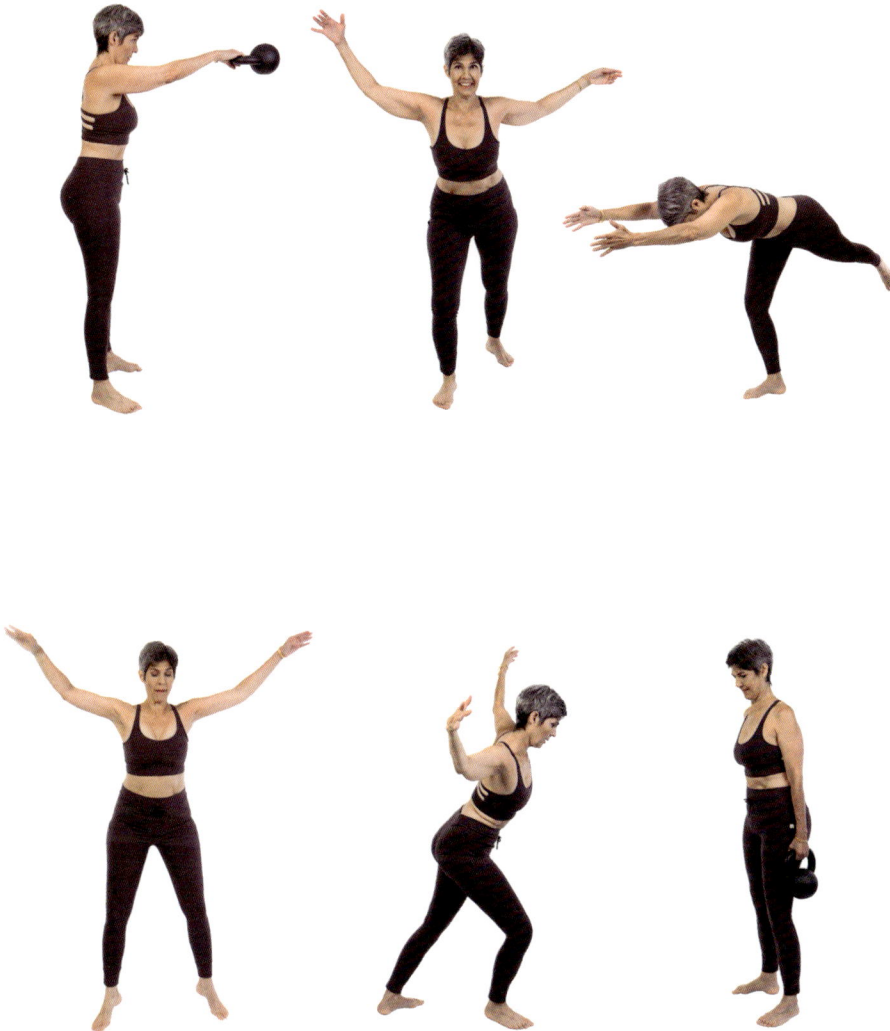

Imagine you are a marionette or doll with a stable torso and freely moving limbs.

You may feel a bit like a marionette; the torso is relatively still and stable, while the limbs are available for movement.

EXAMPLE OF MOVING THE LIMBS WHILE KEEPING THE TORSO TALL AND STABLE

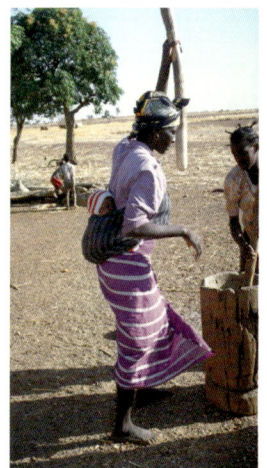

Grinding millet (Burkina Faso)

8 PRACTICE RELAXING AND ENGAGING THE INNER CORSET MUSCLES REPEATEDLY

With time and practice you will no longer need to use your arms to find this action. Your body will learn to do it very quickly when needed.

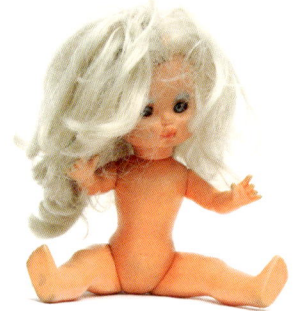

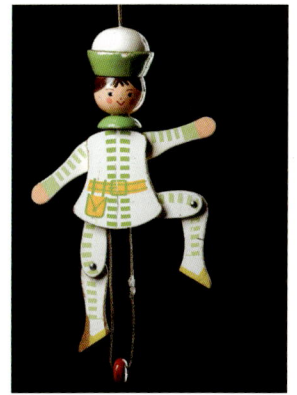

EXAMPLES OF ENGAGING THE INNER CORSET:

EXERCISING

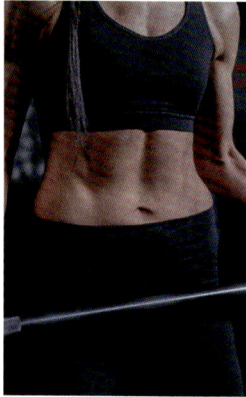

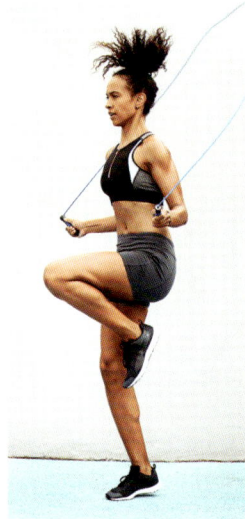

(Portugal)

(Denmark)

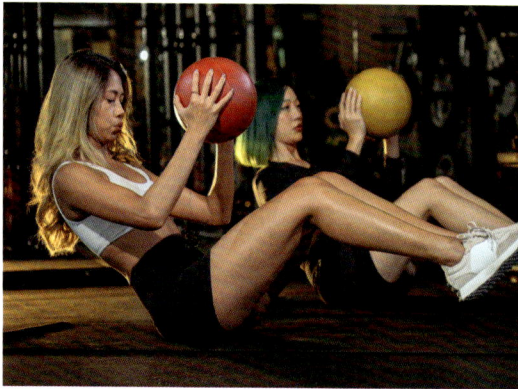

(Thailand)

PERFORMING MANUAL LABOR
(Brazil)

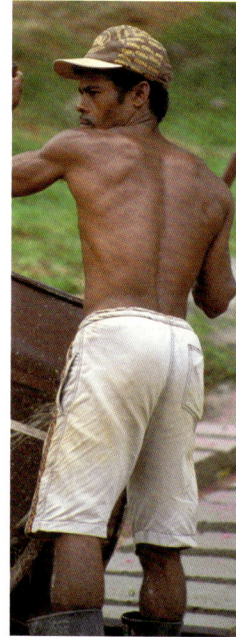

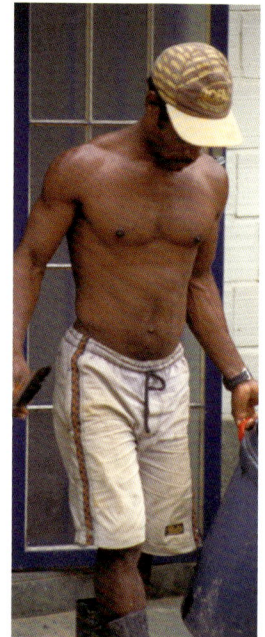

"PLAYING" CAPOEIRA, A CHALLENGING MARTIAL ART
(Brazil)

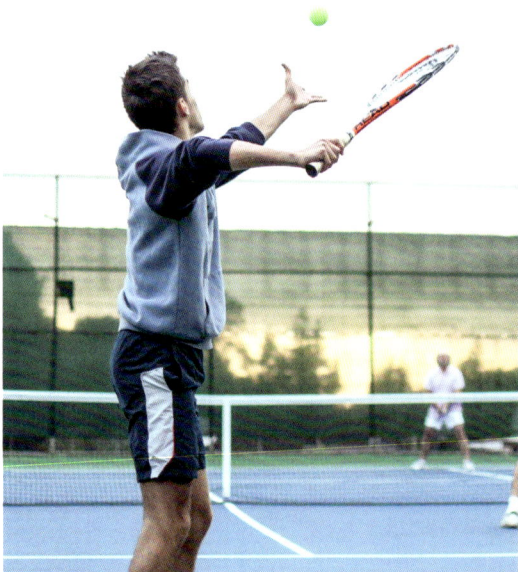

(Germany)

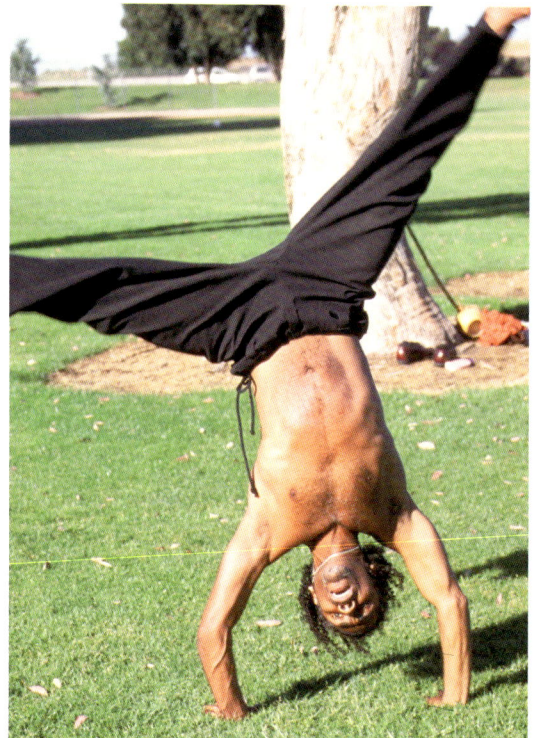

INDICATIONS OF IMPROVEMENT

Using the inner corset can be difficult to learn because your abdominal muscles may not be strong, you may not be used to isolating them, and the long muscles of your back (*erector spinae*) may resist the action due to chronic tightness. With practice, as your inner corset muscles get stronger, and as your long back muscles become more limber, the pattern will be easier to maintain. You will also no longer need any arm action to help engage the inner corset.

Once you start using your abdominal muscles during your daily activities, they become toned very quickly. After some time, you may be able to see their contours on your abdomen even when you are not flexing your muscles (fig.5-9).

fig.5-9

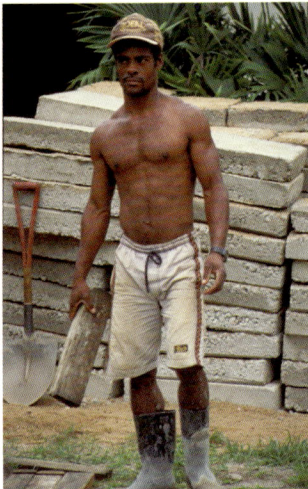

The contours of this worker's abdominal muscles are apparent even when he is relaxed (Brazil).

TROUBLESHOOTING

SWAYING THE LOWER BACK

This is the most common mistake when learning to elongate your torso (see page 120). Keeping your ribs anchored and monitoring your spinal groove with one hand as you start to lengthen your back will help you detect any sway and prevent it from happening. If your abdominal muscles need strengthening, you will find suitable exercises in Appendix 1. I recommend doing those exercises regularly until your abdominal muscles reach a threshold level of strength.

DIFFICULTY BREATHING

If you are accustomed to breathing with your abdomen and not your chest and back, you may find it difficult to breathe while engaging your inner corset. As part of your inner corset, your abdominal muscles are contracted and resist abdominal expansion during inhalation. But your long back muscles (*erector spinae*) may be tight and the muscles between your ribs (*intercostals*) may be stiff from a lack of action in the past, and resist back lengthening and chest expansion during inhalation. You will therefore be hampered in your ability to inhale easily. With rib anchor practice, your long back muscles will relax and lengthen. For your intercostal muscles, force a few deep inhalations to stretch them; this will make your subsequent inhalations easier. Soon you will be able to breathe easily while engaging your inner corset.

FURTHER INFORMATION

WHEN TO USE YOUR INNER CORSET

Although using your inner corset may seem like a contrived action, you automatically use it whenever your spine is subject to extreme stress. For example, when you jump down from a significant height, you instinctively tighten your inner corset to protect your spine (fig.5-10).

fig.5-10

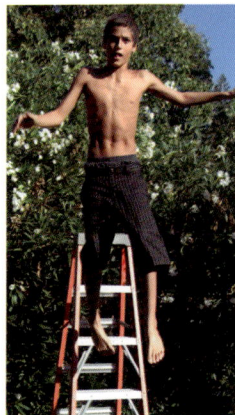

The inner corset muscles automatically contract in high-stress situations like jumping.

In situations of moderate stress, however, such as carrying laundry baskets, weeding, or twisting, most people do not have the instinct to use the same protective mechanism. Failure to do so can lead to cumulative damage of spinal structures—damage that we have come to consider a normal part of aging. By learning to use the inner corset in these situations, you will protect your back from this damage. At the same time, you will be exercising your abdominal muscles. We used to teach that the inner corset is needed only when the spine is subjected to moderate or high-level stress. However, over the years, seeing that people are showing up with less and less abdominal tone, we've changed our guidelines; we now teach to use the inner corset at 10–20% capacity throughout the day. When faced with additional challenge, ramp up the inner corset engagement correspondingly.

REACHING ABOVE YOUR HEAD

A conventional guideline for patients with lower back pain is to avoid reaching above the head, as when reaching for a glass on a high shelf or placing luggage in an overhead compartment. If done carelessly, this is indeed a dangerous maneuver. However, by anchoring the rib cage and engaging the inner corset, you can reach up more safely with the additional benefit of strengthening the abdominal muscles.

PROTECTING YOUR NECK

Just as the inner corset protects the vulnerable lumbar discs, engaging the *longus colli* muscles protects the fragile cervical discs. People in traditional cultures do this when they carry significant weight on their heads. To learn this action, place a soft, light weight, such as a folded towel or Gokhale® Head Cushion, on the crown of your head (fig.6-14 on page 144). A common mistake is to place the weight too far forward on your head, causing the chin to rise and the neck to compress (fig.6-14c). Imagine this weight is heavy and actively push up against it (fig.6-14b). Be moderate in this pushing action and only sustain the push for a few seconds at first.

USING AN EXTERNAL CORSET

Many people assume that corsets are uncomfortable and unhealthy. In fact, some corsets, such as those used in the 18th century, protected and supported the back (fig.5-11). It is true that in Victorian times, some corsets became extreme and unhealthy (fig.5-12). Yet a moderate corset remains a healthy device; weightlifters regularly wear back support belts, as do workers who carry heavy

objects (fig.5-13). The medical profession also prescribes corsets for back pain patients to correct distortions or protect damaged tissues. Simple versions of these are available at medical supply stores and can be useful if you are injured.

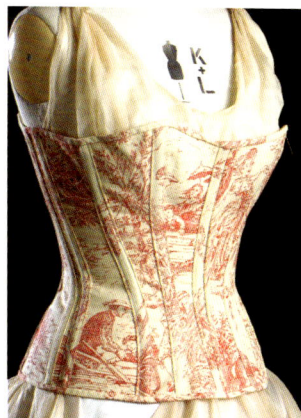

fig.5-11

This early corset is moderate and healthful.

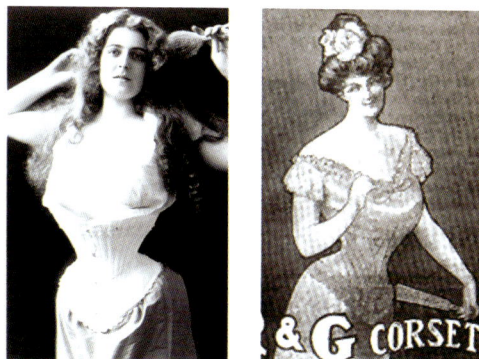

fig.5-12

Some corsets in the Victorian era (19th century) became extreme and compromised health.

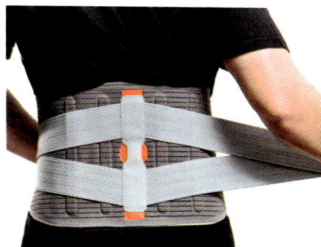

fig.5-13

Modern back belts provide support for performing heavy manual labor or in case of injury.

With inner or external corsets, some people fear loss of flexibility and spinal health. Interestingly, among the Dinkas of South Sudan, young people wear corsets with rigid metal ribbing to show their status (fig.5-14). These corsets are worn day and night for years until the person marries. The only way to remove a Dinka corset is to cut it, which is done only when a larger size is needed. The corsets permit no appreciable flexion, extension, lateral bending, or twist in the spine. The excellent physique of the Dinka is testimony to how little spinal movement is truly needed to preserve good musculoskeletal health.

Note that the Dinka corset stops at the level of the L5-S1 disc. It is interesting to contrast the Dinka corset with some of the more extensive modern medical corsets and devices. In my experience, most people, if they need a corset at all, do best with a corset that leaves the pelvis free to settle in an anteverted position. Unfortunately, many of the available medical devices, such as the TLSO body cast (fig.5-15), not only restrict movement of the pelvis, but fix it in a retroverted position. The TLSO has failed to demonstrate any substantial positive outcome in preventing surgery.

fig.5-14

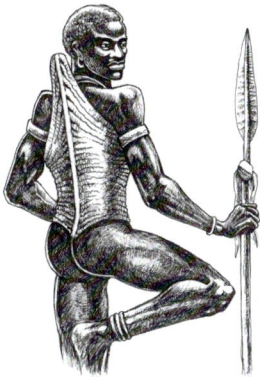

A Dinka corset from Sudan. These are worn day and night for years. Note that the L5-S1 area is allowed to assume its normal curvature.

An interesting case study from my teaching involves K, who became my student at age 13. She suffered from *kyphoscoliosis*, a condition in which her spine had excessive curves, both side-to-side and front-to-back. Her father, a physician, had been proactive in arranging care for his daughter. However, after seven months of physical therapy and two custom TLSO body casts supposed to be worn 20 hours a day for two years proved unsuccessful, doctors recommended surgery. The family was not keen on this route. I taught K how to sit, lie, stand, bend, and walk in the ways described in this book. Reestablishing pelvic anteversion and learning to hip-hinge were particularly important elements in her training.

The immediate feedback in comfort and improved appearance motivated her strongly. Within two months, her outlook was radically different (fig.5-16). There was no further talk of surgery or body casts. Now a grown woman, K is thriving and has given me a standing offer to be a spokesperson for the Gokhale Method.

fig.5-15

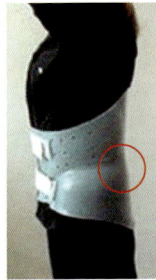

An example of a TLSO, a body cast used for children with scoliosis. Notice the flattening effect on the L5-S1 area.

fig.5-16

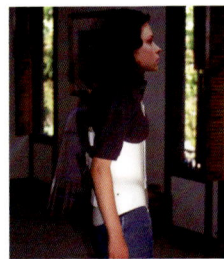

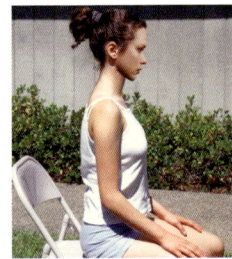

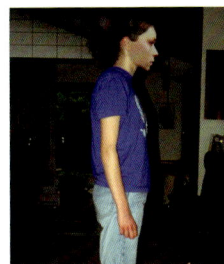

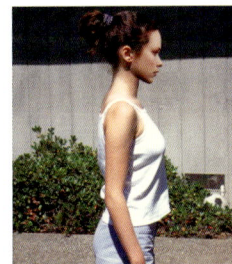

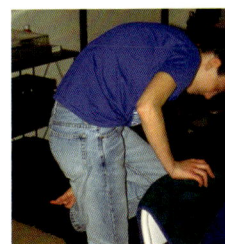

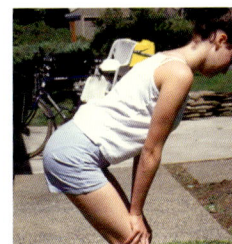

K (age 13 and disguised) with TLSO body cast not producing satisfactory results.

K after three months of training with much-improved appearance and outlook (note the slight sway in the second photograph that she subsequently corrected).

ADDRESSING SCOLIOSIS

If scoliosis persists into adulthood, the effects of gravity and increasing strain and muscle fatigue can cause the curvature to become more pronounced over time. The Gokhale Method teaches how to elongate and straighten the spine in both passive positions (see Chapters 1, 2, and 4) and actively, using the inner corset. This elongation can lessen the severity of scoliotic curvature (fig.5-17) and prevent it from becoming more exaggerated over time.

fig.5-17

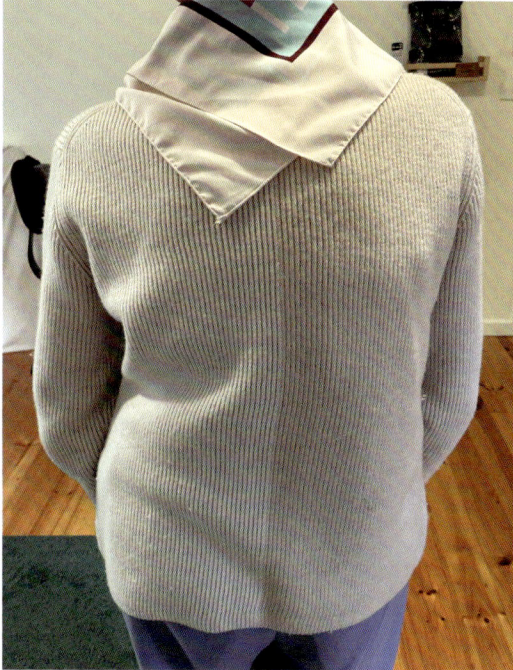

a. Without inner corset

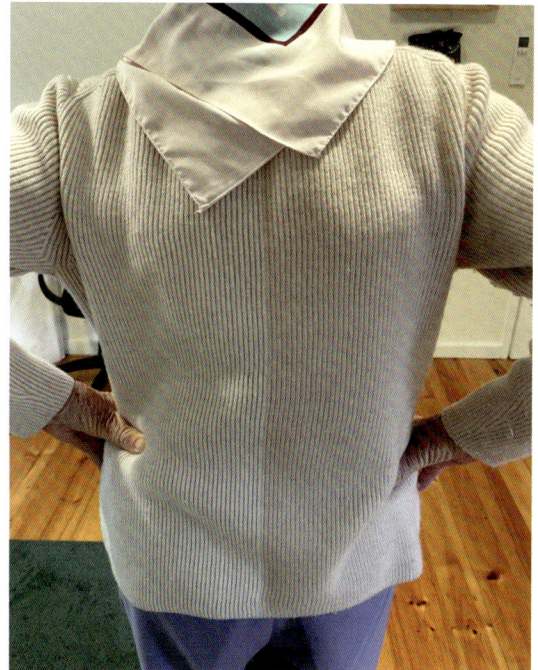

b. With inner corset

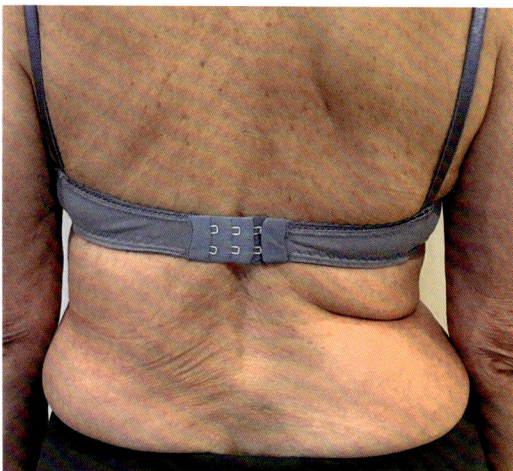

c. Without inner corset

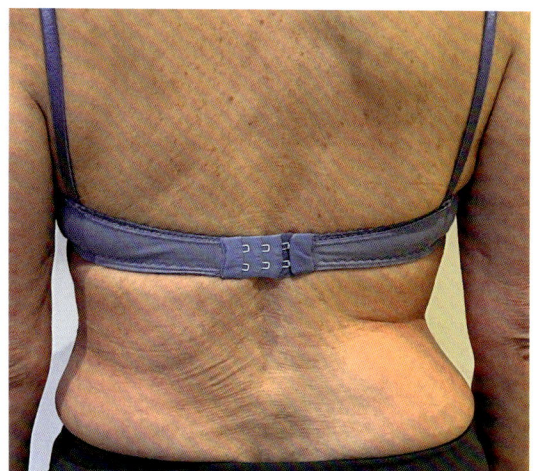

d. With inner corset

Engaging the inner corset muscles can have an instantaneous and profound effect on scoliotic curvature.

RECAP

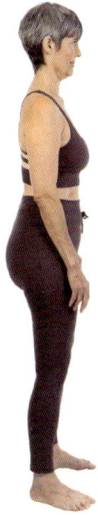

a. **Start with soft knees and bean-shaped feet**

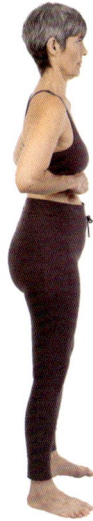

b. **Anchor ribs**

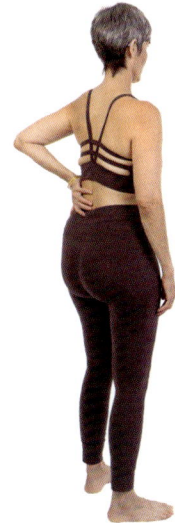

c. **Monitor spinal groove while…**

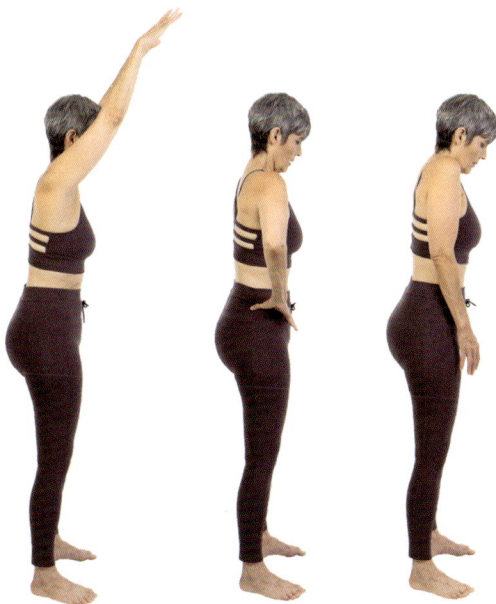

d. **…lengthening torso by:**
- reaching up or
- pushing against the pelvic rim or
- imagining entering cold water

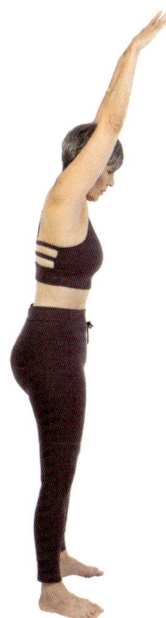

e. **Engage inner corset muscles**

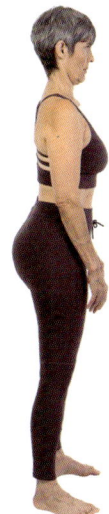

f. **Relax unnecessary tension in rest of body**

6
TALLSTANDING

Stacking your bones

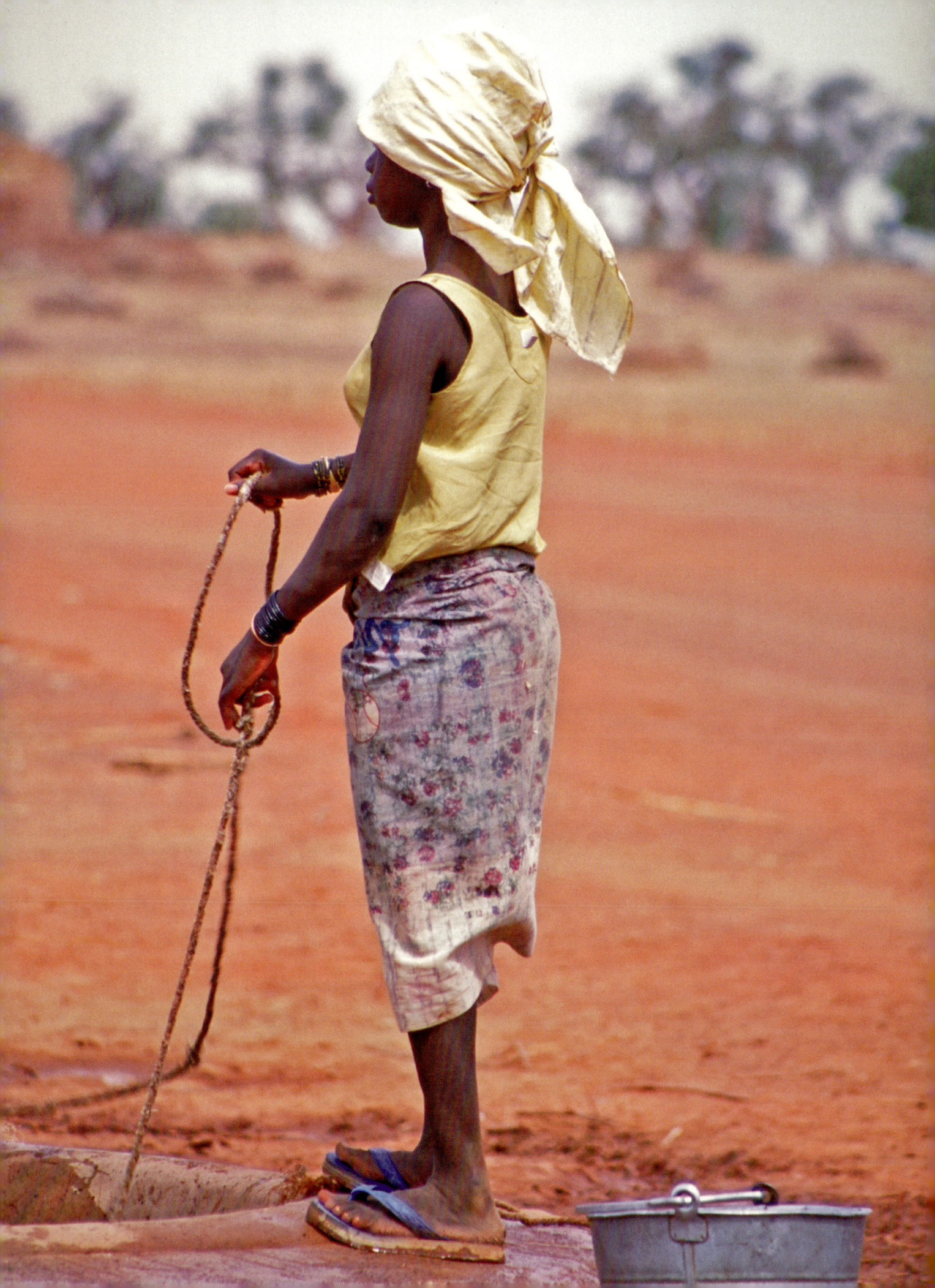

Many people are uncomfortable standing for long periods of time. If they go to a museum, their backs hurt; if they go to a party, their feet hurt. Yet many others stand comfortably all day to earn their living. A few, like the Inuit seal hunters, stand without moving at all for long periods.

By learning how to tallstand, you will be able to stand for long periods without feeling fidgety or uncomfortable. Just as with healthy sitting, healthy standing requires an anteverted pelvis and stacked vertebrae. The hips align over the heels, which carry most of the body weight, and the knees and groin area remain soft (fig.6-1). The position facilitates healthy blood flow to and from the legs. Standing becomes a comfortable, even restful, position.

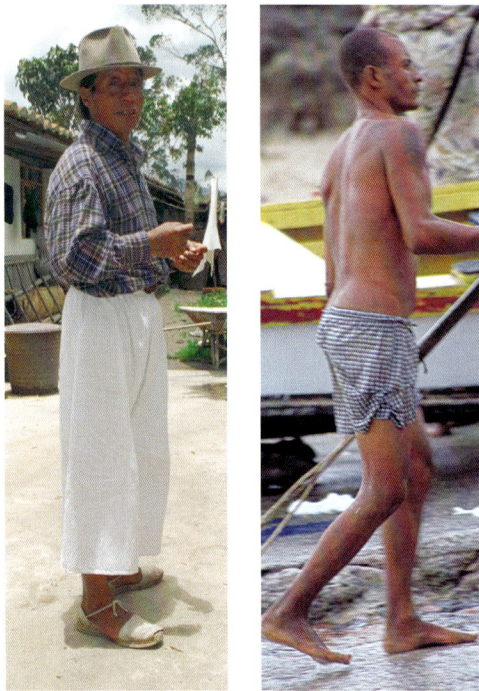
fig.6-1

(Ecuador)   (Brazil)

Healthy erect posture involves an anteverted pelvis and well-stacked vertebrae and leg bones.

People who stand poorly often tuck their pelvis and park their hips forward, impinging the femoral artery and vein, and reducing blood flow to and from the legs (fig.6-2). Reduced blood flow slows the repair of any leg injuries and contributes to such problems as cold feet, Raynaud's syndrome, and varicose veins.

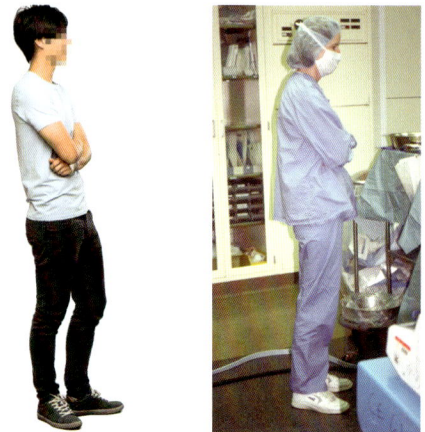
fig.6-2

Poor standing often involves a tucked pelvis that is thrust forward, impinging the femoral arteries, veins, and nerves.

Thrusting the hips forward is usually accompanied by excessive curvature in the spine, which strains the vertebrae, and places inappropriate stresses on the hip joints (fig.6-3). It displaces the weight forward onto the delicate joints in the front of the foot, distorting the foot from its natural arched shape, and contributing to problems like bunions, plantar fasciitis, and arthritis of the foot (fig.6-4). The stance also creates a tendency to lock the knees, which strains the knee ligaments and predisposes people to arthritis of the knee (fig.6-5).

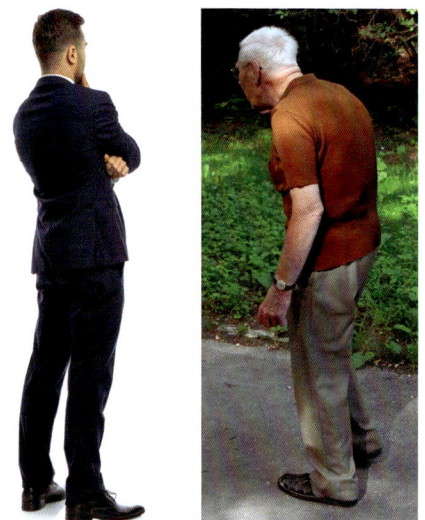
fig.6-3

A tucked pelvis often results in excessive curvature throughout the spine.

fig.6-4

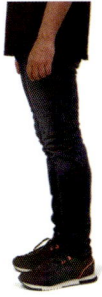

A pelvis thrust forward displaces body weight forward, putting excessive pressure on the delicate structures in the front of the foot.

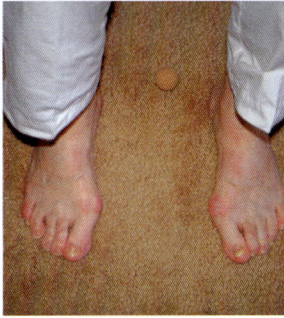

Excessive pressure on the front of the foot may result in bunions and other pathologies.

fig.6-5

Standing with locked knees predisposes people to knee problems.

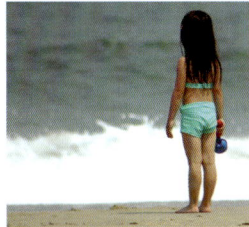

Another common pattern of standing incorrectly is to sway the lower back in an effort to "stand up straight" (fig.6-6). This strains the lower back muscles and over time causes them to adapt to having a shorter baseline length. Strained lower back muscles cause compression in the lower back (*lumbar*) discs and poor circulation in the lower back in general.

fig.6-6

The directive to "stand up straight" often results in a swayed lower back.

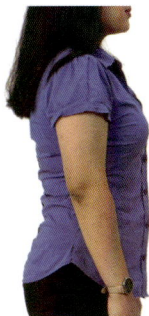

The secret to standing comfortably is a healthy vertical stacking of the body's weight-bearing bones coupled with healthy foot and leg alignment (fig.6-7, fig.6-8). Stacking provides a necessary and healthy stress for the bones, helping to prevent osteoporosis. Stacking also allows the muscles around the joints to relax. The bones get the stress they need, and the muscles are relieved of stress they *don't* need. Because the muscles can relax, they allow good blood circulation.

fig.6-7

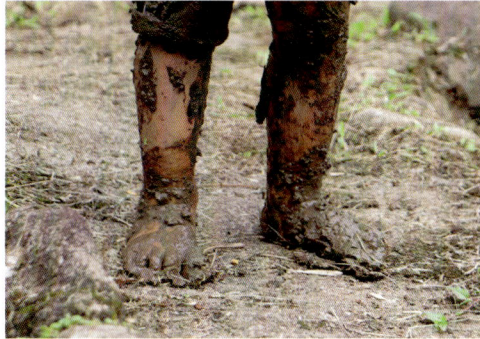

Healthy foot and leg alignment is an important part of healthy standing.

BENEFITS

- Prevents wear and tear on the feet, knees, and hips

- Reduces back pain from tight back muscles or compressed discs

- Enables standing for long periods without fatigue, pain, or damage

- Introduces healthy stress to the weight-bearing bones and helps prevent osteoporosis

- Improves blood circulation in the legs and feet

I was waiting in the checkout line... and almost automatically my body went into a tallstanding posture. I went from wondering how long it was going to take me to get through the line, to being content in the present.

Ted Gulick, Atlanta, GA

131

fig.6-8

PELVIS ANTEVERTED   LOWER BACK STRAIGHT

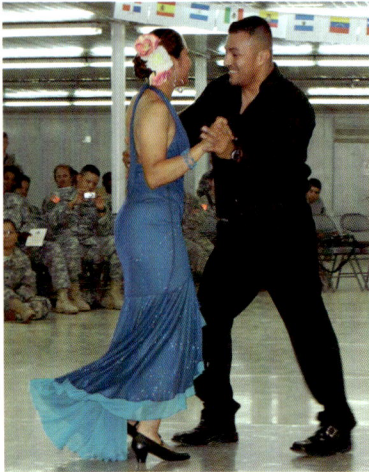

(USA)

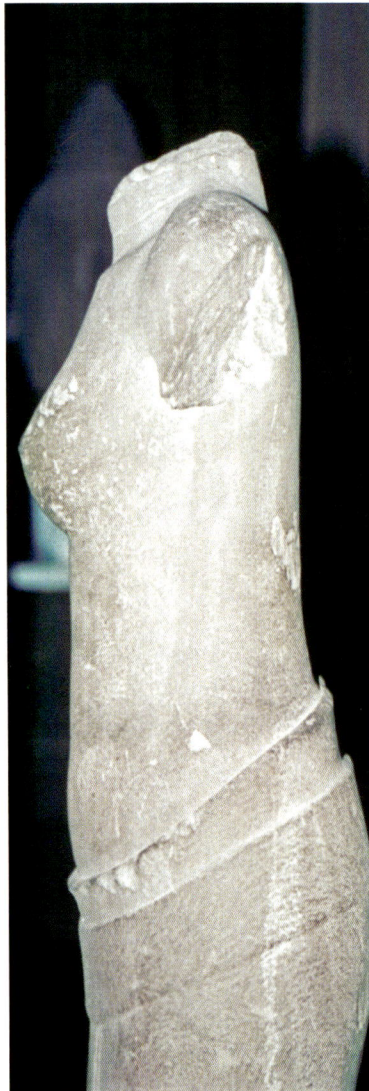

(Brazil)

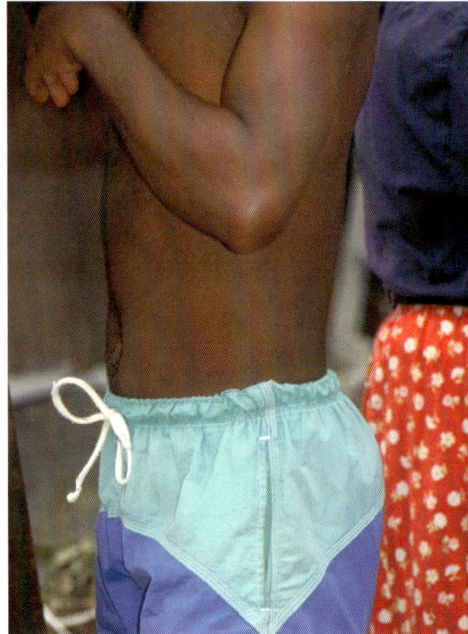

(Brazil)

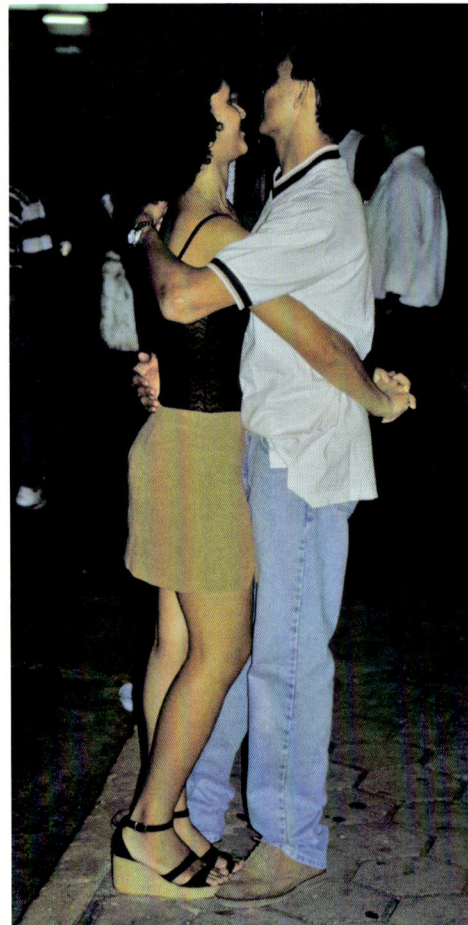

(USA)

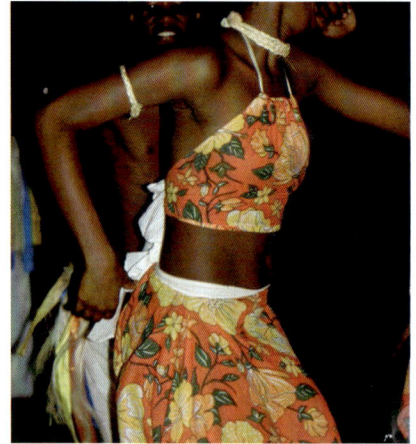

(Cambodia)

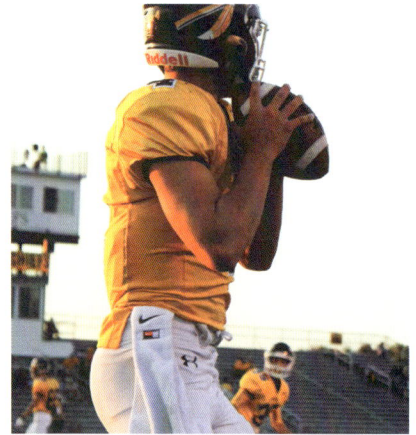

(Brazil)

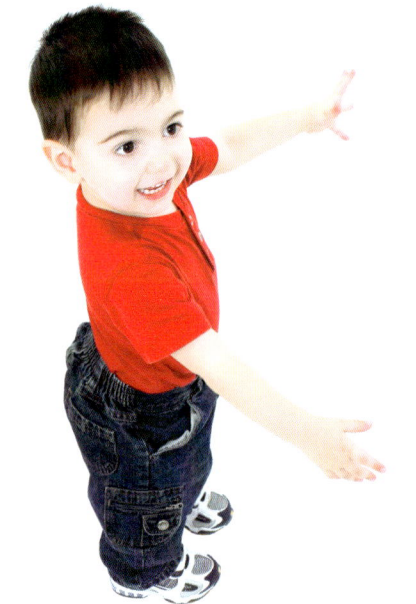

(USA)

fig.6-8 (continued)

UNIFORM DEPTH OF SPINAL GROOVE

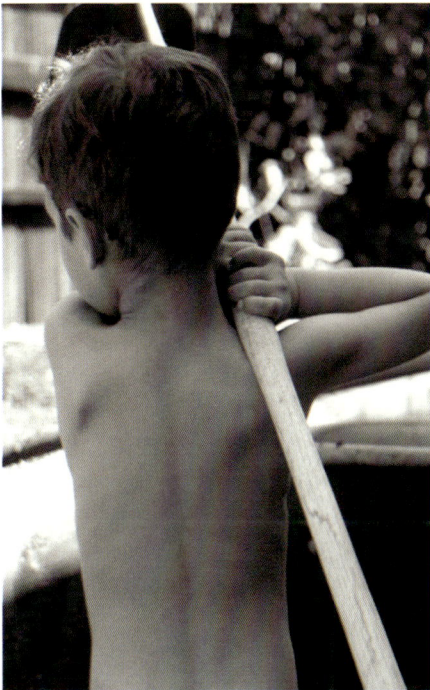

(USA)

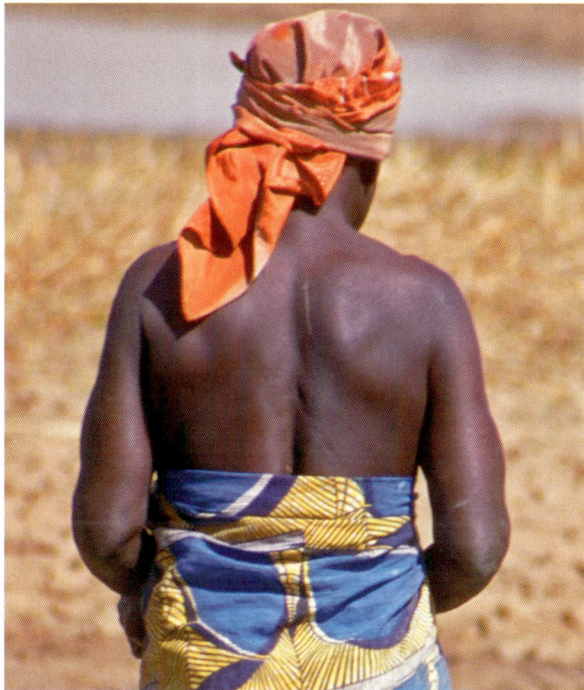

(Burkina Faso)

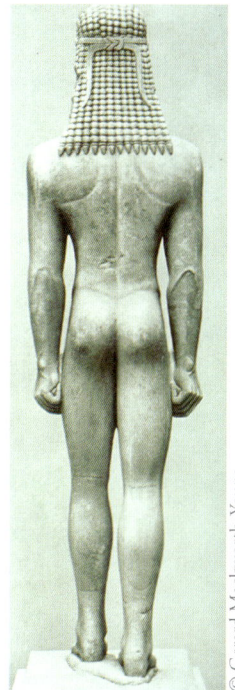

© Gerard Mackworth-Young

(Greece)

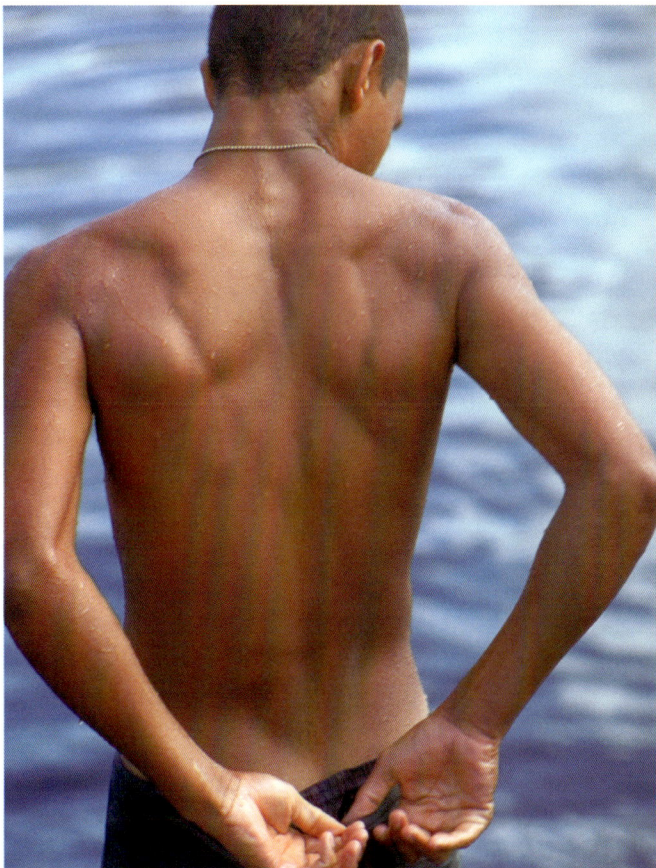

(Brazil)

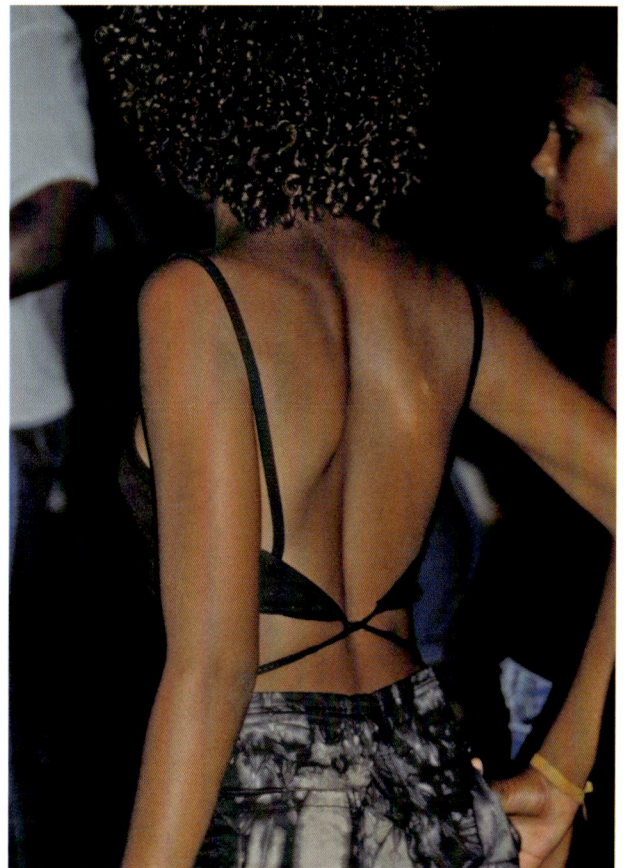

(Brazil)

EQUIPMENT

You will need a full-length mirror or device with a camera.

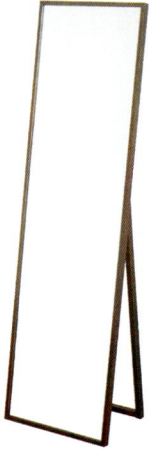

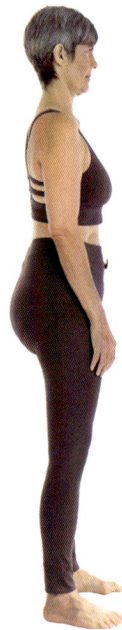

1 STAND IN PROFILE TO A FULL-LENGTH MIRROR OR DEVICE WITH A CAMERA WITH YOUR FEET HIP-WIDTH APART

Because your feet are your foundation when you stand, it is important that they be arranged well. You will kidney bean "shape" them in the next few steps.

KIDNEY BEAN-SHAPED FEET

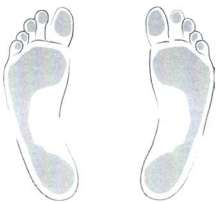

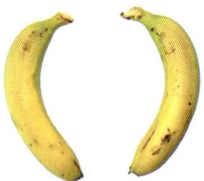

2 RELEASE THE WEIGHT ON YOUR LEFT FOOT AND RAISE THE HEEL SLIGHTLY

Leave your foot muscles relaxed as you do this.

Kidney bean-shaped feet are the foundation of comfortable standing. They are defined by pronounced arches and curvature from the big toe to the heel.

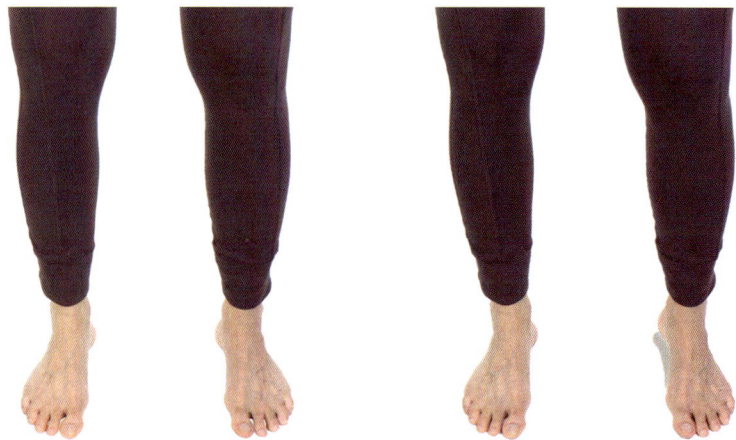

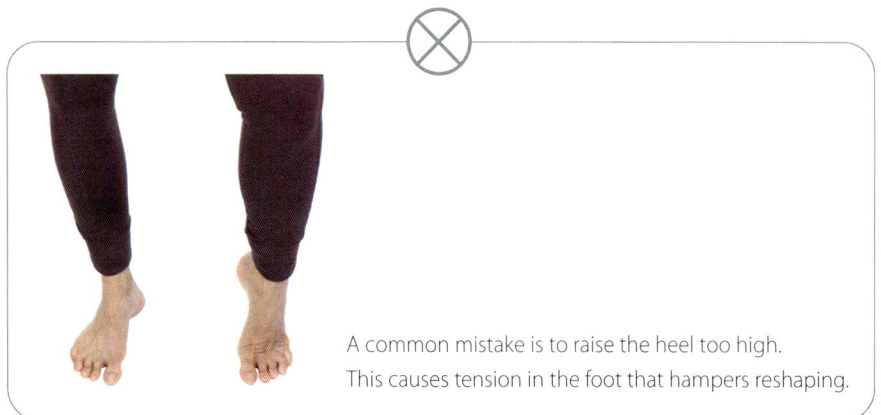

A common mistake is to raise the heel too high. This causes tension in the foot that hampers reshaping.

3 WITH YOUR TOES AND BALL OF THE FOOT FIXED IN PLACE ON THE FLOOR, PIVOT THE HEEL INWARD BEFORE PLANTING IT FIRMLY ON THE FLOOR

Note that this action emphasizes the inner arch of your foot, creating a "kidney bean" shape. Also note that your legs will turn outwards ("externally rotate") in this step. In fact, focusing on externally rotating your knees can help you create a kidney bean shape in your foot.

EXAMPLES OF KIDNEY BEAN-SHAPED FEET

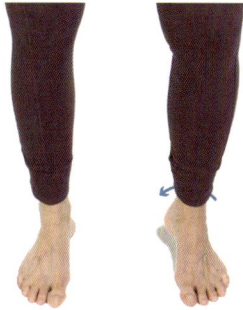

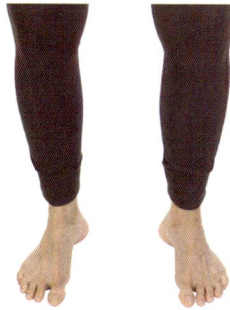

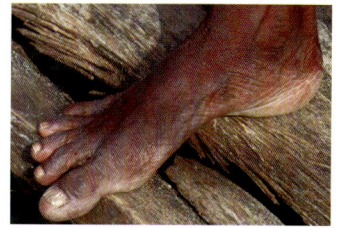

(India)

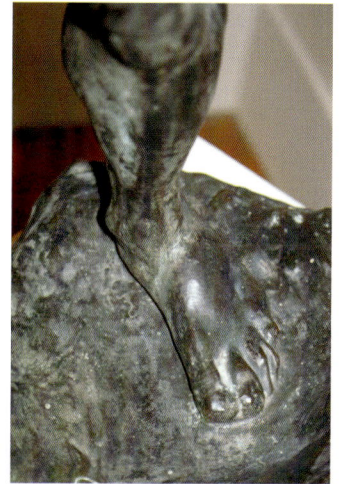

(France)

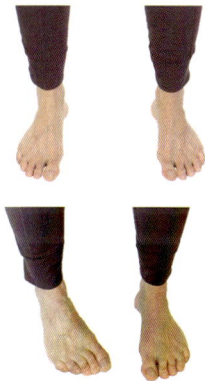

A common mistake is to pivot the front of the foot inward rather than the heel. This easily results in a "pigeon-toed" stance.

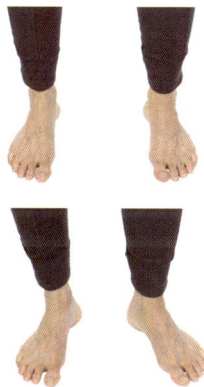

Another common mistake is to let the ball of the foot pivot outward as the heel moves inward. This simply increases the outward angle of the foot rather than changing its shape.

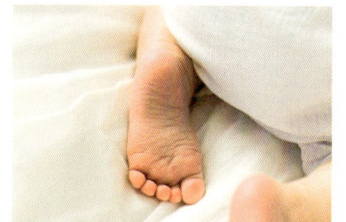

(USA)

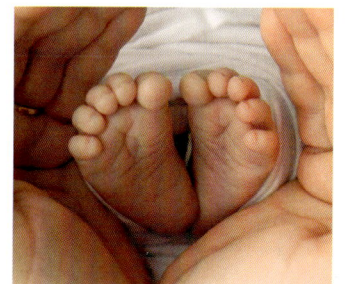

(Georgia)

Kidney bean-shaped feet are a function of strong tibialis anterior muscles (See Appendix 1 for exercises to strengthen this muscle).

4 IF NECESSARY, USE YOUR HANDS TO GUIDE THE MOVEMENT

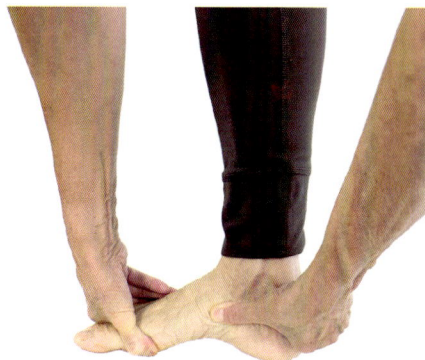

Steady the front of the foot with one hand. Grasp the heel with the other hand, lift the heel from the floor, and firmly guide it inward.

EXAMPLES OF HEALTHY FOOT STRUCTURE FROM AROUND THE WORLD

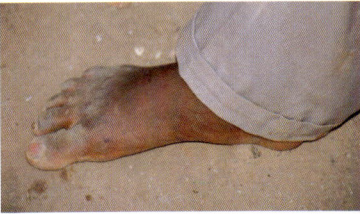

(Burkina Faso)

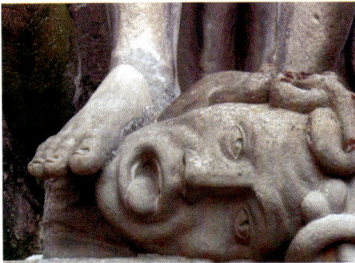

(Germany)

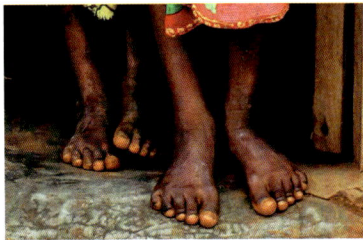

(Nigeria)

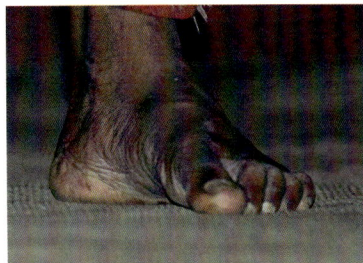

(Kathakali dancer, South India)

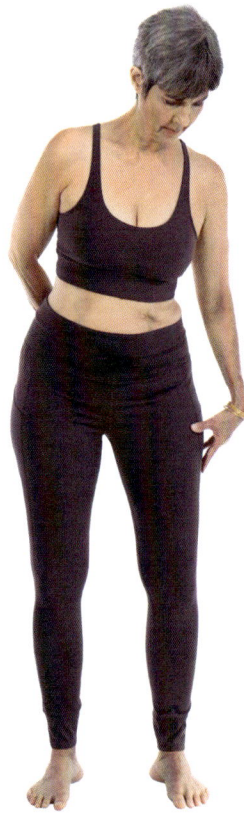

5 CHECK THAT YOUR LEFT FOOT IS NOW POINTING 10–15° OUTWARD AND YOUR WEIGHT IS EVENLY DISTRIBUTED BETWEEN THE INSIDE AND OUTSIDE OF THE FOOT.

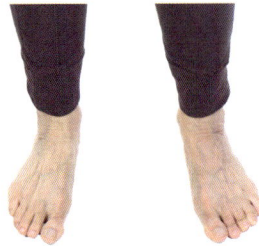

A common mistake is to *pronate* the foot. If you cannot prevent this, use an insole (see page 146).

Another common mistake is to place excessive weight on the outside of the foot. This can be corrected by adjusting the alignment of your ankle.

6 REPEAT STEPS 2 THROUGH 5 WITH THE RIGHT FOOT

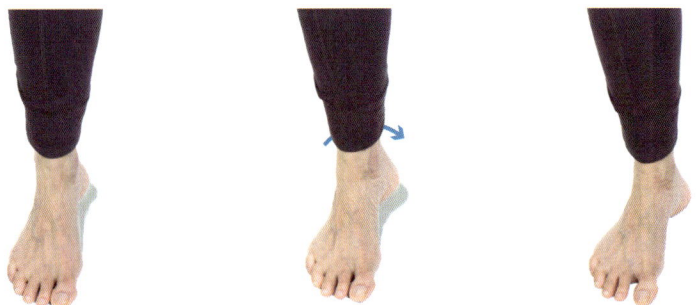

7 CHECK THAT YOUR KNEES AND LEGS ARE ROTATED 10–15° OUTWARDS

Bend your knees a little and check that your knees and feet are aligned. Imagine that a line runs outward from your heel through the second or third toe. Your knee should point along this line.

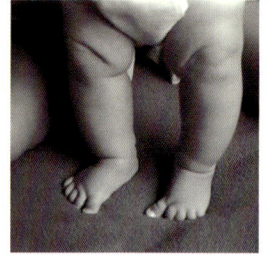

(USA)

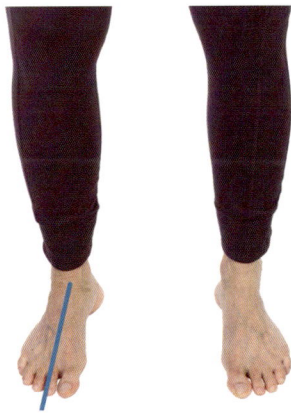

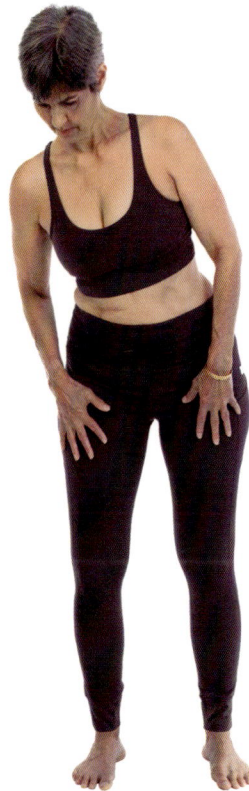

You may have to shift your head over your knee to get a straight-down, centralized, aerial view of the alignment.

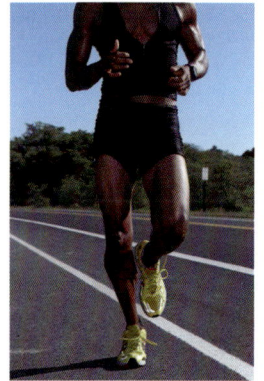

(USA)

If necessary, "wrap" your leg muscles to rotate your legs outward

This action involves your gluteal and leg muscles (see sidebar).

EXTERNAL LEG ROTATION

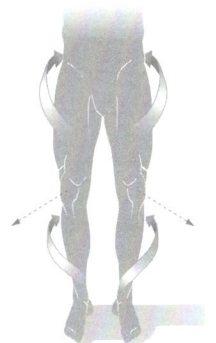

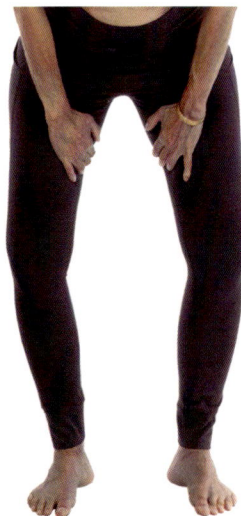

"Wrapping" your leg muscles outward externally rotates the entire leg, resulting in healthy alignment of the hip, knee, and ankle joints, and recreation of the inner arch of the foot. Two key muscles involved in this action are tibialis anterior (on the shin) and gluteus medius (see Appendix 1 for strengthening exercises).

137

HEALTHY STANDING
POSTURE FROM
AROUND THE WORLD

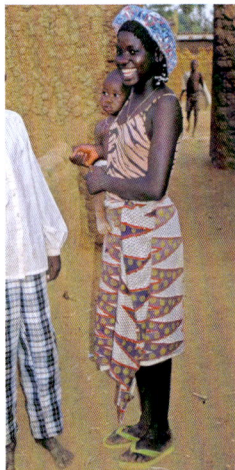

(Burkina Faso)

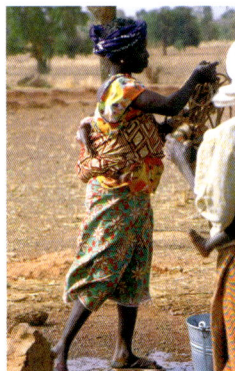

(Burkina Faso)

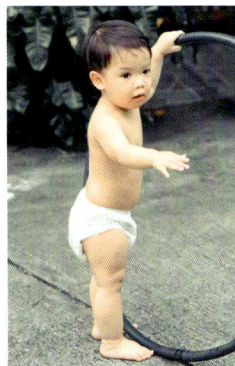

(Thailand)

8 REARRANGE YOUR WEIGHT TO FALL OVER YOUR HEELS

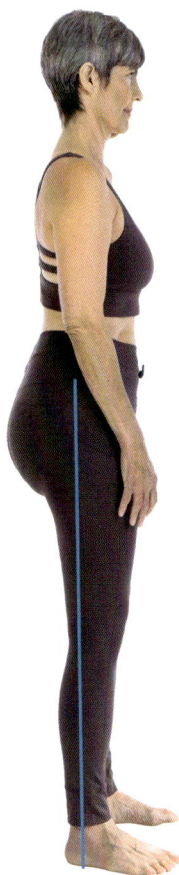

Stand in profile to a full-length mirror. Imagine a plumb line dropping from your hip joint to your feet. The plumb bob should fall close to the heel. If it does not, shift your hips back. Simultaneously bring your torso forward (bend at the hip, not the waist) so as not to topple backwards.

⊗

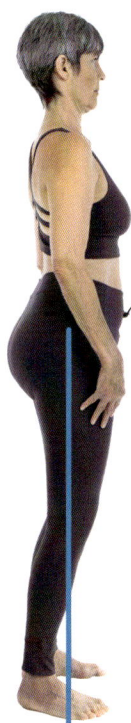

A common mistake is to place a significant amount of your weight on the front of the feet. In this case, the plumb bob would fall in front of your heel.

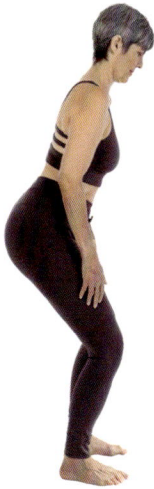

9 SOFTEN THE KNEES AND GROIN AREA AND ANTEVERT THE PELVIS

Bend equally at the knees and hip joints in a zigzag fashion. Note that your torso is now parallel to your lower legs, and your pelvis "nests" between your legs. This action allows gravity to passively antevert the pelvis (i.e., without back muscle tension).

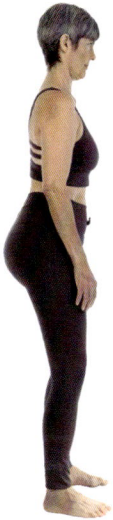

Leaving the weight on your heels, slowly straighten your torso and legs, but stop just short of locking the knees or the groin. Your behind will now be behind you. Resist any urge to use muscle tension to stick it backward or to hold it in place; let it relax into its new position.

For several days, you may feel as though you are leaning forward; a glance in the mirror will reassure you.

10 CHECK THE GROIN CREASE FOR SOFTNESS

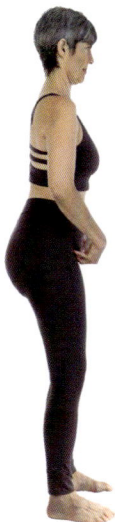

Place your fingers where the top of the legs hinge at the hip. You would like to feel some "give" in the soft tissue before reaching bone.

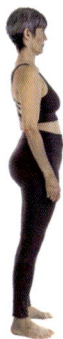

⊗ Common mistakes include letting your weight return to the front of your feet and locking your knees or groin crease as you straighten up. Perform Step 9 again slowly.

HEALTHY STANDING POSTURE FROM AROUND THE WORLD

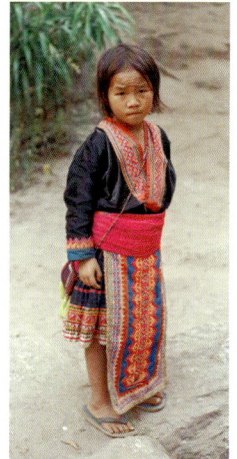

(Thailand)

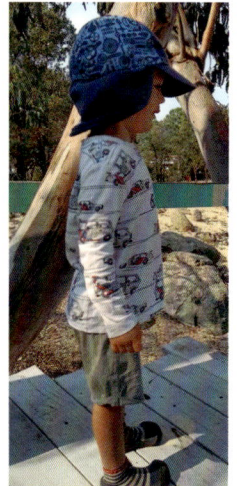

(Australia)

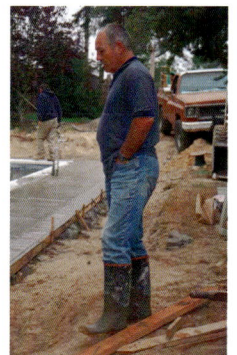

(USA)

139

ROTATING THE RIB CAGE FORWARD

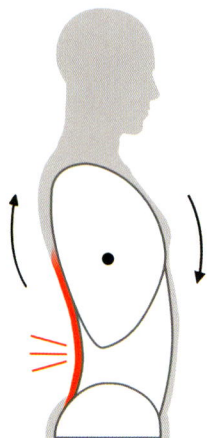

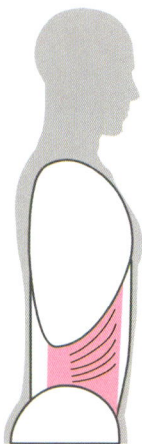

The rib anchor technique involves pivoting around an axis running from side to side roughly through the middle of the rib cage.

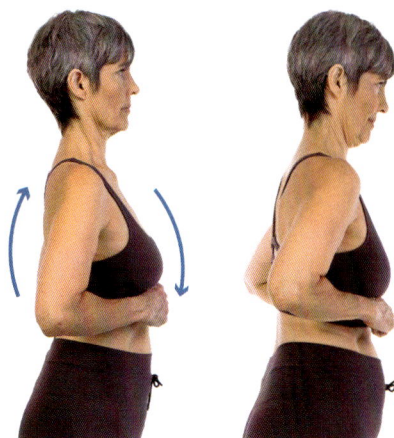

11 PERFORM THE RIB ANCHOR

Rotate your rib cage forward. The front of the rib cage will move downward; the back will move upward. Note that the bottom of the rib cage in the front becomes flush with the contour of the abdomen, rather than flaring.

For now, you will "anchor" the rib cage in this new position via contraction of the *abdominal oblique* muscles; as these muscles gain tone and your lower back muscles gain length, you will find your rib cage will better default to this position.

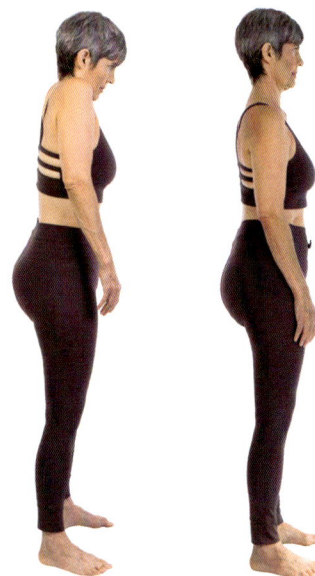

RIB ANCHOR
VIDEO

12 RELAX THE MUSCLES IN YOUR LOWER BACK

To check that your lower back muscles are relaxed, breathe deeply. If your lower back is relaxed, you can feel it lengthen upwards and/or expand gently outwards as you inhale.

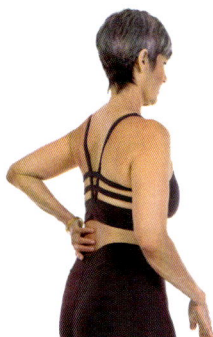

Use your fingertips to check for uniform depth of the midline groove along the lumbar spine.

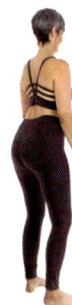

A common mistake is sticking your bottom back in an attempt to achieve anteversion. This results in an unhealthy sway and tight back muscles. Repeat Step 9, which uses gravity to achieve true anteversion.

13 PERFORM A SLOW SHOULDER ROLL WITH EACH SHOULDER, SETTLING IT IN ITS DOWN-AND-BACK POSITION

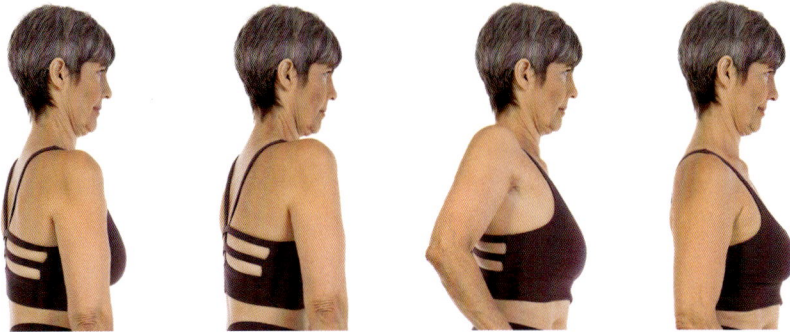

Keep your rib anchor engaged. Be sure you don't unwittingly tighten and sway your lower back as you roll and settle your shoulders.

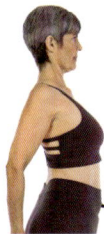

A common mistake is to sway the back when doing a shoulder roll.

14 LENGTHEN YOUR NECK; CHECK FOR AND RELEASE ANY TENSION

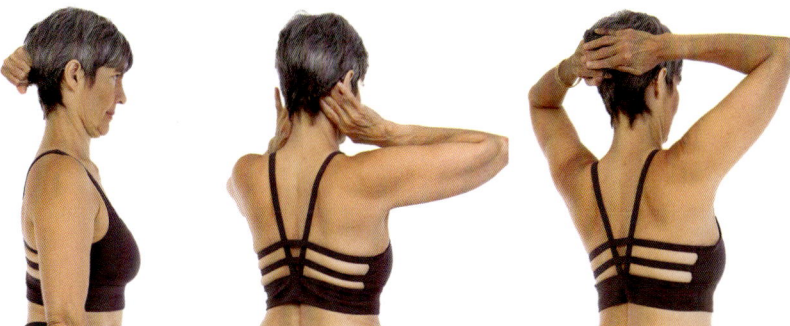

Your head should settle into its natural position with the chin angled slightly downward.

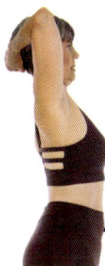

A common mistake is to sway the lower back while lengthening the neck.

EXAMPLES OF POSTERIOR SHOULDERS IN TALLSTANDING

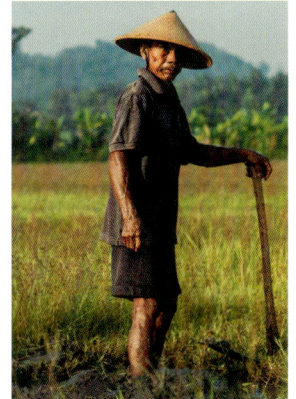

(Indonesia)

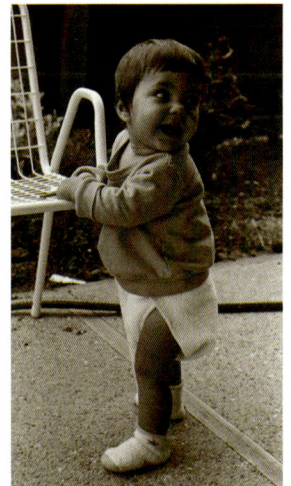

(USA)

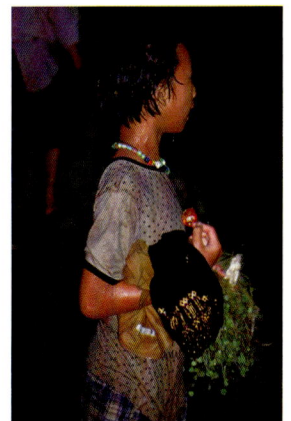

(Thailand)

141

INDICATIONS OF IMPROVEMENT

If you are used to standing with your hips thrust forward, your groin and knees locked, and your torso leaning backwards to maintain balance, you may feel like a chimpanzee in this new stance. Stand sideways to a mirror and look at your profile, especially from the shoulders down. This will reassure you that you are in fact vertically aligned. Give your brain time and repetition to reset; soon the awkwardness will fade.

As you alter your stance, you will notice these specific changes in your feet (fig.6-9):
- Each foot maintains a kidney bean shape and has strong musculature.
- Each foot has well-developed inner, outer, and transverse arches.
- At rest, your feet naturally angle outward 10°–15°.

fig.6-9

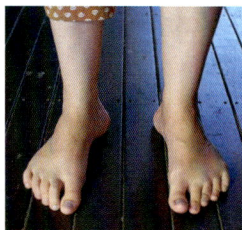

(Australia)

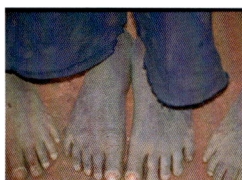

(Burkina Faso)

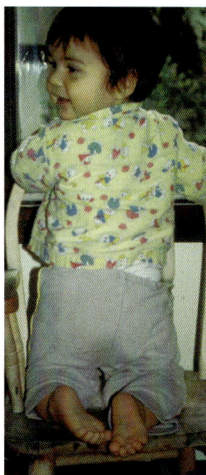

(USA)

As you change your stance, you will notice the following features in your feet: kidney bean shape, pronounced arches, and a 10º–15º outward angle on the floor.

TROUBLESHOOTING

FEELING THAT YOU ARE LEANING FORWARD
Many people are used to standing with their hips parked forward and their spines arched backward to compensate. Tallstanding can thus feel significantly, and sometimes absurdly, leaned forward. If this is your case, a glance in the mirror will reassure you that from the shoulders to the feet, you are quite upright. It may be that your head is somewhat forward of your torso due to rigidity in the upper thoracic area. This is something that will rectify with time, but needs a little patience.

UNABLE TO CONTRACT THE FOOT ARCH MUSCLES
If you have difficulty attaining a kidney bean shape in your feet, even when you use your hands, you may need someone's help (fig.6-10). You will soon be able to do it on your own. If you have considerable rigidity in your feet and ankles, consider using massage to help increase flexibility.

If it is comfortable for you to rest a foot across your other knee, self-massage and reshaping your foot can be an easy activity while watching TV or listening to a podcast.

fig.6-10

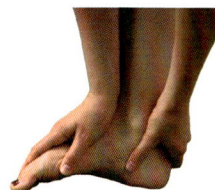

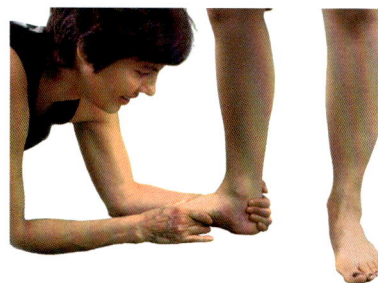

If it is difficult to make your feet kidney bean shaped, use your hands, or get help from someone else.

When learning this action, many people experience tension around the toes. Be patient; with time, you will isolate your arch muscles better, releasing the tension in your toes.

UNEVEN DISTRIBUTION OF WEIGHT
If you find your weight is concentrated over the inside or outside of your foot, rather than evenly distributed, roll your ankle slightly outward or inward, respectively. If you cannot prevent your foot from pronating (ankle rolling excessively inward), use an insole (see page 146).

DIFFICULTY SHIFTING WEIGHT ONTO HEELS

Here is a simple way to shift your weight onto your heels: Very slowly bend forward and then backward at the groin (fig.6-11). Try to use a minimum of muscular effort. Gradually decrease the amplitude of your forward and backward bends until you settle at a balance point. You will discover that your weight is now mainly on your heels.

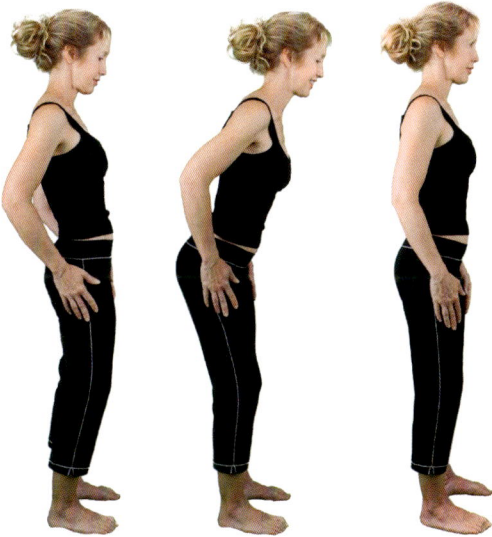

fig.6-11

Shifting the hips forward and back helps locate a balance point.

If you still find it challenging to shift your weight to your heels, try placing a small ball (about 1/2 inch or 1 cm in diameter) under the transverse arch of each foot (fig.6-12). These will help you identify where your weight falls. If you carry your weight forward over the arches of your feet, the balls will feel very uncomfortable.

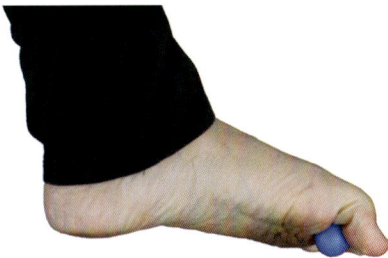

fig.6-12

Placing a small superball under the transverse arch of each foot (behind the toes) can help train you to leave your weight on your heels. This can also help strengthen your foot arch muscles.

PROBLEMS ALIGNING THE SHOULDERS

Sometimes it is helpful to use an aid for shoulder alignment. Have a friend gently tie your upper arms behind you. Use a long piece of cloth or small sheet and fold it several times to make a thick band. Then run it under your arms and tie the ends so that the shoulder blades are drawn close together behind you (fig.6-13). Make sure you are comfortable, that your circulation is not compromised, and that you are not allowing your ribs to jut out in the front. This puts your shoulders in better alignment than you can achieve on your own, and gives you one less body part to monitor.

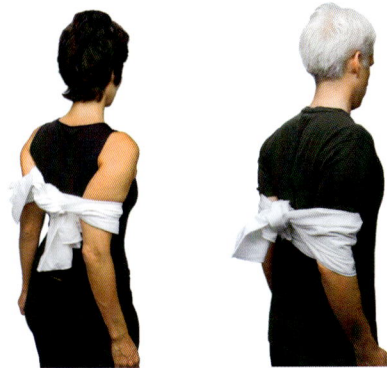

fig.6-13

Having your arms tied behind your back can help you experience good shoulder alignment without strain.

DIFFICULTY SENSING YOUR VERTICAL AXIS

You may be unsure whether you have successfully learned to tallstand. If you want to sense your new vertical axis, place a light weight, such as a folded hand towel or Gokhale Head Cushion, on the crown of your head (fig.6-14). This will help you find a good alignment and make you aware of any habitual or excessive movements that pull you out of alignment.

To move even closer to your ideal vertical axis, you can push upward and engage the *longus colli* muscles (just in front of your cervical spine) (fig.6-14b). People who carry significant weight on their heads use this action to protect their spines (fig.6-15). You can also use this technique when learning to sit well and walk well (see Chapters 3 and 8, respectively). Note that until your neck is well-aligned and your neck muscles strong, you should not try to place a heavy weight on your head.

fig.6-14

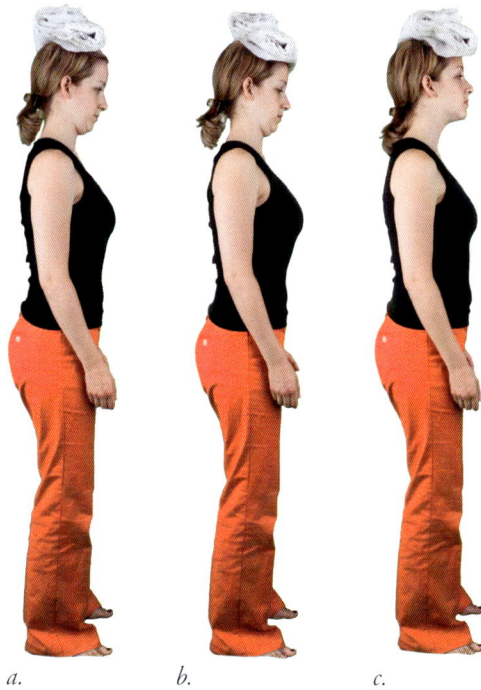

a.   b.   c.

a) Placing a light weight (that will not hurt you if it falls) on the crown of your head can help you locate your vertical axis. b) Push up against the weight to engage your longus colli muscles. c) A common mistake is to carry the weight too far forward on your head.

fig.6-15

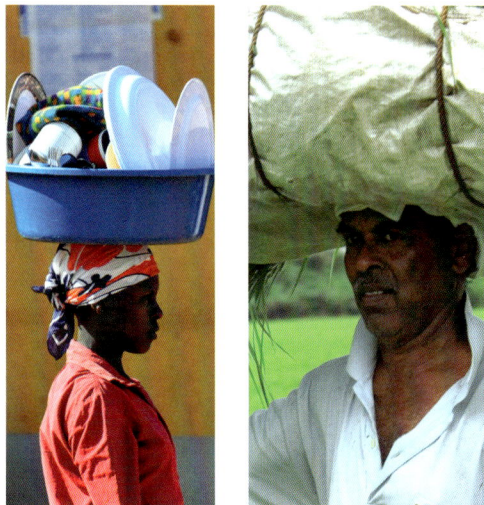

(Uganda)   (India)

People who carry weight on their head push up against the weight using their neck (longus colli) muscles as well as their inner corset. In this way, they sustain no damage from the weight.

FURTHER INFORMATION

ARM POSITION

When standing for an extended period of time, people in traditional cultures usually rest their arms on some part of their bodies (fig.6-22 on page 148). In all the photographs, the shoulders retain a healthy alignment. This is even true when the arms are folded across the front. (Beginners should avoid this position because it can easily lead to hunched shoulders.)

Notice that when the arms do hang by the side of the body (fig.6-16), they hang to the back of the torso and the thumbs face forward or, when carrying, are externally rotated (fig.6-17).

fig.6-16

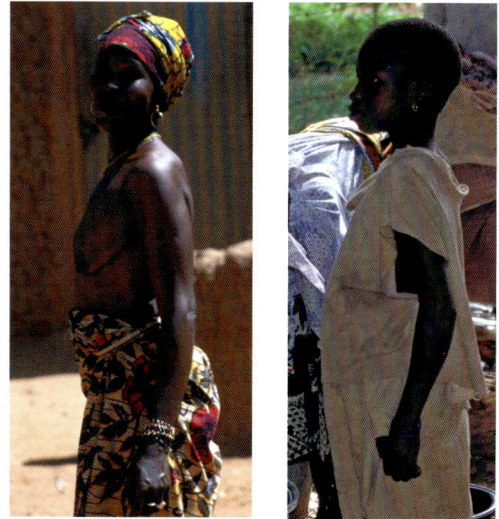

(Burkina Faso)   (Burkina Faso)

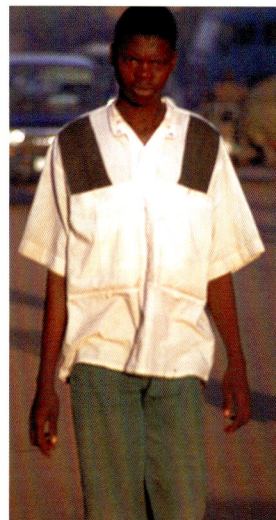

In traditional cultures, when the arms hang at the sides, they align well back along the torso with the thumbs facing forward.

(Burkina Faso)

fig.6-17

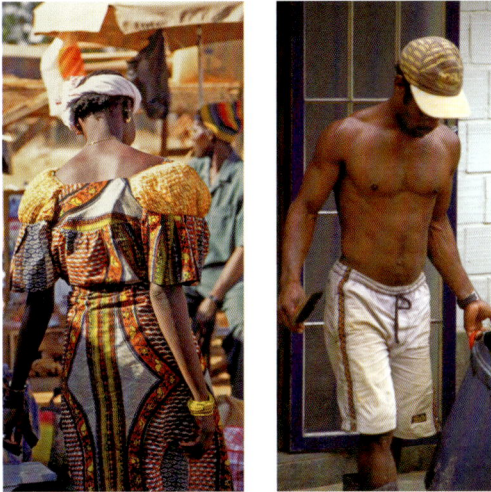

(Burkina Faso)   (Brazil)

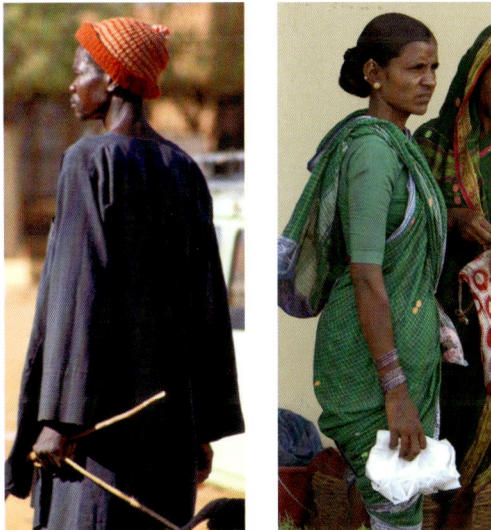

(Burkina Faso)   (India)

People in traditional cultures carry objects with their arms somewhat externally rotated (thumbs facing forward) or very externally rotated (palms facing forward).

WEIGHT ON THE HEELS

When we evolved from being quadrupedal to bipedal, the foot changed significantly. In comparing our feet with those of our primarily quadrupedal primate relatives, one of the striking differences is the sturdiness of the human heel bone. The bones towards the front of our feet remain relatively delicate, but the heel bone is enlarged and constructed with cross-grain reinforcement for weight-bearing (fig.6-18). In our bones we have compelling evidence of how we are designed to stand: primarily on our heels.

fig.6-18

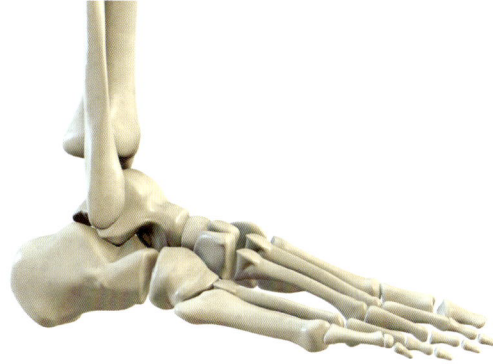

The heel bone in our species is a sturdy bone adapted for weight-bearing. The bones in the front of the foot, by contrast, are delicate and not constructed to bear the weight of the body as a baseline.

NATURAL ARCHES OF THE FEET

Tallstanding gives your arches (inner, outer, and transverse) a chance of staying intact (fig.6-19). Collapsed arches usually reflect significant postural distortion throughout the body, and they also cause a set of problems of their own, especially in the bones, joints, and ligaments of the feet. Flat feet appear to be far more common now than in earlier times, when they were considered enough of a disability to make a man unfit for military service. Now, flat feet are so common that the military cannot afford to exclude people on this basis.

fig.6-19

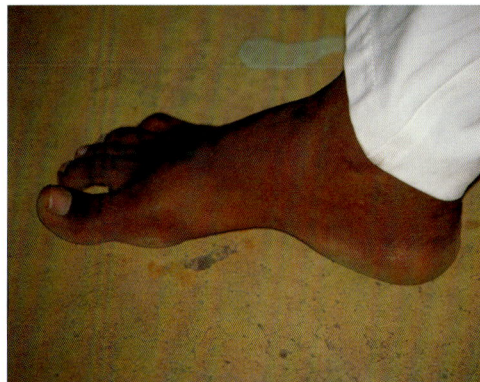

Healthy foot with intact arches (Brazil).

BARE FEET

A frequent question is whether it is healthy to go without shoes. The answer depends on the condition of your arch muscles, the alignment of your body, and the surface on which you stand and walk. If your feet and alignment are healthy, going barefoot on softer surfaces, such as grass, dirt, or sand, gives your foot muscles a healthy workout. If you have weak arch muscles, even a casual stroll on the beach can further distend your ligaments. Don't go barefoot without maintaining your weight over your heels and actively engaging your arch muscles while walking (see Chapter 8, Glidewalking). Even if your arches are in good shape, it is never advisable to go barefoot for any length of time on hard surfaces such as concrete or asphalt.

PREGNANCY

Pregnancy is a time when it is especially important to have healthy posture. Pregnant women are prone to damaging the ligaments in their feet. The hormone relaxin, circulating through their system to relax the pelvic joints in preparation for delivery, relaxes all ligaments, including those in the feet. The additional weight of the baby, especially if carried on the front of the feet, can permanently overstretch the foot ligaments. Some women experience a dramatic increase in foot length, sometimes as much as one or two shoe sizes.

SHOES

Good shoes are especially important, given the harsh and unnatural surfaces on which we walk, and the corresponding damage and underdevelopment in our feet. Most consumers and many manufacturers are ignorant of what constitutes a health-promoting shoe. Here are some characteristics of a good shoe (fig.6-20):
- Somewhat kidney bean-shaped, with a wide toe box
- Some degree of shock absorption, particularly in the heel, but not excessive cushioning, which hampers feedback to the nervous system
- Arch supports for all three arches of the feet

Since I first published this book, there are far more shoe brands offering kidney bean-shaped shoes, with wide toe boxes. This is heartening to see. Often these are barefoot-style shoes. If your

arches are not already well-defined, it is important to use insoles in such shoes until your foot muscles are stronger.

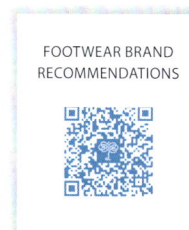

fig.6-20

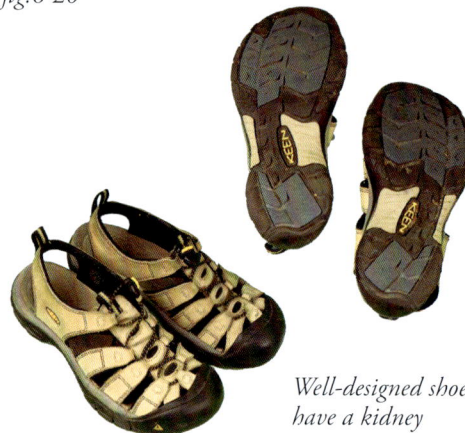

Well-designed shoes have a kidney bean-shaped sole, pronounced arch supports, and shock absorbency.

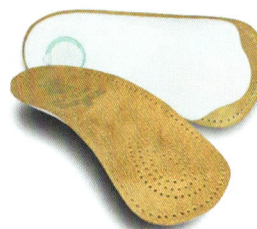

Well-designed insoles, like these ones made by Pedag®, support the inner, outer, and transverse arches of the foot.

INSOLES

For people with flat arches, it is useful and, in fact, important to use an insole. Engagement of the foot muscles cannot (and should not) always maintain the shape of the feet. When these muscles are relaxed, healthy ligaments fulfill this role. However, when foot ligaments have been overstretched, an insole can provide the necessary support and prevent your foot from spreading. Select an insole that supports all three arches of the foot. Used passively, it will prevent further distortion of your foot. Used as a training device, it can remind you to use your foot muscles to maintain your arches.

Most commercial arch supports provide some protection and support for the most important arch of the foot, the inner arch. If you have little or no arch on the inner edge of your foot, commercially available arch supports may be adequate at first.

However, after a few months of doing the foot-strengthening exercises in Appendix 1, you should probably add support for the outer and transverse arches as well. Such supports may be part of an insole or sold separately as pieces to be attached to a shoe or insole. You may have to look a little harder to find the best insoles for your foot, or have them custom-made. Transverse arch supports, also called metatarsal arch supports, are often sold separately as pieces to be attached to a shoe, insole, or arch support. Some podiatrists prescribe custom "orthotics." These tend to be fairly rigid and expensive, and are usually constructed to reflect the existing shape of the patient's foot. This assumes that the shape of the foot will not change through time.

In fact, there is a lot that people can and should do to modify their foot shape. For specifics, see the foot exercises in Appendix 1.

SPINE CONTOUR CONFUSION

As a novice posture student, you may wonder why the profiles of certain muscular individuals (including a lot of Greek statues), that otherwise exhibit good posture, appear to be rounded in the upper spine (fig.6-21). These individuals have large muscles around their shoulders. Because the shoulders are placed back along the spine where they belong, they give the appearance of a rounded upper back. Yet the spine, buried especially deeply between the shoulder blades, remains straight.

fig.6-21

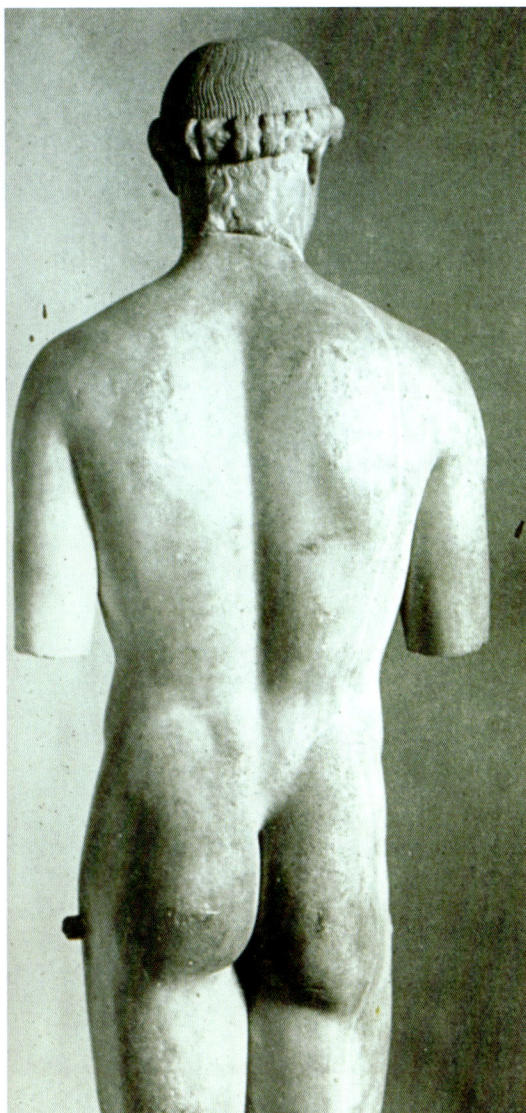

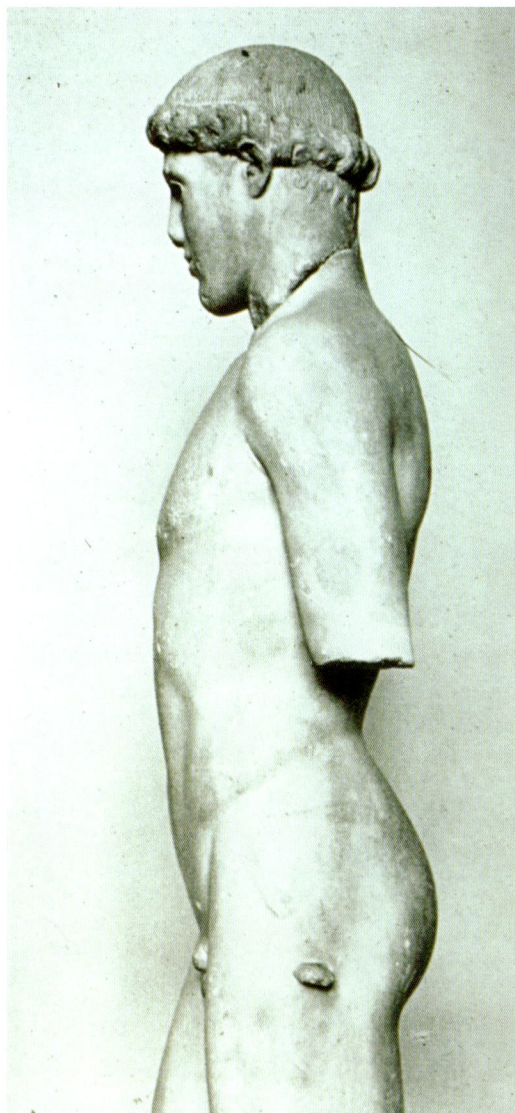

© Gerard Mackworth-Young

The straight thoracic spine is hidden behind large upper back muscles in these statues.

fig.6-22

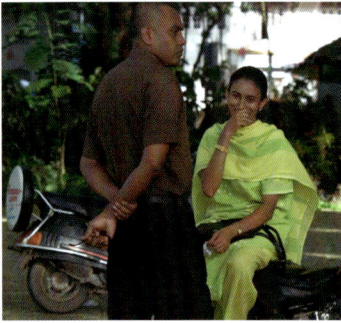

(India)

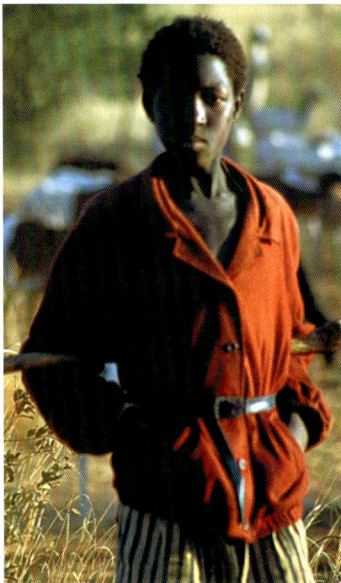

(Burkina Faso)

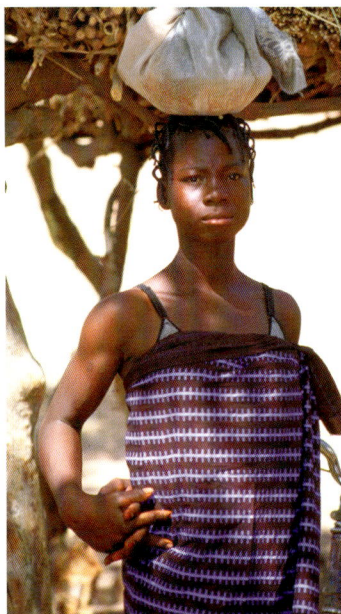

(Burkina Faso)

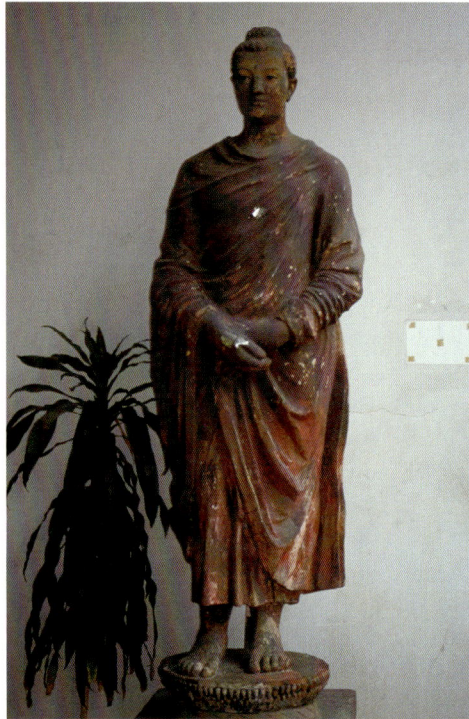

(Thailand)

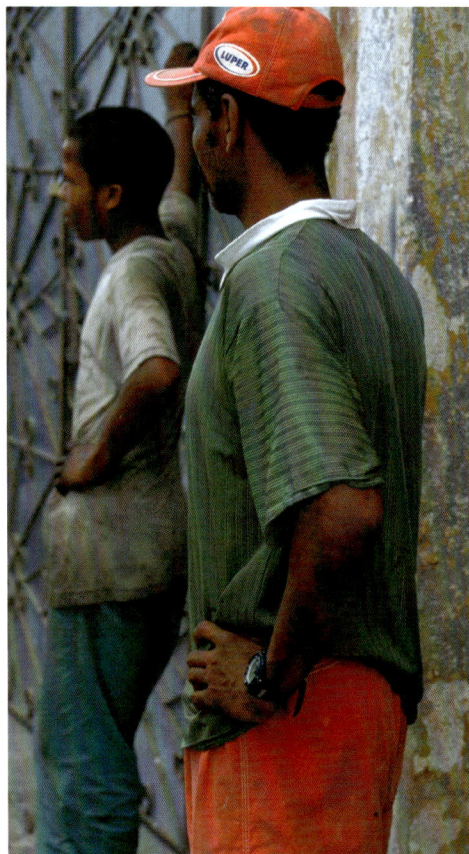

(Brazil)

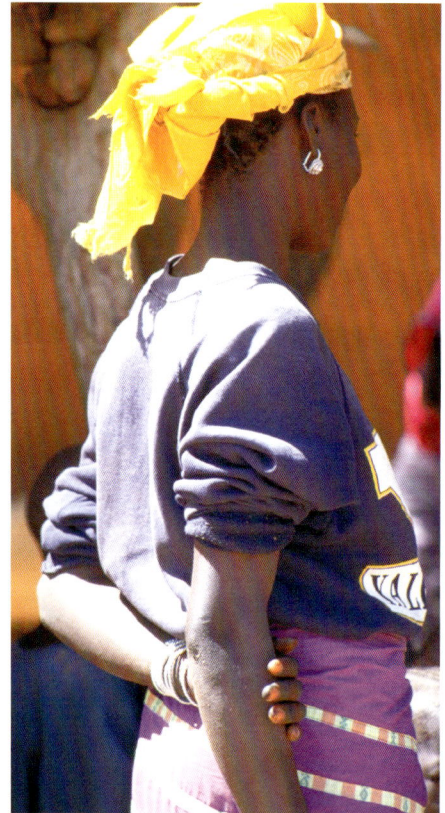

(Burkina Faso)

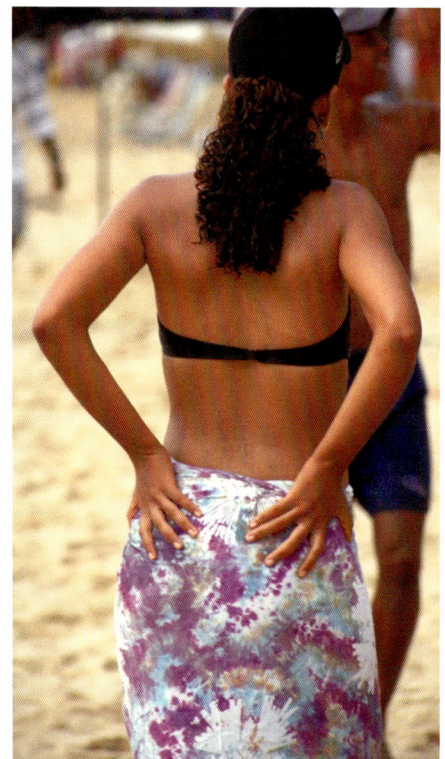

(Brazil)

People in traditional cultures often rest their arms on some part of their bodies.

RECAP

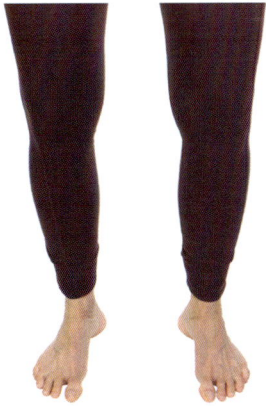

a. Form a kidney bean shape with each foot

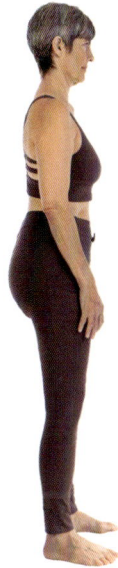

b. Shift most of your weight to your heels

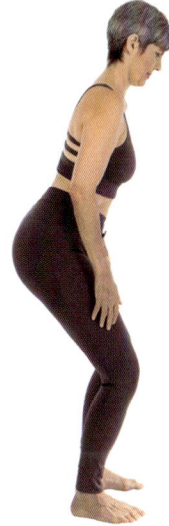

c. Bend at knee and hip joints and relax abdomen to enable pelvic anteversion

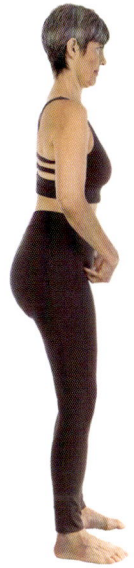

d. Return to being more upright, but leave softness in knees and groin crease

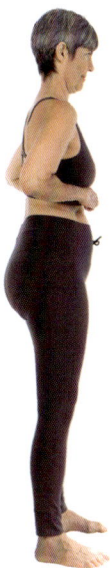

e. Establish rib anchor

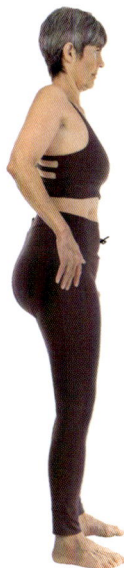

f. Perform shoulder rolls and lengthen back of neck

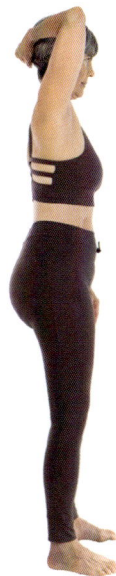

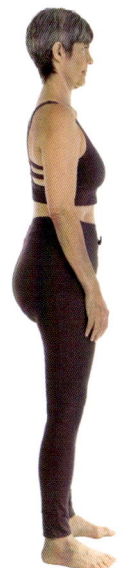

g. Maintain rib anchor and relax rest of body

7

HIP-HINGING

Hinging at the hips to bend

This older Burkinabé woman was gathering water chestnuts while I photographed and filmed her for hours. She spends most of the time bent over, rising every 10–15 minutes for a very short time and then going back to her bent position. She does this every day for seven to nine hours and reports no pathology in her back (though she says she would prefer to sit in a chair all day!). Notice her flat back, the even groove overlying her spine, the well-developed musculature alongside her spine, and her shoulder blades positioned back and down relative to her spine (the same as they would be in standing).

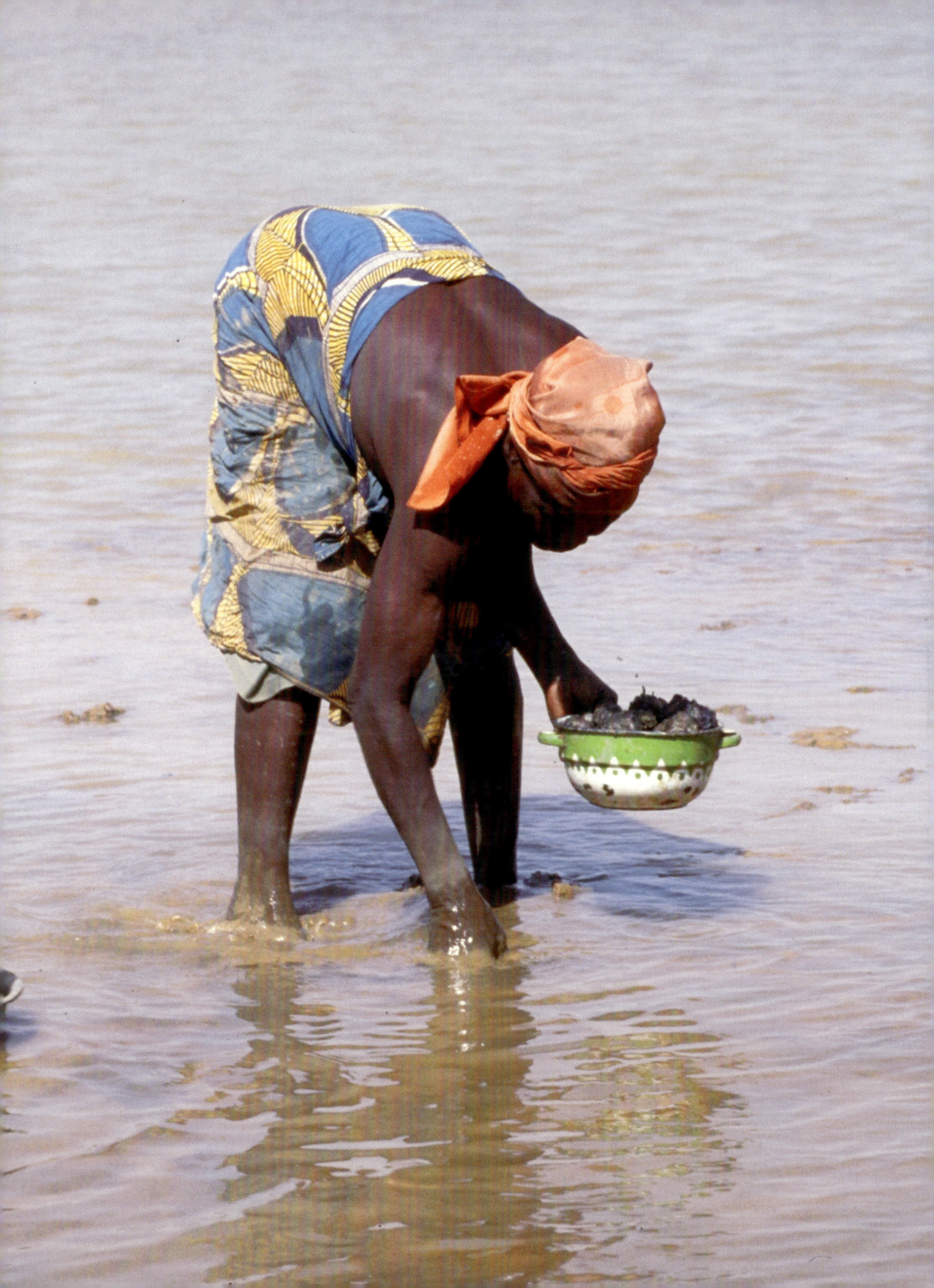

If there is one action that makes or breaks a back, it is bending. People who bend with a straight spine usually enjoy good back health (fig.7-1); people who bend with a rounded spine often develop back pain (fig.7-2). Furthermore, by watching people bend, a skilled observer can predict where tension or pain is likely to occur (fig.7-3).

To learn how to bend well, we need to observe populations with little incidence of back pain: people in nonindustrial cultures, as they bend over their rice paddies or gather water chestnuts all day (fig.7-5), ancestral populations, and young children the world over. These people bend for long hours without a problem, while many of us in industrialized cultures cannot bend for even five minutes without pain.

fig.7-1

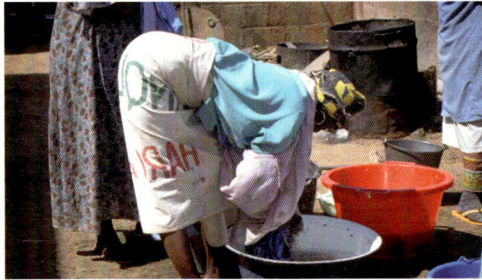

Woman bending well while washing clothes (Burkina Faso)

fig.7-4

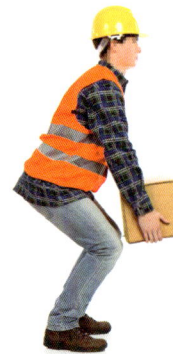

Most people are taught to bend and lift with an upright torso and bent knees (USA).

fig.7-2

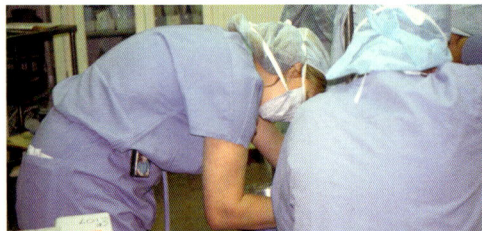

Woman bending poorly, resulting in pain (USA)

fig.7-5

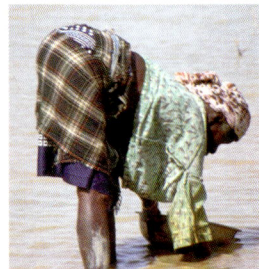

Example of healthy bending from the hips with a straight back (Burkina Faso)

fig.7-3

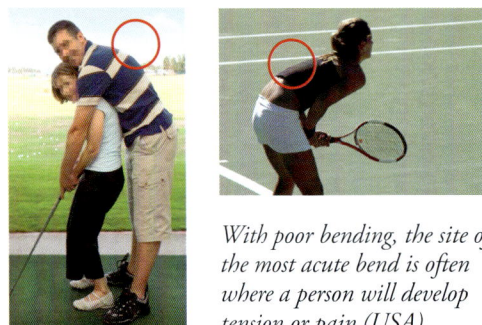

With poor bending, the site of the most acute bend is often where a person will develop tension or pain (USA).

Successful bending requires a healthy baseline back contour that you preserve as you bend. By now, you have achieved that baseline:

- You have learned to tip your pelvis forward in anteversion to restore your natural lumbosacral angle.
- You have lengthened the muscles that run longitudinally on either side of your spine, so they no longer draw your spine into the shape of an overstrung bow.
- You have reset your shoulder blades further back, so their weight and the weight of your arms no longer curve your spine forward.
- You have resettled your head further back to crown the spine so that its weight no longer causes your upper spine to curve forward.

Of all our common daily activities, bending is the one that is least often done right, and the one that most experts teach inadequately (fig.7-4).

- You have learned to use the abdominal muscles of your inner corset to preserve the natural shape of your spine and, when necessary, lengthen it.

In this chapter, you will learn how to bend without undoing all that fine work.

ANATOMY OF A BACKACHE...

Most people round their backs as they bend, compressing the front (anterior) part of certain discs and squeezing the contents to the back (posterior) part (fig.7-6). This causes wear on the fibrous exterior at the back of the disc, the worst possible site. Because the spinal cord and emerging nerves lie directly behind the discs, a disc that bulges or herniates in the posterior direction is likely to impinge on the nerves behind it, causing pain, numbness, tingling, and loss of muscle function anywhere along the pathway of that nerve.

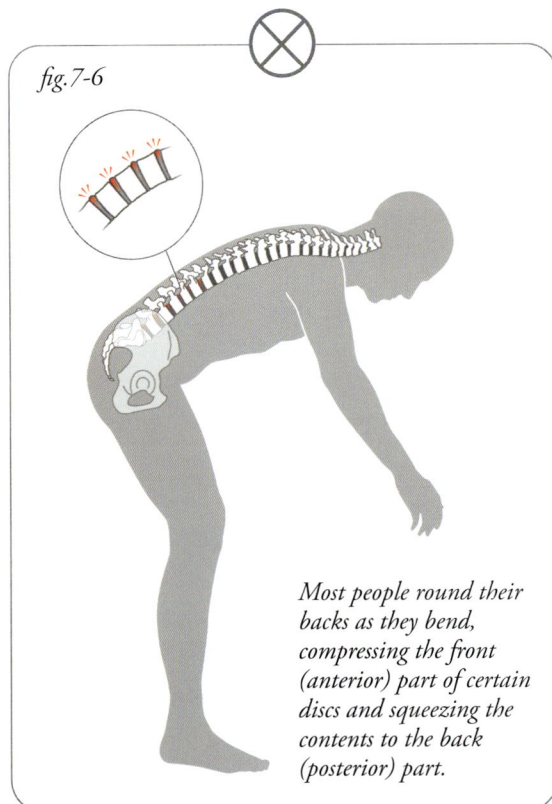

fig.7-6

Most people round their backs as they bend, compressing the front (anterior) part of certain discs and squeezing the contents to the back (posterior) part.

In addition, rounding the back stretches some of the ligaments in the rounded part. Since ligaments are not elastic, repeated stretching at the same site can cause them to become lax and lose their function of limiting spinal distortion. Ligament

distension can result in abnormal forward curvature (*kyphosis*) even when standing upright (fig.7-7). An extreme case is the "dowager's hump," where flaccid ligaments permit an extreme curvature in the thoracic spine.

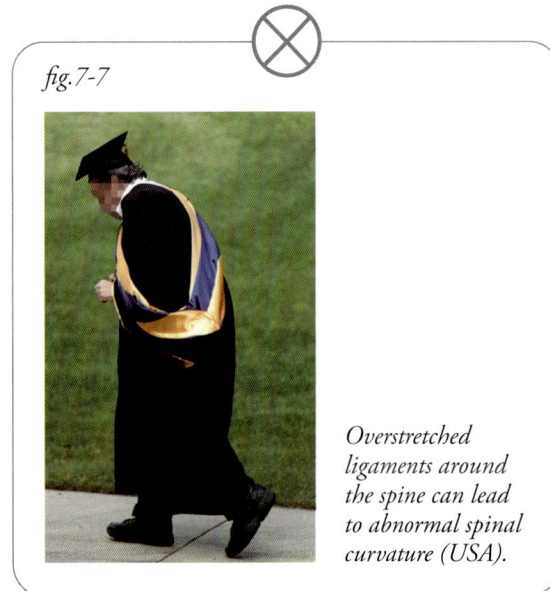

fig.7-7

Overstretched ligaments around the spine can lead to abnormal spinal curvature (USA).

... AND HOW TO AVOID IT

Healthy bending involves hinging at the hip joint rather than elsewhere in the torso, preserving the shape and length of the back throughout the bend. The advantages of bending this way are many. No discs are compromised and no back ligaments are strained. The knees are spared and the back muscles benefit from a healthy challenge. Whereas improper bending is indeed a threat to the back, healthy bending through hip-hinging is a beneficial exercise (fig.7-8).

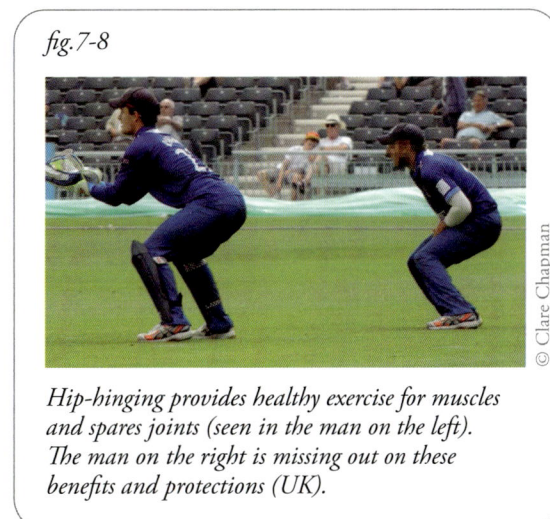

fig.7-8

Hip-hinging provides healthy exercise for muscles and spares joints (seen in the man on the left). The man on the right is missing out on these benefits and protections (UK).

With hip-hinging, the *erector spinae* muscles work to keep the back aligned, rather than rounded forward in response to the pull of gravity (fig.7-9). This strengthens the muscles and is, in fact, an ideal way to train them: the different fibers of the muscles develop exactly as needed to keep the back straight.

fig.7-9

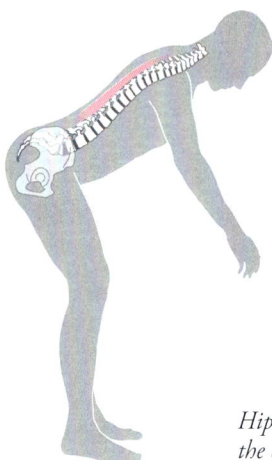

Hip-hinging strengthens the erector spinae muscles.

Hip-hinging stretches the hamstring muscles with every bend (fig.7-10). Indeed, periodic bending increases flexibility in these muscles, which is key to healthy pelvic anteversion. In contrast, tight hamstrings pull on the sitz bones (*ischial tuberosities*), forcing the pelvis into retroversion (fig.7-11). Note that if your hamstrings are tight, you can ease the demands on them by bending your knees as needed. But don't bend your knees unnecessarily, as this puts undue pressure on the knee joints.

fig.7-10

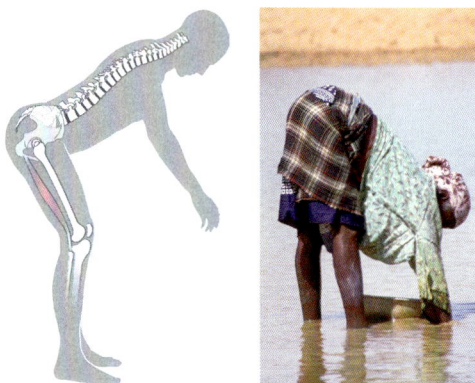

Hip-hinging stretches the hamstring muscles, increasing their flexibility over time.

fig.7-11

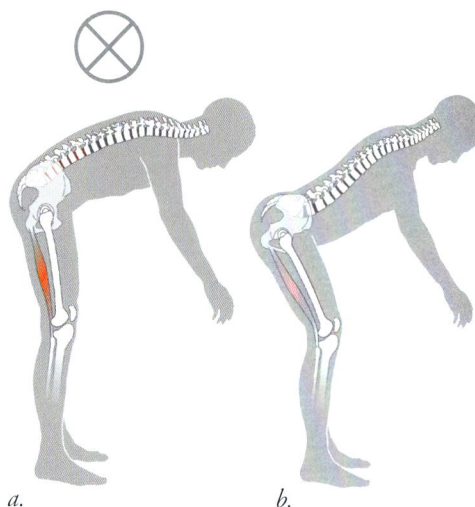

a.   *b.*

Tight hamstring muscles pull on the sitz bones (ischial tuberosities), making it difficult to tip the pelvis forward for hip-hinging (a). Bending the knees compensates for tight hamstring muscles and facilitates hip-hinging (b).

When you bend well, the rhomboid muscles, which run between the inner borders of the shoulder blades and the thoracic spine, work to prevent the shoulder blades from slumping forward (fig.7-12). The extra strength they develop during bending helps their resting function. The stronger and more toned they are, the better they can peg your shoulder blades back and in toward your spine. In a modern lifestyle, there are not many opportunities to strengthen the rhomboids, as we do not draw water from wells or haul in fishnets. Bending well is one of the few ways of challenging these muscles.

fig.7-12

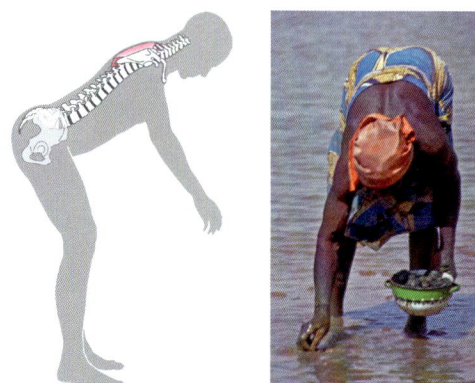

In good bending form, the rhomboid muscles grow strong as they work against the pull of gravity.

People are often taught to bend with their knees to preserve their backs. Although this does preserve the back, it stresses the knees a great deal, and eliminates opportunities to lengthen the hamstring muscles and strengthen the back muscles (fig.7-13). It is also impractical for many tasks. You should reserve bending with your knees for those tasks that would overchallenge your back muscles (for example, when lifting objects that are unusually heavy) and for when your back is injured.

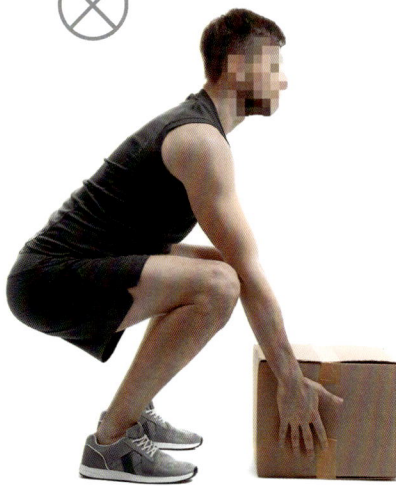

fig.7-13

a. The way to bend that is usually recommended can cause excessive wear and tear to the knees and is impractical for many tasks (USA).

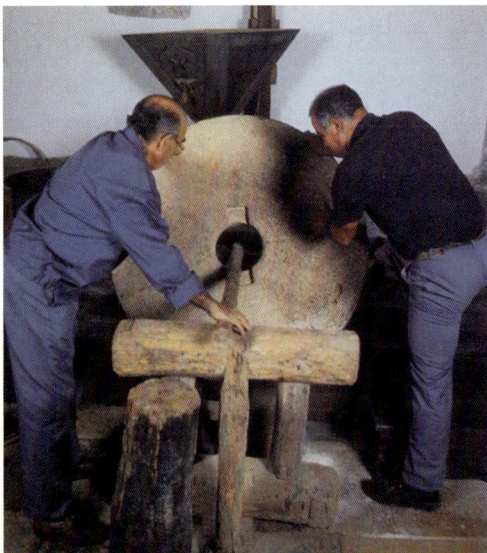

b. Hip-hinging spares the knees and is very practical (Portugal).

BENEFITS

- Avoids compressing or compromising the spinal discs

- Avoids distending the ligaments around the spine

- Strengthens key back muscles

- Stretches hamstrings, glutes, and external hip rotators

- Strengthens rhomboid muscles

COMPARING DIFFERENT BENDING STYLES

The following table summarizes the positive and negative effects of three bending styles. Hip-hinging is the only style that has no negative effects.

EFFECT ON	HIP-HINGING	BENDING WITH A ROUNDED BACK	BENDING WITH THE KNEES
DISCS	Preserves	Damages	Preserves
LIGAMENTS	Preserves	Distends	Preserves
KNEES	Preserves	Preserves	Wears
BACK MUSCLES	Strengthens	Does not strengthen; perhaps stretches	No effect
HAMSTRINGS	Stretches	Minimal to no stretch	No effect
RHOMBOIDS	Strengthens	Does not strengthen; perhaps stretches	No effect

I am still marveling at my newfound ability to access objects at floor level without incurring pain.

Sebastian Randerson,
New South Wales, Australia

EQUIPMENT

You will need a full-length mirror.

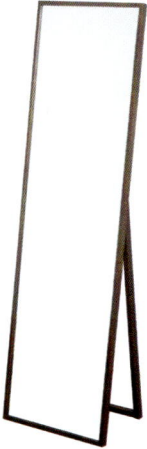

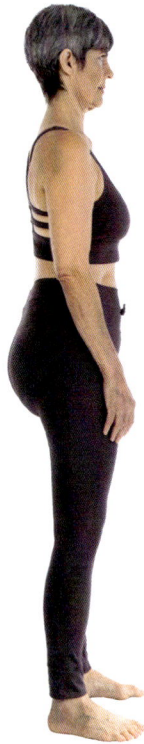

1 BEGIN BY TALLSTANDING

Stand with your feet pointed outward about 10º–15º with each in a kidney bean shape. Check that the groove over the midline of your lower back has an even depth from top to bottom.

To bend just a little, place your feet about hip-width apart. To bend deeply, use a wider stance.

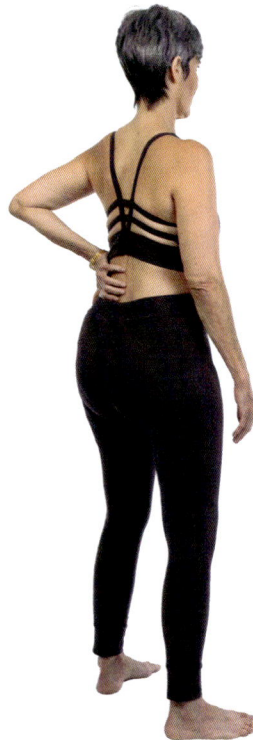

PREPARING FOR A DEEP BEND

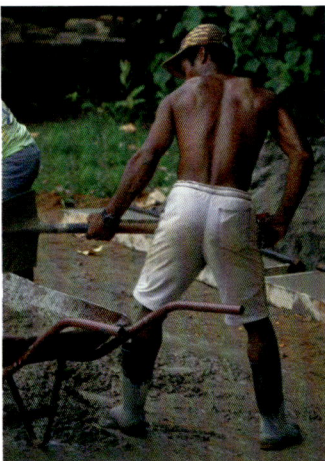

2 PLACE ONE HAND ON YOUR LOWER BACK WITH THE FINGERTIPS ON YOUR MIDLINE GROOVE

This hand will monitor your groove as you bend.

Notice wide stance and well-aligned legs (Brazil).

3 SOFTEN YOUR KNEES; DO NOT LOCK THEM

This allows your knees to bend as needed to accommodate tight hamstrings.

4 START TO BEND YOUR TORSO FORWARD FROM THE HIP JOINTS

Rotate your pelvis forward on the heads of the thigh bones (*femurs*). Your pelvis initiates the movement and your back moves in sync. When the pelvis stops moving, the back stops moving. While your fingertips may feel the midline groove deepen as you bend, its depth should remain uniform along its length. If the groove deepens in one area, engage your rib anchor. If instead you feel the groove disappear, straighten up and proceed again with care. See pages 162-163 for more detailed guidance.

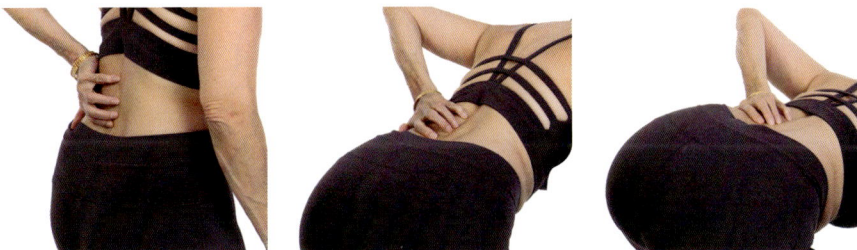

Bending with a healthy back (hip-hinging)

Bending with a rounded back

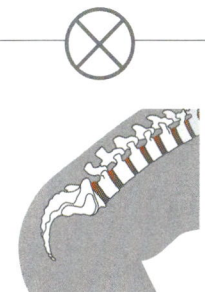

Bending with a swayed back

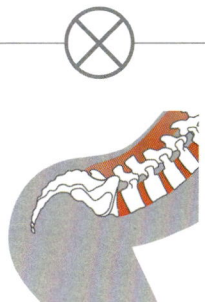

IDEAL AND COMPROMISED WAYS TO BEND

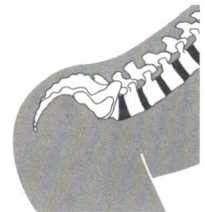

Hip-hinging does not threaten the discs.

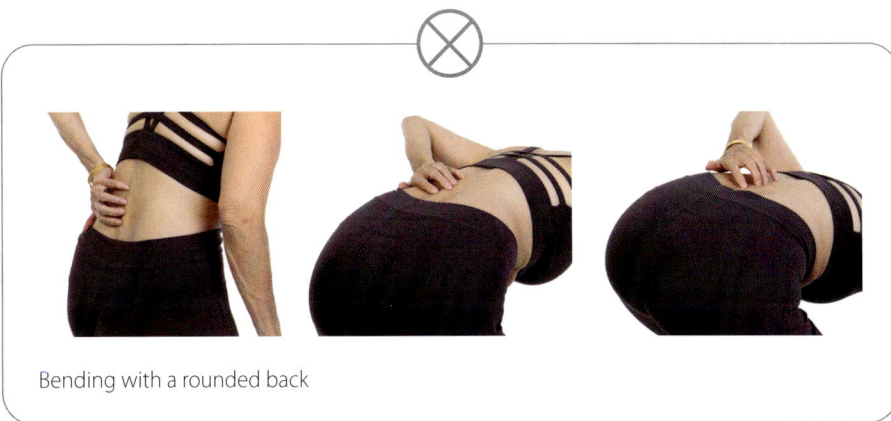

Rounding the back while bending compresses the spinal discs in a particularly dangerous way.

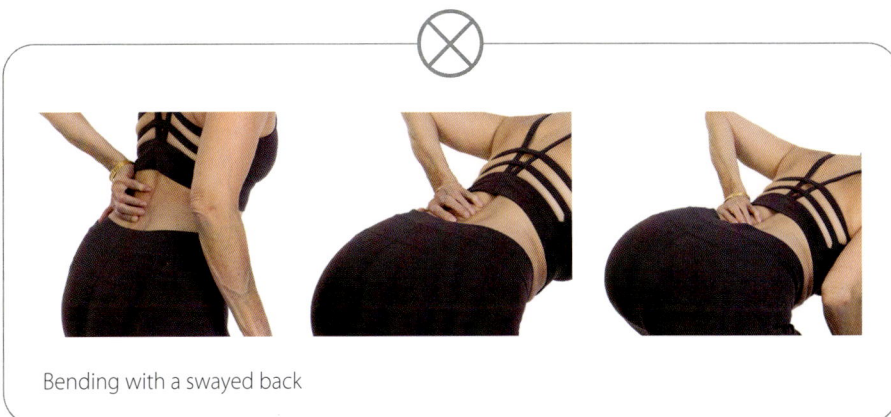

Swaying while bending generally compresses the spine.

157

DEGREE OF HAMSTRING FLEXIBILITY INFLUENCES BENDING FORM

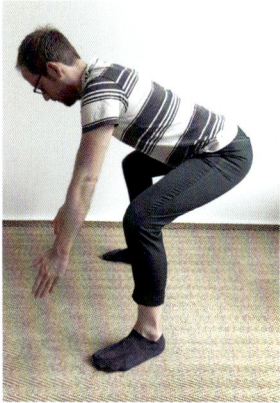

Limited hamstring flexibility necessitates significant bending with the knees while hip-hinging (Germany).

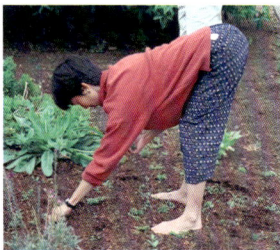

Good hamstring flexibility permits hip-hinging with slight bending at the knees (USA).

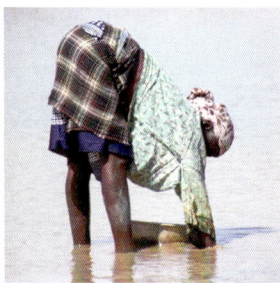

Extreme hamstring flexibility allows for hip-hinging with straight legs (Burkina Faso).

5 IF YOUR HAMSTRINGS ARE TIGHT, BEND YOUR KNEES AS NEEDED TO PRESERVE THE SHAPE OF YOUR BACK

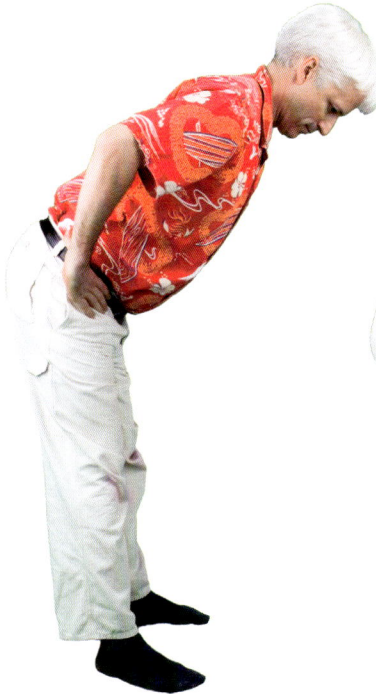

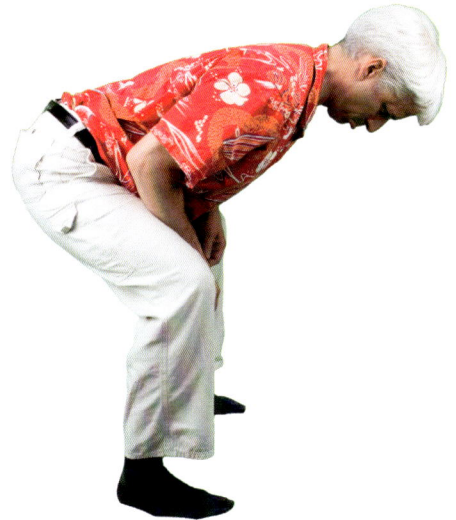

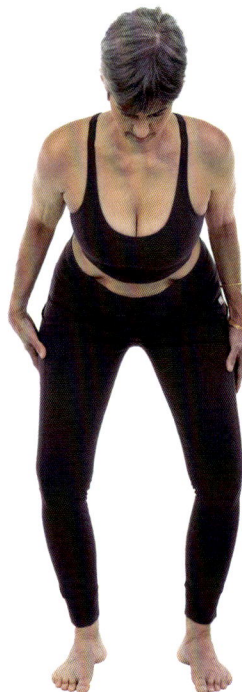

Be sure the knees point in the same direction as the feet, and the bend is smooth and coordinated.

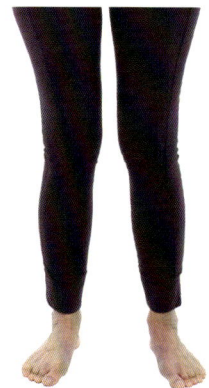

A common mistake is to let the knees turn in. Fashioning the feet into a more exaggerated kidney bean shape usually solves this problem. Some people may find it necessary to also use their hands and/or their hip and leg muscles to rotate their legs outward and align their knees (see page 137).

6 DURING THE BEND, KEEP YOUR HEAD, NECK, AND SHOULDERS IN THE SAME RELATIONSHIP TO YOUR TORSO AS WHEN STANDING UPRIGHT

Think of your neck as an extension of your spine. Engage the muscles at the back of the neck to keep your head and neck from protruding forward. Engage the rhomboid muscles to prevent your shoulders from slumping forward.

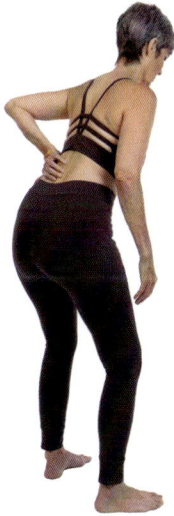

a.

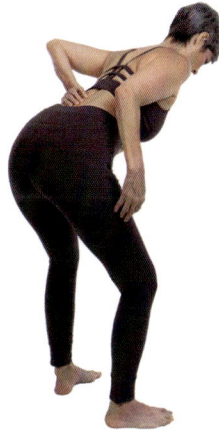

b.

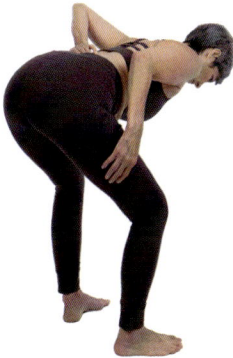

c.

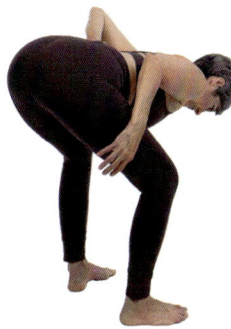

d.

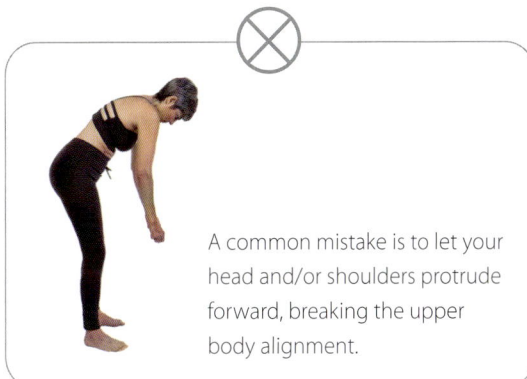

A common mistake is to let your head and/or shoulders protrude forward, breaking the upper body alignment.

DRINKING BIRD

This familiar toy provides a useful image to help you hip-hinge.

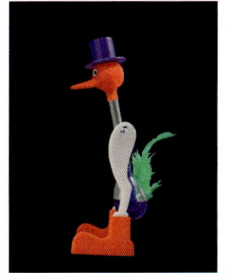

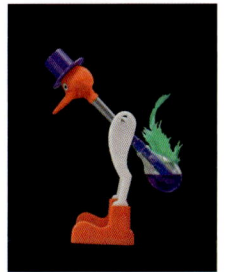

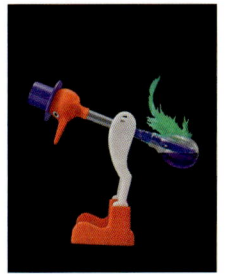

MECHANICAL TOYS

Old-fashioned mechanical toys often exhibit a traditional bending form.

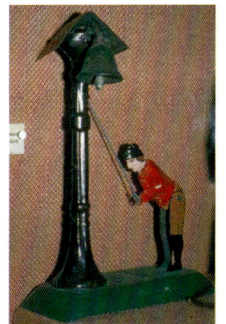

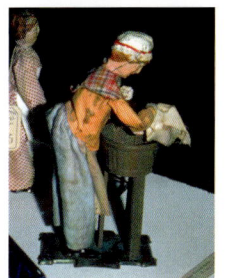

"BIRD'S BEAK"

Nesting the pelvis between the legs results in an acute angle between the legs and torso, called a "bird's beak" in Portuguese culture.

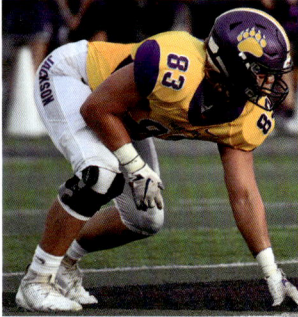

Football player in line of scrimmage (USA)

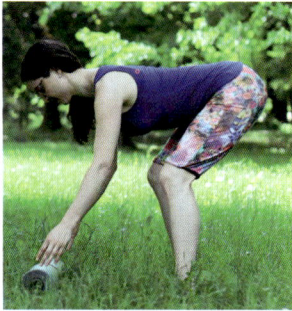

Reaching for a yoga mat (Slovenia)

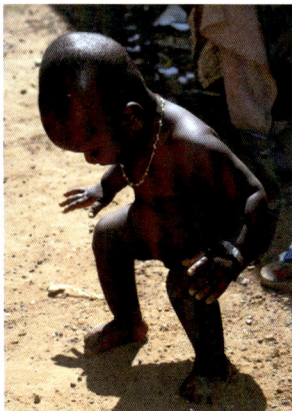

This child's pelvis and belly nest easily between his legs (Burkina Faso)

7 AS YOU GO INTO A DEEPER BEND, NEST THE PELVIS BETWEEN THE LEGS

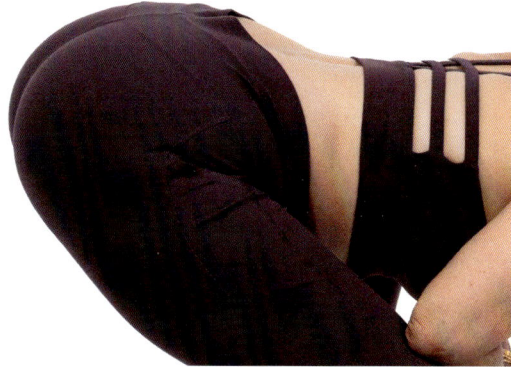

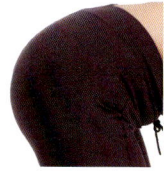

A common mistake is to rotate the pelvis inadequately so it does not nest between the legs

This can only happen if the legs are externally rotated and there is some flexibility in the hip joint. If you cannot find this action now, skip it. As you increasingly gain flexibility around your hip joints, the action becomes easier (see Appendix 1 for an optional stretch to accelerate this process).

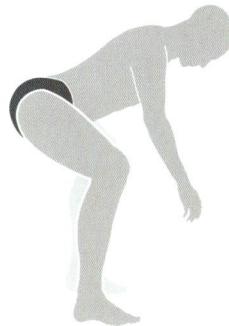

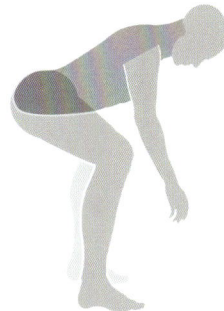

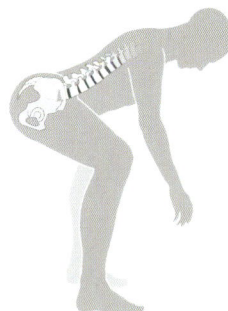

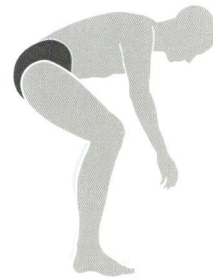

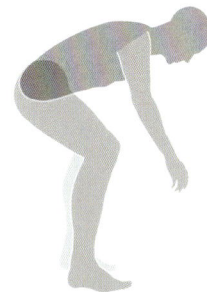

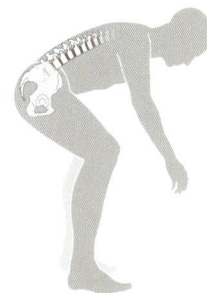

8 WHEN YOU ARE READY TO STRAIGHTEN UP, UNHINGE AT THE HIP JOINT, MOVING THE TORSO AS ONE UNIT

Monitor your groove with your fingertips as you do this. Once again, your goal is to maintain a uniform groove depth throughout the action.

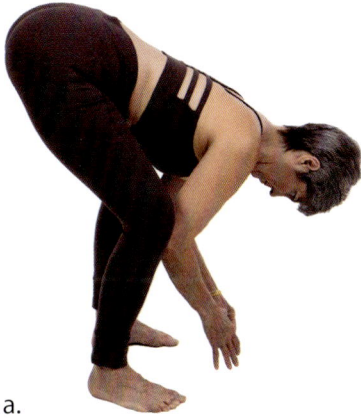

a.

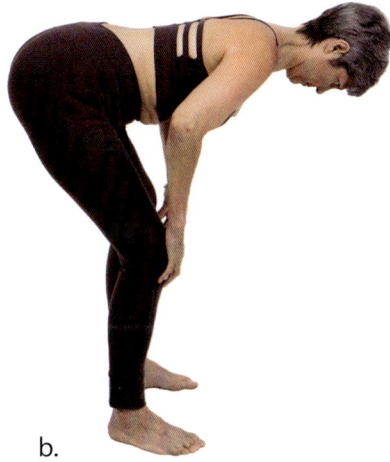

b.

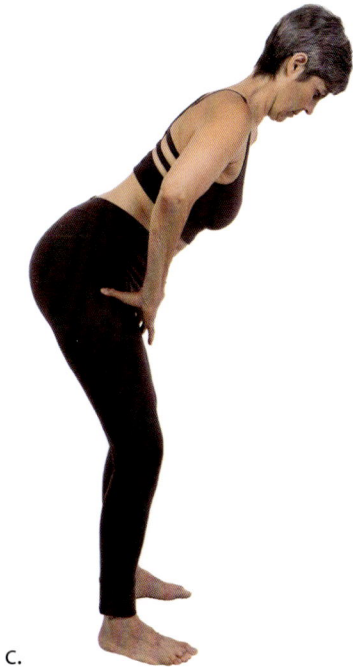

c.

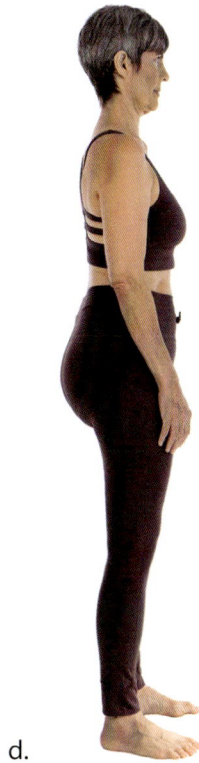

d.

EXAMPLES OF STRAIGHT BACKS WITH HIP-HINGING

As these people bend and unbend, their backs remain straight.

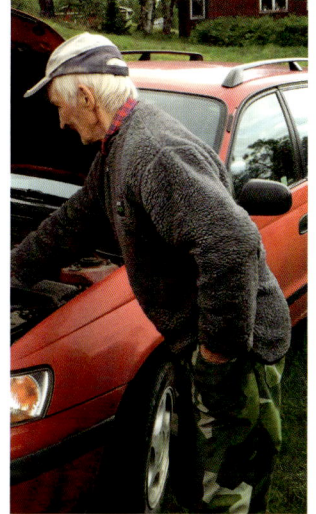

(Sweden)

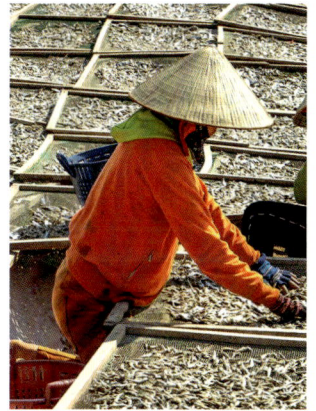

(Vietnam)

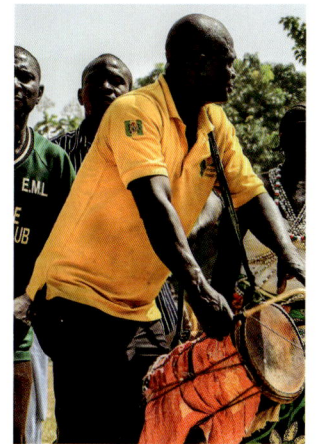

(Nigeria)

161

INDICATIONS OF IMPROVEMENT

At first hip-hinging will require concentration and slow motion. With time you will memorize this movement pattern and be able to do it as quickly and automatically as your old way of bending.

The muscle strength and flexibility you create by hip-hinging will in turn facilitate improved bending form. Over time you will find it easier to bend deeply, stay in a bent position longer, and bend your knees less (fig.7-14). As you perfect the form and combine it with engaging your inner corset (see Chapter 5), you will feel confident about combining bending and lifting (fig.7-15).

fig.7-14

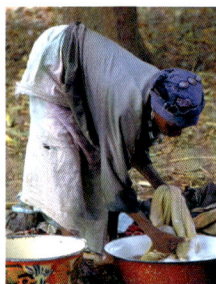

Hip-hinging will allow you to bend deeper, for longer periods of time, with straighter legs (Burkina Faso).

fig.7-15

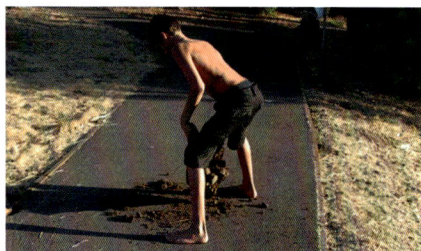

With practice, you will gain the confidence to lift heavier objects while hip-hinging. Do not attempt this before your form is excellent (USA).

TROUBLESHOOTING

BENDING IS PAINFUL
Perhaps your back muscles are in spasm from a recent injury. Because this way of bending uses your back muscles, it may be better to bend using just your knees until your back is further healed. Perhaps the pain is caused by rounding or swaying your back as you bend. If so, try engaging your inner corset before you begin to bend. This helps

you maintain your torso as a single unit. If you are still having trouble, try bending your knees more.

THE GROOVE IN YOUR LOWER BACK DISAPPEARS AS YOU BEND
This problem is very common when people are learning to hip-hinge. It is difficult (for some people, very difficult) to rotate the pelvis forward as a part of bending. It takes patience. Keep in mind that you have a deeply ingrained subroutine in your brain that is triggered when you bend. You are now trying to edit this subroutine.

Place your fingertips on your midline groove to give you feedback as you very slowly try to bend by rotating your pelvis forward. If you feel any change in the groove, return to the point where the groove is restored. Practice bending just a little way while keeping your groove intact. Soon you will be able to bend further with your groove intact. Looking at your profile in a mirror is another way to get useful feedback. It sometimes helps to reach back and around to your sitz bones and pull them up to help this action (fig.7-16).

Remember that tight hamstrings will limit how far forward you can bend with straight legs without losing your groove. An easy solution is to bend the knees as needed. Tight *external hip rotator* muscles can restrict your pelvis from nesting between the legs, causing the back to round during a deep bend. In both cases, exercises to lengthen the muscles are beneficial. See Appendix 1 for exercises that target these muscles.

fig.7-16

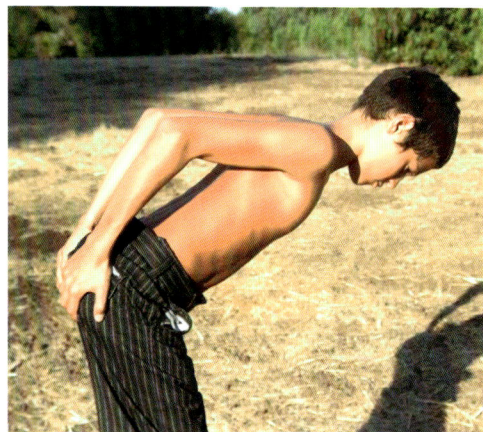

Pulling up on your sitz bones can be a helpful guide to tipping your pelvis forward into anteversion (USA).

THE GROOVE IN YOUR LOWER BACK GETS DEEPER AS YOU BEND

As you bend, the demands on your back muscles increase to resist the pull of gravity. Ideally, the *erector spinae* muscles contract just enough to keep the shape of your spine constant throughout your bend. If the muscles overcompensate, the groove in your back deepens. You may be overcontracting the muscles of your lower back out of habit. It takes patience and feedback from your fingertips to eliminate this excess tension from your bending routine.

If you still cannot keep the groove from deepening, try to engage your inner corset as you bend (see Chapter 5). This will help you move your torso as a unit and learn the new movement pattern. Later, when you have learned the pattern, you will no longer need to use your inner corset for normal bending, but can reserve it for when you need to lift heavy objects.

FURTHER INFORMATION

In this chapter you have learned the ideal way to bend with no distortion in the back. A healthy back can accommodate small distortions in bending, particularly in the upper *(thoracic)* spine, without incurring damage. The shape of the lumbar spine, however, should not change throughout the bend.

HAMSTRING FLEXIBILITY

Village African women, who spend long hours bending or sitting with outstretched legs (fig.7-17), tend to have especially flexible hamstring muscles and frequently bend with completely flat backs (fig.7-1,fig.7-5). The men, who spend less time in these two positions, have less hamstring flexibility and often round their thoracic spines slightly as they bend. They do, however, preserve a healthy shape in their lumbar spines (fig.7-18).

The degree of flexibility in the hamstring muscles also dictates how much the knees must bend to preserve a straight back in hip-hinging (see photos on page 158).

fig.7-17

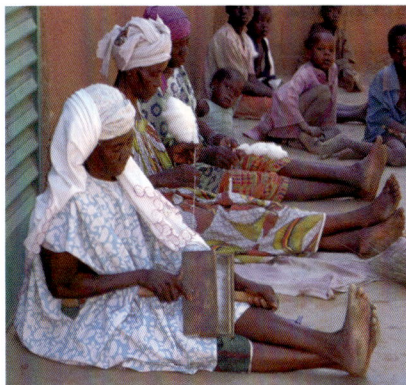

Weavers spend many hours sitting with outstretched legs, resulting in very flexible hamstring muscles (Burkina Faso).

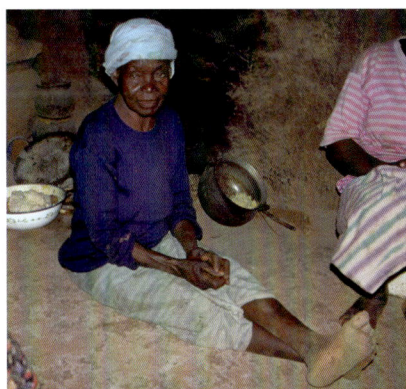

Flexible hamstring muscles are one result of doing household chores while sitting with outstretched legs (Burkina Faso).

fig.7-18

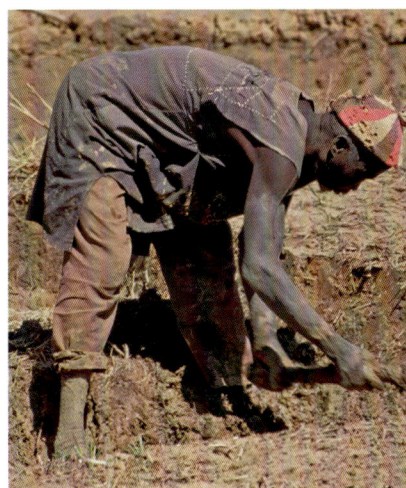

A slightly less "perfect" bending form that includes some curvature in the thoracic, but not the lumbar spine (Burkina Faso).

BENDING FOR EXTENDED PERIODS

When bending for long periods of time, as when weeding a garden, it is natural to rest a forearm, elbow or hand on the corresponding thigh (fig.7-19). This is more restful for your back muscles.

fig.7-19

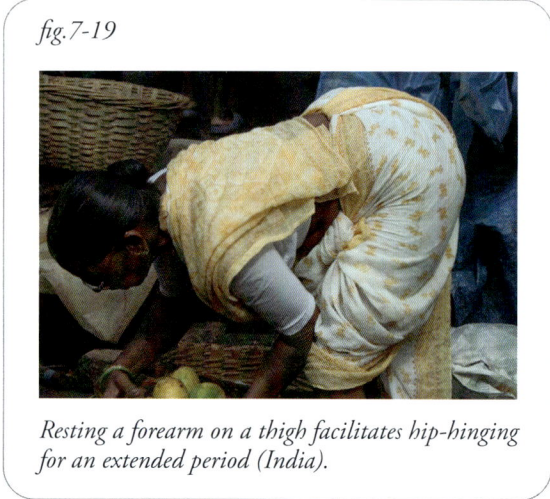

Resting a forearm on a thigh facilitates hip-hinging for an extended period (India).

BENDING WHILE SITTING

The same principles for bending apply whether sitting or standing (fig.7-20).

fig.7-20

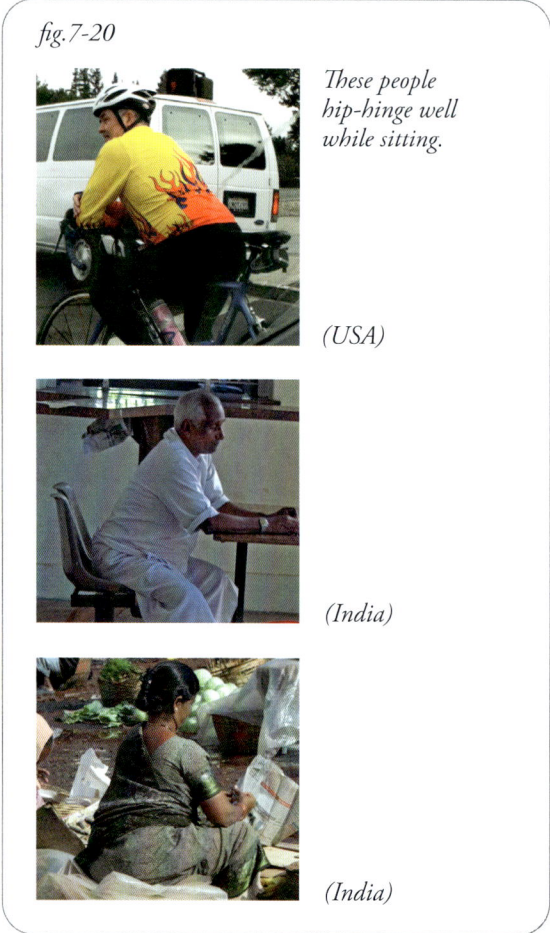

These people hip-hinge well while sitting.

(USA)

(India)

(India)

EXTRA WEIGHT

Full-bodied people often bend well (fig.7-21), perhaps because the downside of bending poorly would be extreme and immediate.

fig.7-21

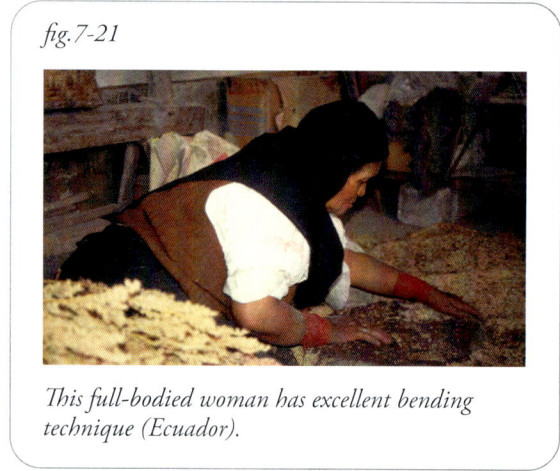

This full-bodied woman has excellent bending technique (Ecuador).

HIP-HINGING FOR ATHLETIC ADVANTAGE

Hip-hinging puts your entire body in a position of mechanical advantage to optimize performance in most sports. The shoulders remain in their baseline position, increasing the range of motion of the arms and optimizing the blood circulation to and from the arms. The pelvis is anteverted, putting the muscles in the lower limbs in a position of mechanical advantage. In addition, hip-hinging is easy on your joints, enabling you to play your sport with fewer injuries for more years.

The photo below (fig. 7-22) shows my son on the right winning a Bay Area wrestling tournament over from an opponent widely regarded as stronger than he. Notice that his form gives him more reach, better arm position and better buttock position, all of which are important in most sports.

fig.7-22

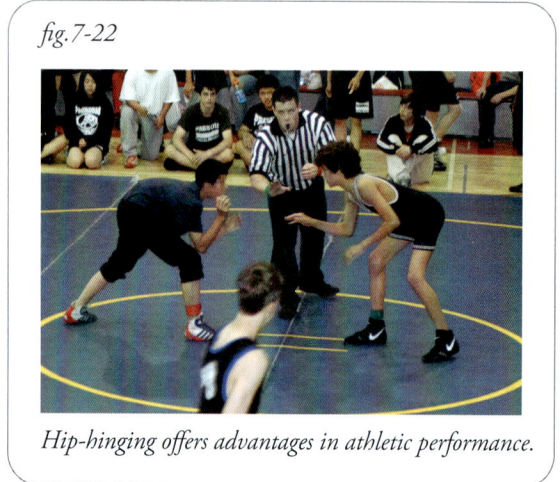

Hip-hinging offers advantages in athletic performance.

TRAINING CHILDREN TO HIP-HINGE

It is important to handle infants in ways that preserve the alignment of their spines (see figs. F-14 and F-15 on page 13). Doing so helps the child learn to use the torso as a unit (fig. 7-23), rather than distort it too readily when performing actions with the arms or legs. Additionally, providing good models helps children develop and maintain healthy movement patterns.

fig. 7-23

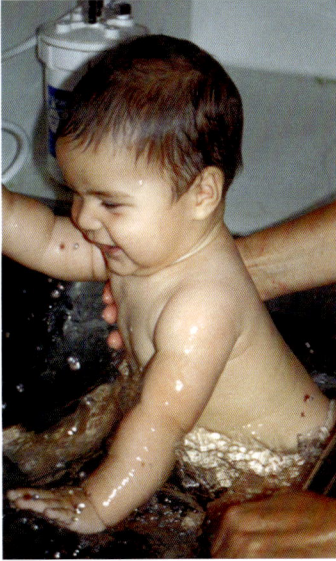

(USA)

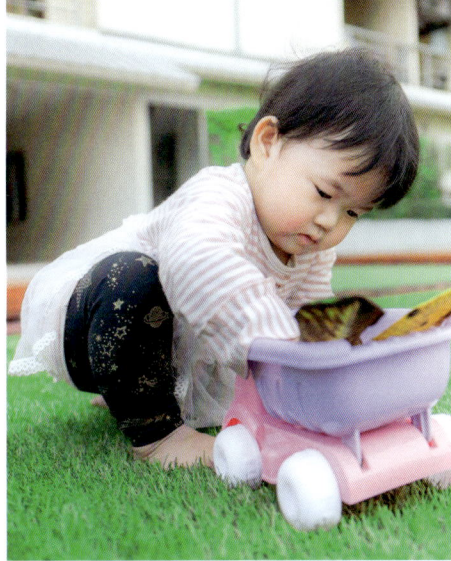

(China)

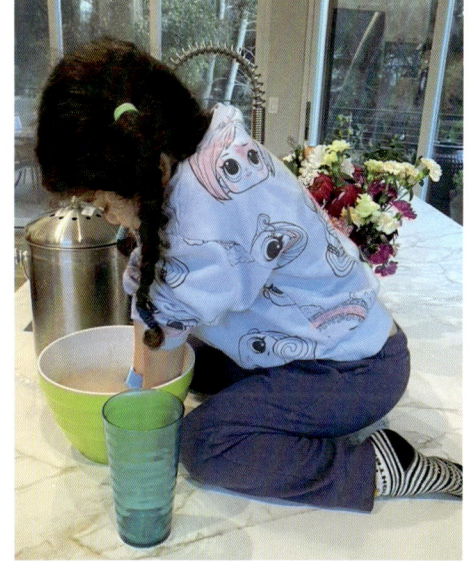

(USA)

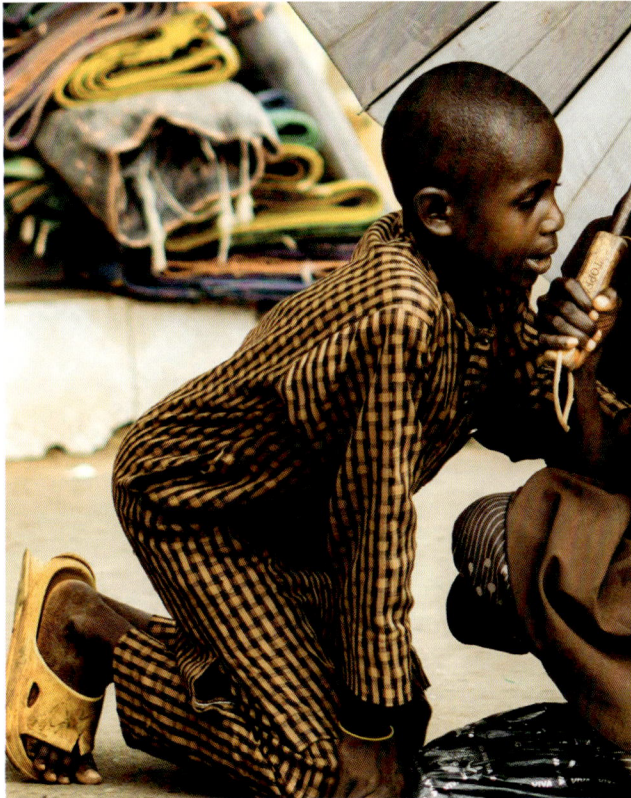

(Nigeria)

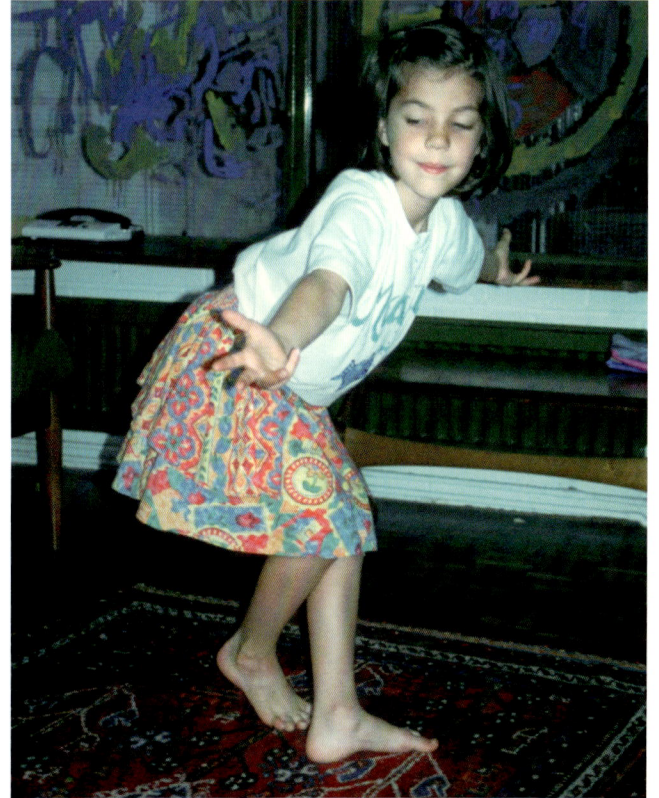

(USA)

Babies that have been carried and handled well tend to bend by hip-hinging.

EXAMPLES OF HIP-HINGING

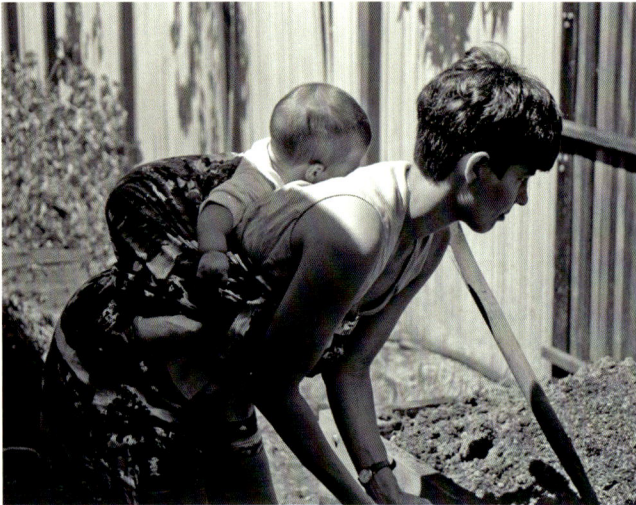

(USA)

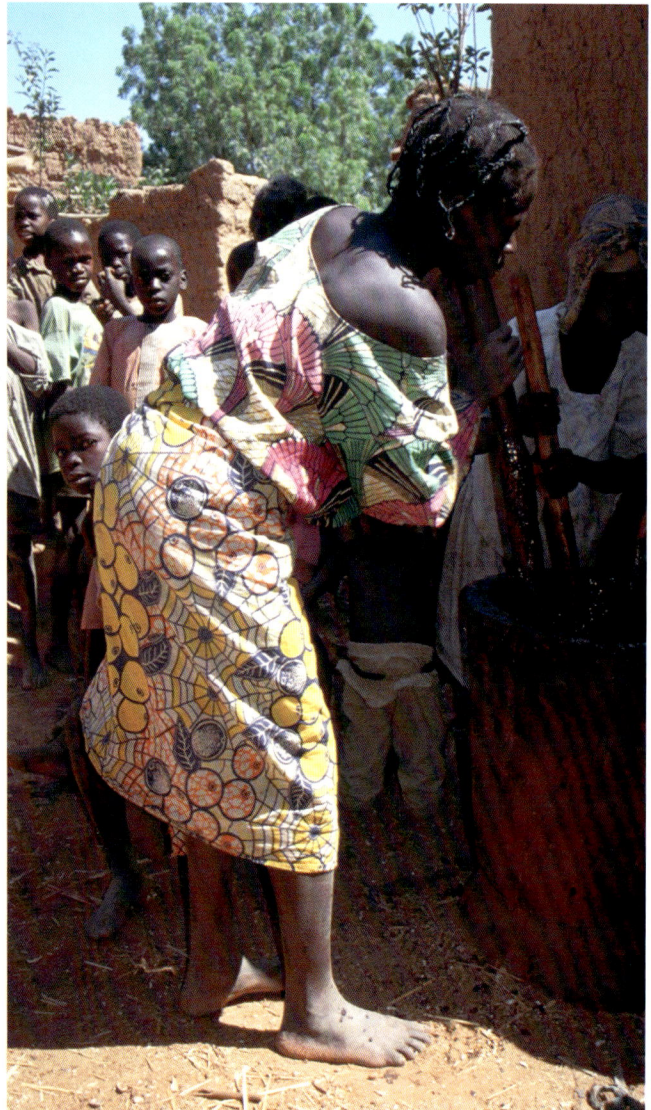

(Thailand)

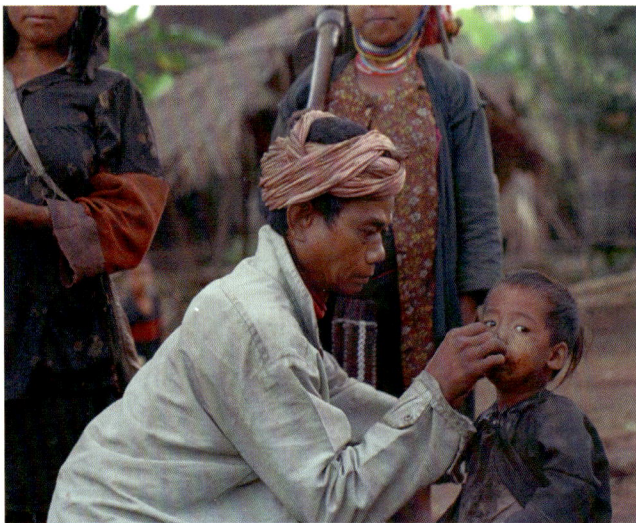

(Burkina Faso)

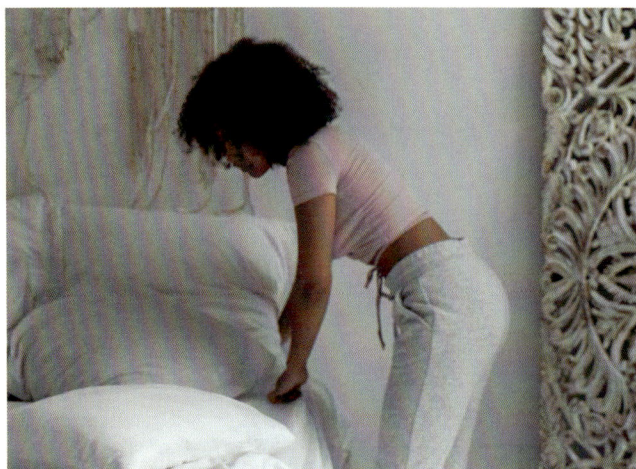

(Russia)

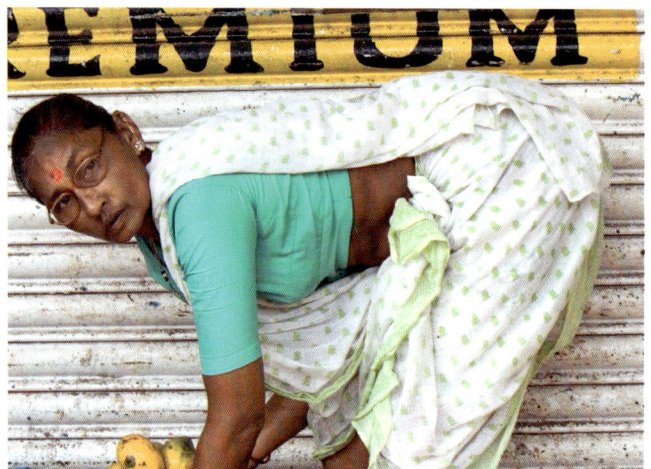

(India)

RECAP

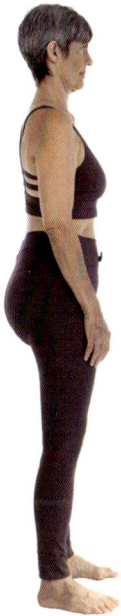

a. **Set up tallstanding**

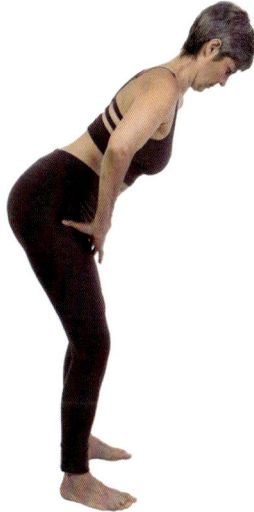

b. **Hinge at hip joint, not at waist or upper back**

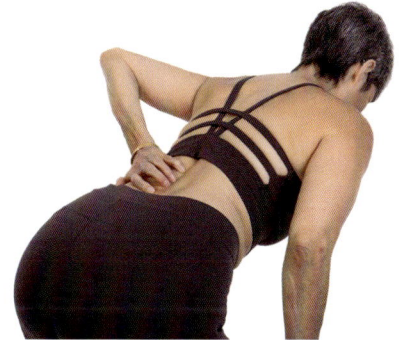

c. **Maintain an even depth in spinal groove**

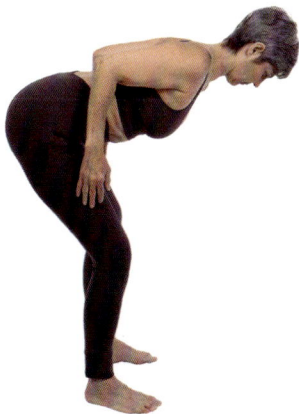

d. **Keep shoulders and head in line with spine**

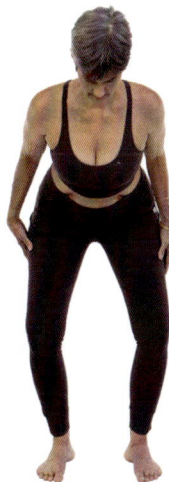

e. **Ensure knees point outward**

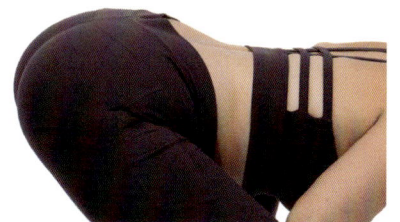

f. **For a deep bend, nest pelvis between legs**

8

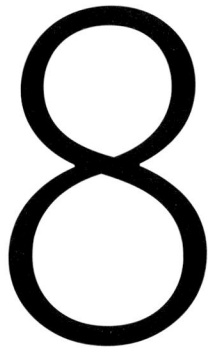

GLIDEWALKING

Walking as a series of forward propulsions, not falls

This Burkinabé woman is walking back from hanging her laundry to dry. Notice her pronounced lumbosacral angle, the development of her buttock muscles, the positioning of her shoulder blades far back relative to her torso, the straightness of her neck, and the downward angle of her chin.

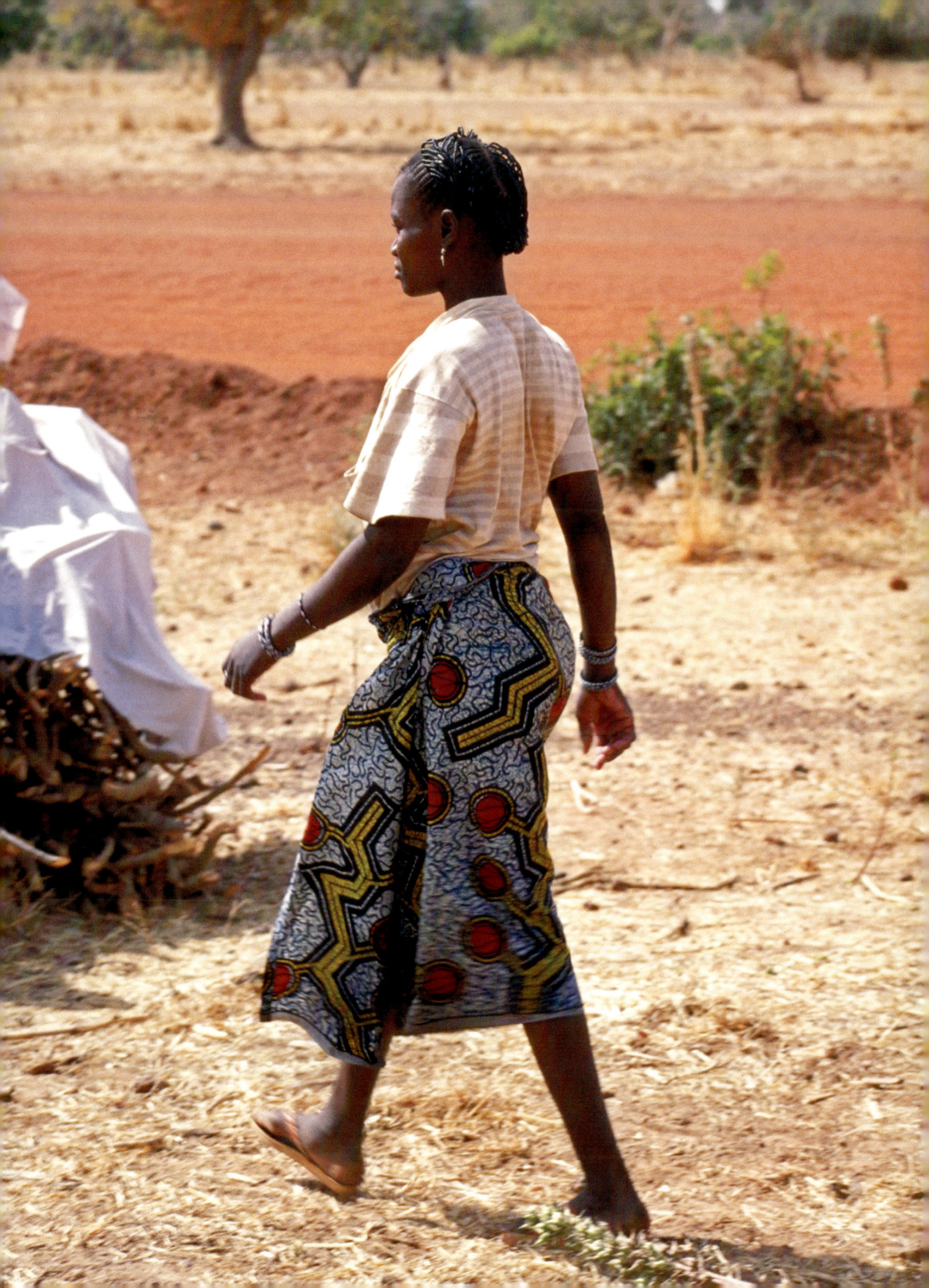

In this chapter, you will learn to walk well. Walking is often hailed as one of the best exercises you can do, and it is! A brisk walk, when done in a healthful way, provides excellent cardiovascular exercise. It also tones and stretches muscles in your lower body with a relatively low risk of injury to joints, bones, or muscles (fig.8-1).

If you walk poorly, however, you may underuse some muscles and overstress your joints, risking injury and degeneration. Many people in industrialized cultures walk in a way that's similar to how they stand—with their pelvis tucked and parked forward, and their weight shifted too far forward on their feet (fig.8-2,fig.8-3). With a tucked pelvis, the gluteal and posterior leg muscles are underused and walking consists of a series of forward falls blocked abruptly by the landing leg (fig.8-4). The back twists, sways, or hunches with each step. The impact of each step is an assault to every weight-bearing joint in the body.

fig.8-2

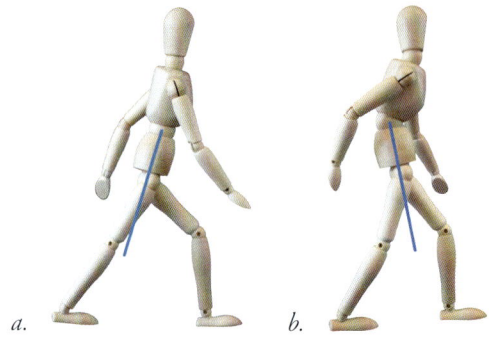

a.   *b.*

The pelvic axis extended downward lines up more toward the back leg in healthy walking (a) and more toward the front leg in unhealthy walking (b).

fig.8-3

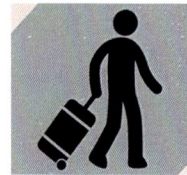 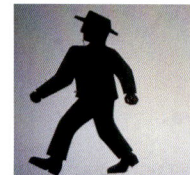

(UK)   *(France)*

Poor walking form is so prevalent in industrial societies that even our signage shows bad form.

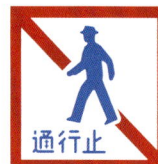 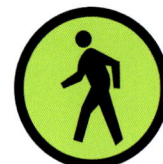

(Japan)   *(Philippines)*

In countries with intact kinesthetic traditions, signs correspondingly exhibit good walking form.

fig.8-1

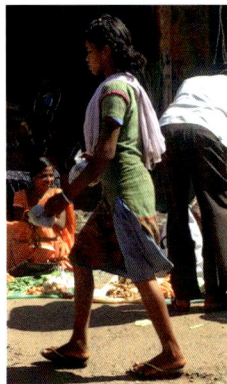 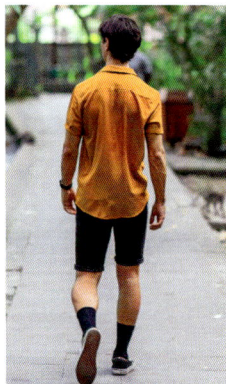

(India)   *(Indonesia)*

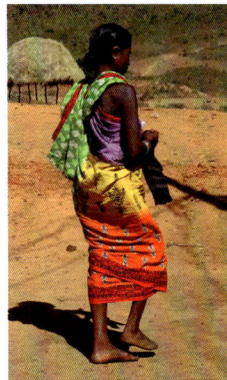 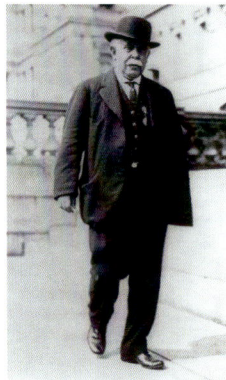

(India)   *(USA)*

In healthy walking, the joints are spared through healthy alignment and gentle footfall, while various muscles are exercised and stretched appropriately.

fig.8-4

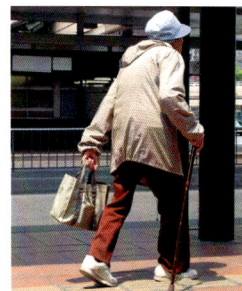 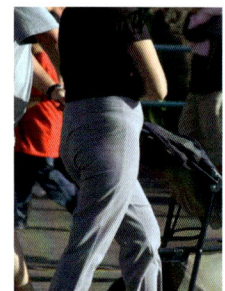

Poor walking form predisposes the hip joint to wear and tear, and underexercises the leg and buttock muscles.

Optimal walking is a series of controlled forward propulsions with cushioned landings, resulting from strong contraction of the buttock, leg, and foot muscles. In this way, these muscles get the exercise they need, and the back is spared unnecessary wear and tear. The front knee is bent at landing, which contributes to cushioning the joints from impact. After landing, the front leg straightens, commencing the forward propulsion. The heel remains grounded until close to the completion of the stride, protecting the anterior part of the foot from pathologies like bunions and plantar fasciitis. All this can only be achieved when the pelvis is anteverted.

Natural gait has become rare enough in our society to merit a special name: glidewalking. The torso keeps its integrity and moves forward smoothly while the *gluteal muscles*, legs, and feet do the work. The arms and shoulders are relatively still except in very brisk walking. The overall sensation is that of gliding forward through space.

Glidewalking provides many benefits. It strengthens the gluteal muscles—every step is a rep (fig.8-5). Strong gluteal muscles support pelvic anteversion, which is key to healthy posture. Strong gluteal muscles play an important role in keeping one's balance and preventing falls. In most people in industrialized cultures, the gluteal muscles are underdeveloped (fig.8-4). This is especially problematic for elderly people, who have a high risk of bone fracture when they fall.

fig.8-5

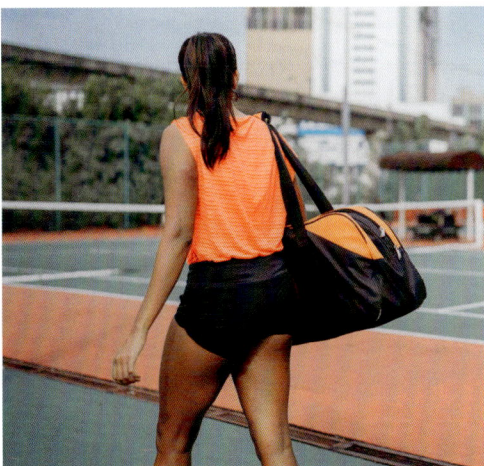

Glidewalking strengthens the gluteal muscles; strong gluteal muscles support pelvic anteversion (Malaysia).

Glidewalking provides one of the few opportunities in daily activity to stretch the *psoas* muscle. Sitting for long periods, as well as emotional stress, can cause psoas muscle tightness; a tight psoas sways the lower back and contributes to back pain. In glidewalking, the psoas gets a beneficial stretch at the moment of push off (fig.8-6).

fig.8-6

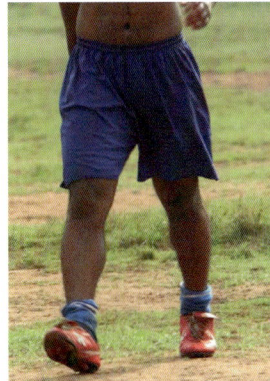 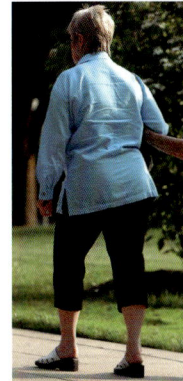

(India)   (USA)

Glidewalking stretches the psoas muscles.

Glidewalking also provides strengthening exercise for the arch muscles of the feet. Most people walk in a way that overly relies on the large muscles of the leg. Ideally, walking also uses the foot arch muscles. If we walked barefoot on natural surfaces, the arch muscles would strengthen as the feet worked to grab and push off the ground. Because of the prevalence of shoes and surfaces lacking much contour, most people use the muscles of their feet merely as padding. In glidewalking, the arch muscles are actively engaged with each step (fig.8-7). This is parallel to skilled cycling where, in addition to the large leg muscles, the arch muscles of the feet augment the power of each "stride."

fig.8-7

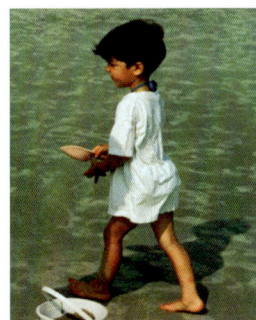

Glidewalking strengthens the arch muscles of the foot; strong arch muscles maintain the baseline shape of the foot as a platform for the work of other muscles (USA).

Glidewalking helps preserve the health of the hip joints in several ways. First, glidewalking strengthens the glutes and stretches the psoas muscles, helping restore pelvic anteversion and normal architecture in the hip joints. Poor alignment in the hip joints (i.e., the pelvis is tucked and/or parked forward) and the resulting stiffness in the surrounding muscles predispose one to arthritis of the hip joints (fig.8-8). Restoring normal architecture in the hip joints stops this process from progressing further and can reverse some of the damage that has happened. Second, glidewalking includes a relaxed "swing phase" in each stride (fig.8-9), which helps restore a healthy joint space between the head of the thigh bone (femur) and the hip socket (acetabulum). For many people, the muscles surrounding the hip joints are tense at all times, causing stress within the hip joints. During the swing phase of glidewalking, the leg hangs like a pendulum from the hip socket, stretching these muscles. Third, the soft impact of glidewalking causes no damage to the hip or other weight-bearing joints. A heavy tread jams the hip joint (and every other weight-bearing joint) with every step. Glidewalking limits the amount of stress in the weight-bearing joints to a healthy level, sufficient to prevent osteoporosis but not so as to cause wear or arthritic changes.

fig.8-9

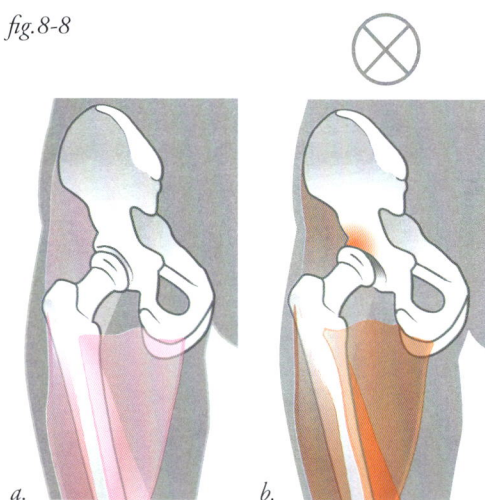

(Brazil)

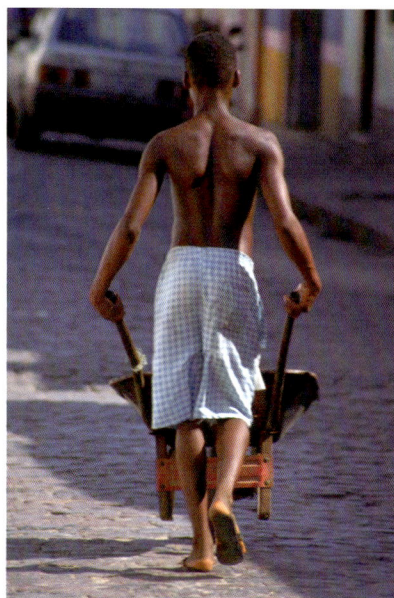

(USA)

With glidewalking, the leg hangs loosely from the hip socket in the passive "swing" phase, reestablishing a healthy space in the hip joint.

fig.8-8

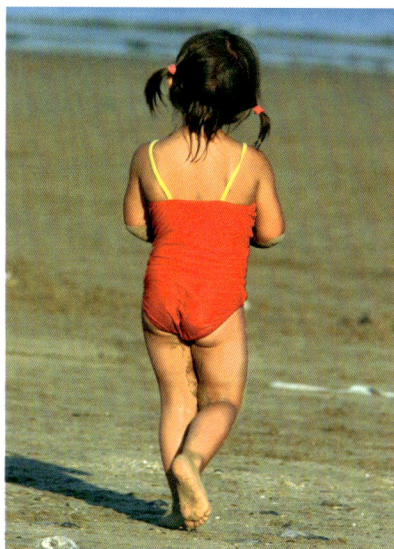

a.   *b.*

When the hip joint is correctly aligned (a), the muscles around the joint can relax appropriately, there is adequate space within the joint, and the fit between the leg and hip bones is correct. With poor alignment at the hip joint (b), some of the surrounding muscles are obliged to remain tense, the space in the joint is jammed, and the poor fit between the leg and hip bones predisposes the joint to arthritic changes.

You will learn this new way of walking in increasing rounds of detail. You may feel you should be able to master all this in a single session, but most people cannot. Remember, it took you about a year to master walking when you first learned, and you started with a clean slate. Now you have to unlearn your old pattern as you master this new way of locomotion. But it won't take forever, because this time you have your intellect to help, and you have explicit instructions.

BENEFITS

- Strengthens the gluteal muscles, improving balance and helping maintain pelvic anteversion

- Strengthens the leg muscles

- Strengthens the arch muscles of the feet

- Mobilizes and strengthens the ankles

- Restores and maintains healthy hip joints

- Stretches the psoas muscles

- Provides appropriate stress to weight-bearing bones, helping to prevent osteoporosis

- Reduces excessive stress to weight-bearing joints, preventing wear and tear

- Stimulates circulation throughout the body, especially in the legs, helping to prevent blood clots, varicose veins, and other problems

Studying this method has enabled me to avoid what would have been my fifth foot surgery. I can now walk again without pain. It has given me a new lease on life.

Honor Rautmann,
Sun River, OR

[The Gokhale Method] has helped me help myself by becoming more in tune with my body and increasing muscle awareness. Glidewalking has been great for me. I am more athletic, I can run better from being more light-footed, I look slimmer to people even though I haven't lost weight. My suggestion to other students: be patient and remind yourself of the overall lesson when you get lost in details. You will definitely see results!

Dev Takle,
Sunnyvale, CA

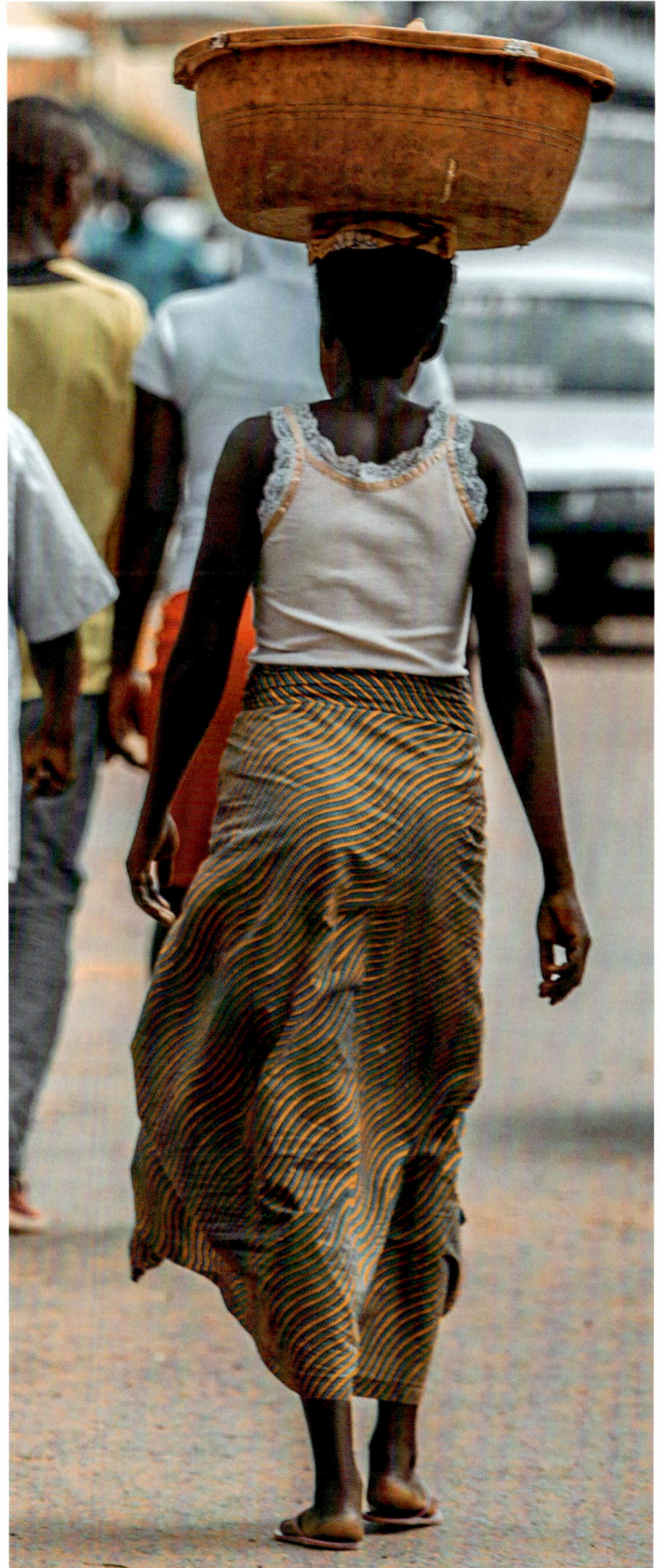

(Burundi)

173

EQUIPMENT

You will need:
- *A full-length mirror*
- *A wall, table, counter, or rolling chair, for balance*

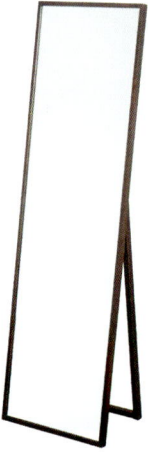

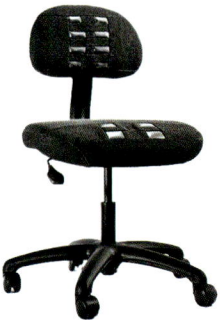

For those of us who have developed less than ideal ways of walking, glidewalking can seem highly complex, encompassing many new actions. I find it works best to break it down into six main phases:

Part A: Assessing Your Habitual Walk
Part B: Practicing the 4-point Checklist Stance
Part C: Breaking Down a Stride
Part D: Active Footwork
Part E: The Passive Phase of Walking
Part F: Putting It All Together: Refining Your Gait

PART A: ASSESSING YOUR HABITUAL WALK

1 TAKE A VIDEO OF YOURSELF WALKING SIDE-ON TO THE CAMERA

Walk at a moderate pace.

2 ASSESS YOUR FORWARD LEAN

Freeze the frame of the video just before your front foot reaches the ground.

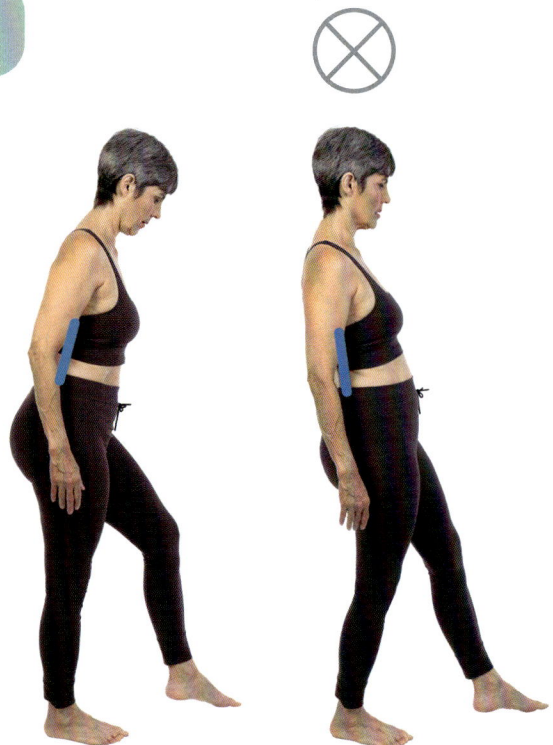

Draw an imaginary line through your lower spine; does it angle slightly forward? If not, you likely have the common tendency to lean backwards rather than forwards, leading with your hips. This undermines most aspects of healthy, natural walking. Even though it will likely feel very awkward, it is important that you learn to shift your hips back (leave your behind behind) and lean more forward when walking.

3 ASSESS FOUR KEY ASPECTS OF YOUR STRIDE

A helpful framework for healthy walking is the 4-point Checklist. The 4-point Checklist is one frame in the motion picture that is natural human gait.

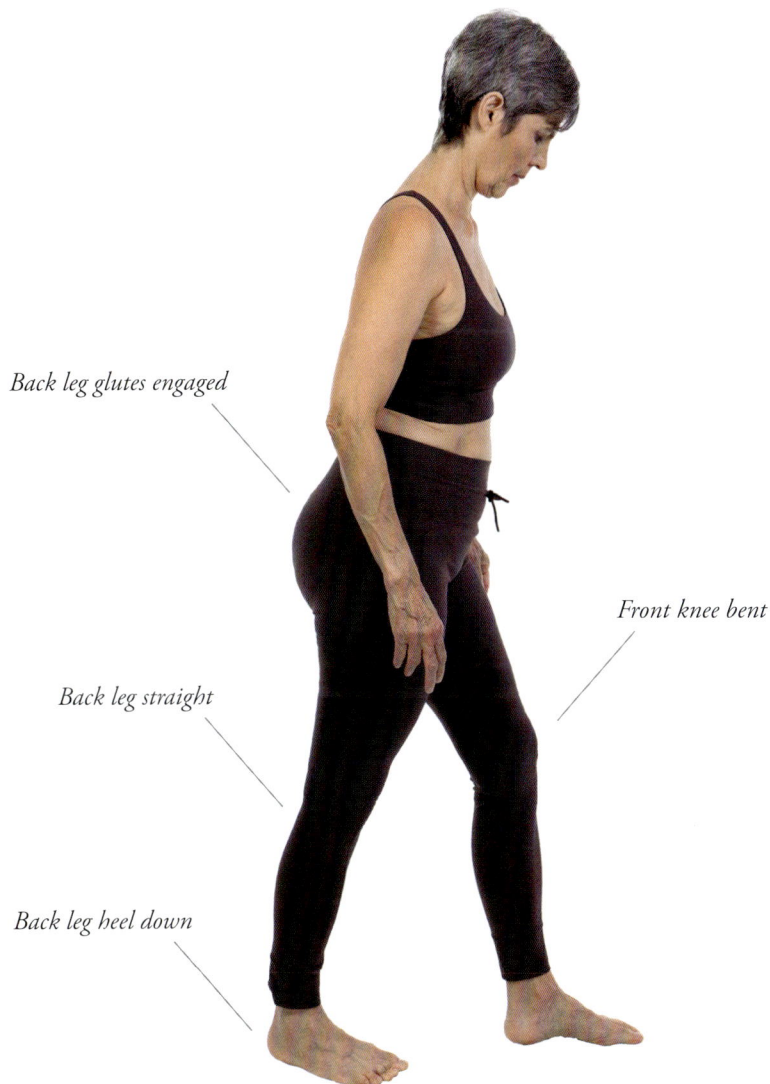

Back leg glutes engaged

Front knee bent

Back leg straight

Back leg heel down

EXAMPLES OF THE 4-POINT CHECKLIST WITH A FORWARD LEAN

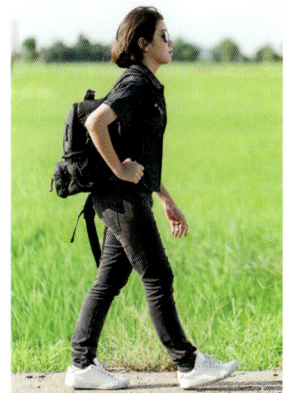

(Thailand)

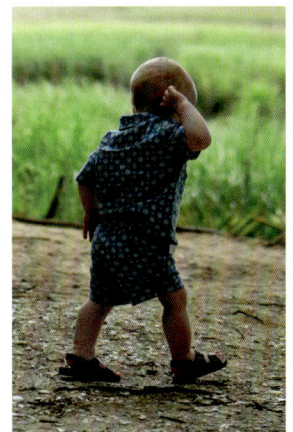

(USA)

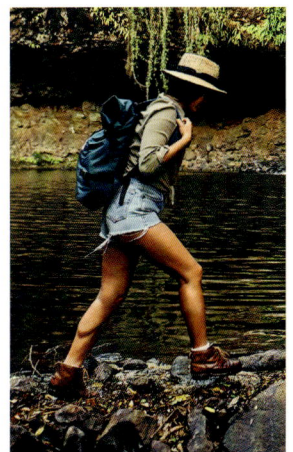

(Australia)

It is natural to lean forward when walking; this facilitates the 4-point Checklist.

Freeze the frame of the video just after your front foot reaches the ground. Assess the 4-point Checklist:

- ☐ Back leg glutes engaged
- ☐ Back leg straight
- ☐ Back leg heel down (or barely lifted)
- ☐ Front knee bent

Most beginners will find they need to work on several or all of these elements.

EXAMPLES OF THE 4-POINT CHECKLIST STANCE

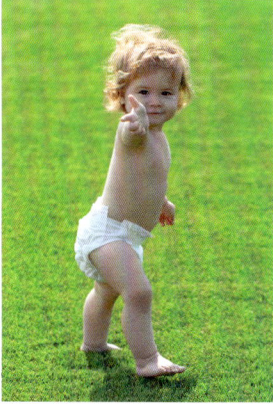

(USA)

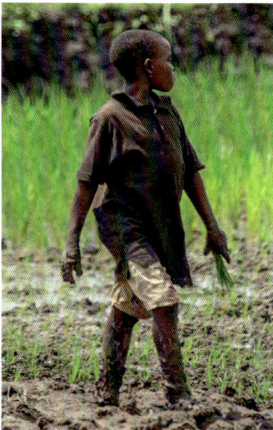

(Burundi)

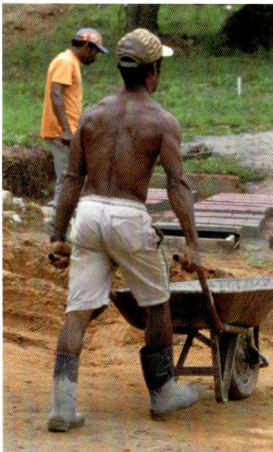

(Brazil)

PART B: PRACTICING THE 4-POINT CHECKLIST STANCE

1 BEGIN BY TALLSTANDING (SEE CHAPTER 6)

It's easier to start with healthy posture and maintain it than try to make corrections while moving. When setting up in tallstanding, pay special attention to the zigzag squat that settles the pelvis into anteversion.

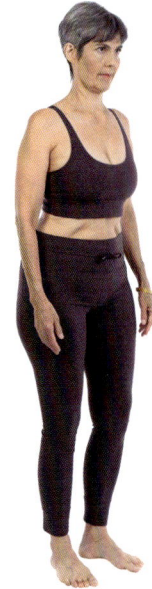

2 LEAN FORWARD FROM THE HIPS (SEE CHAPTER 7)

It's natural in walking for your torso to be more in line with your back leg than front leg. Imagine you are preparing to run; your buttocks move backward and your torso angles forward. This may feel strange for walking—as if you are leaning forward excessively— but is important for facilitating the 4-point Checklist. Glance at your reflection in a mirror and you'll likely see the angle is less marked than it feels.

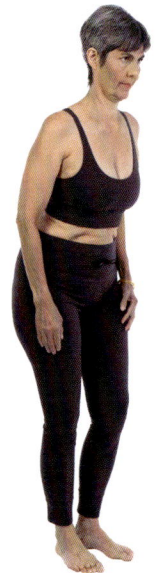

3 STRAIGHTEN ONE LEG AS YOU TRANSFER YOUR WEIGHT TO THAT FOOT, MOSTLY WEIGHTING THE HEEL

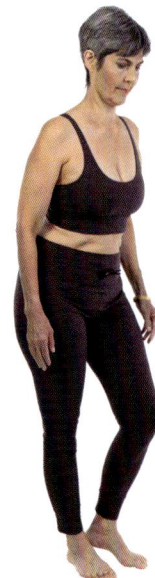

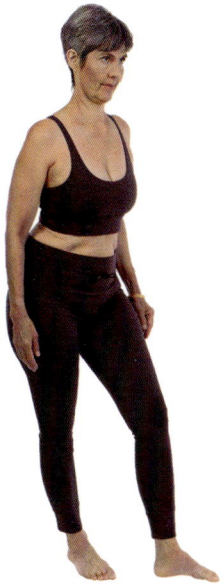

4 LEAVING YOUR HIPS RELATIVELY STILL AND YOUR WEIGHT ON YOUR BACK FOOT, MOVE YOUR OTHER LEG FORWARD

KEEPING THE "BEHIND" BEHIND WHEN WALKING

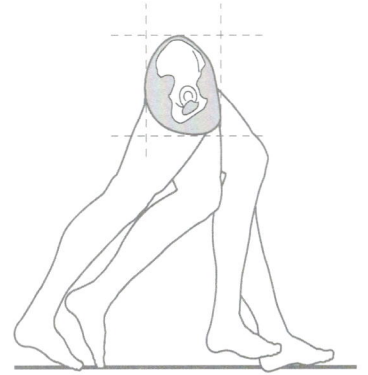

When viewed from the side, the position of the pelvis stays constant throughout the stride.

5 LAND YOUR FRONT FOOT ON THE GROUND AND GO THROUGH THE 4-POINT CHECKLIST

Adjust your body as needed.

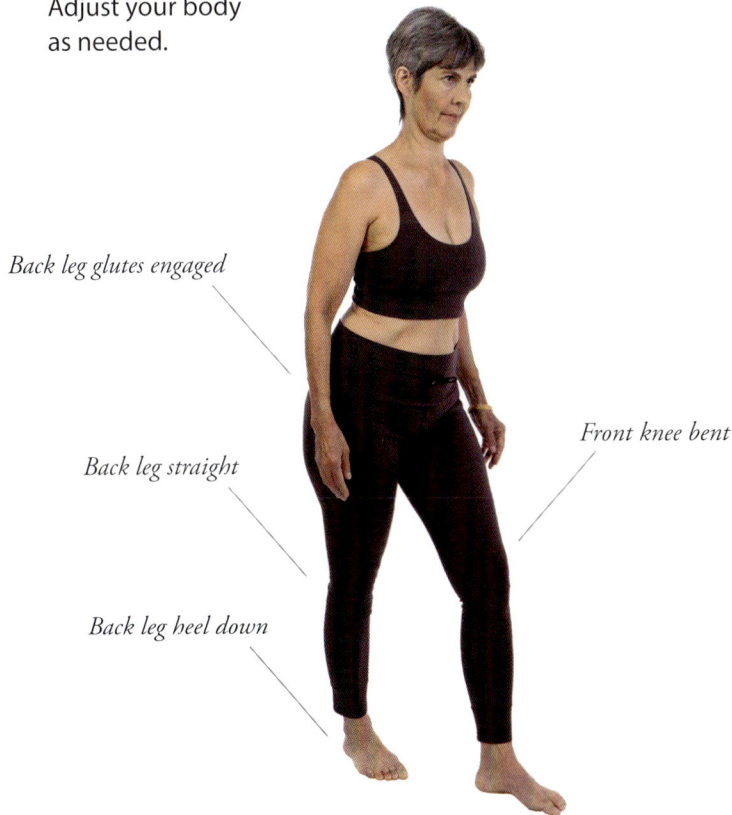

Back leg glutes engaged

Front knee bent

Back leg straight

Back leg heel down

6 REPEAT STEPS 4 AND 5, ADJUSTING FOR THE 4-POINT CHECKLIST AT THE END OF EACH STRIDE

EXAMPLES OF GLIDEWALKING

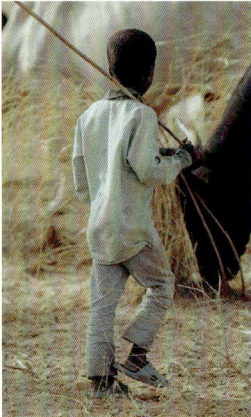

(Nigeria)

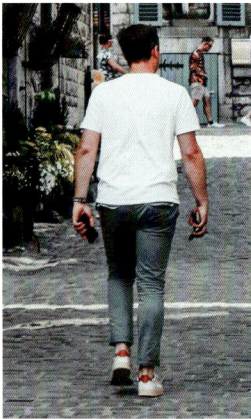

(Belgium)

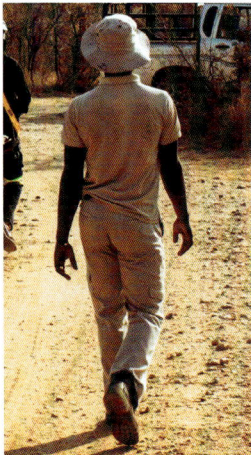

(Botswana)

7 NOW CHALLENGE YOURSELF TO LAND DIRECTLY IN THE 4-POINT CHECKLIST STANCE WITHOUT NEEDING ANY ADJUSTMENTS AFTER LANDING

It is helpful to pause and adjust for the 4-point Checklist just before landing: freeze frame your body when your front foot is about an inch (2.5cm) off the ground.

A common mistake is to tuck and/or lead with the pelvis.

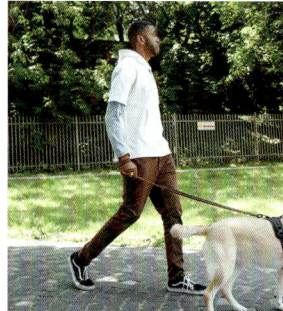

Migrate your hips back and lean forward from your hips so your weight is over your back heel. Pushing a chair on wheels, or imagining leaning into a hill or walking against a strong headwind may help.

DRILL: WALKING BACKWARDS

You may find that walking backwards reaching your back heel to the ground encourages elements of the 4-point Checklist to happen more easily.

1 START IN TALLSTANDING

2 ADOPT A ZIGZAG SQUAT, BENDING AT THE HIPS AND KNEES

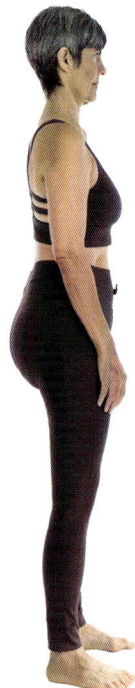

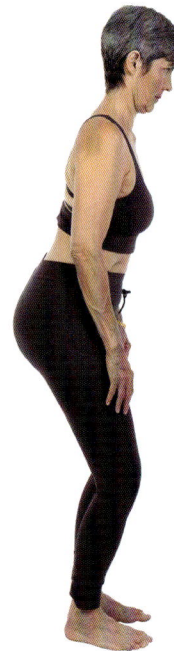

3 EXTEND YOUR LEFT LEG BACKWARDS, REACHING YOUR HEEL TO THE GROUND

Notice your left glutes engage and your left leg straightens while your right knee bends.

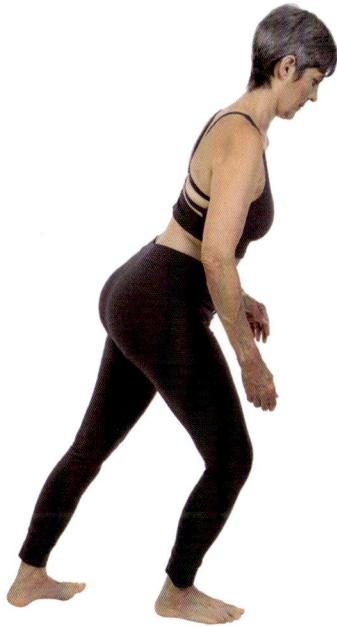

EXAMPLES OF THE 4-POINT CHECKLIST STANCE

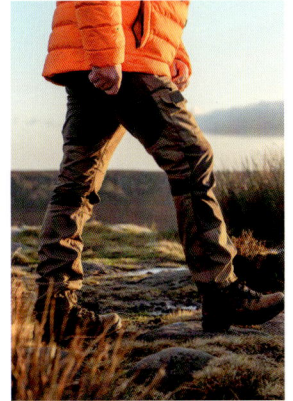

(UK)

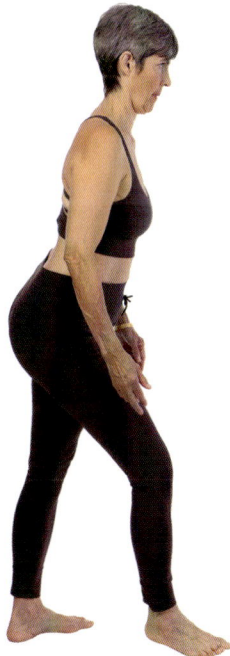

4 TRANSFER MOST OF YOUR WEIGHT TO YOUR LEFT FOOT

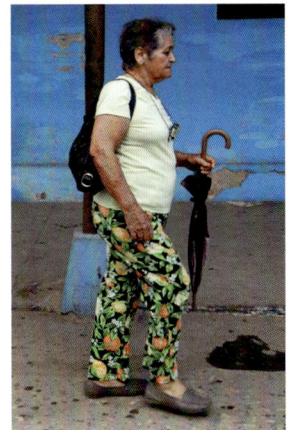

(Turkey)

5 GO THROUGH THE 4-POINT CHECKLIST, ADJUSTING AS NEEDED

☐ Back leg glutes engaged
☐ Back leg straight
☐ Back leg heel down (or barely lifted)
☐ Front knee bent

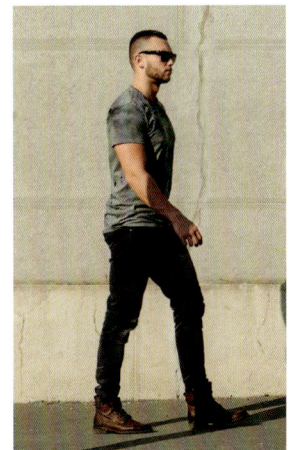

(Serbia)

A HEALTHY STRIDE

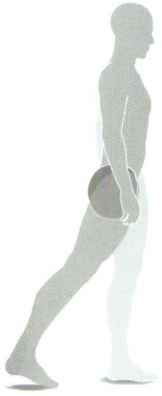

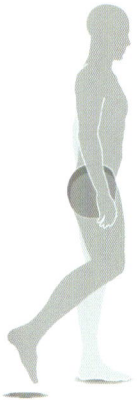

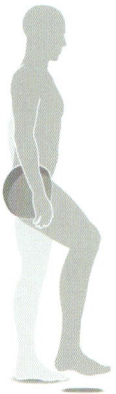

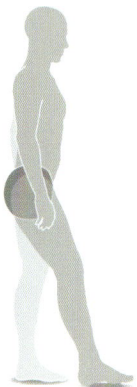

6 REPEAT STEPS 2–5, EXTENDING THE RIGHT HEEL BACKWARDS AS YOU CONTINUE TO LEAN FORWARDS

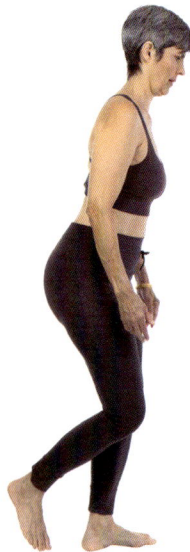

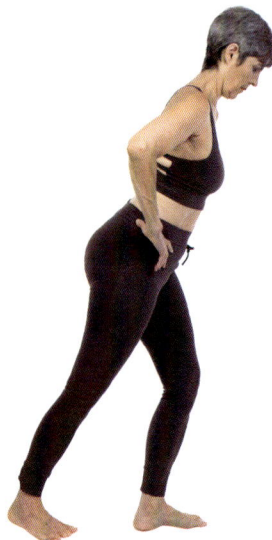

A common mistake is to not lean forward enough.

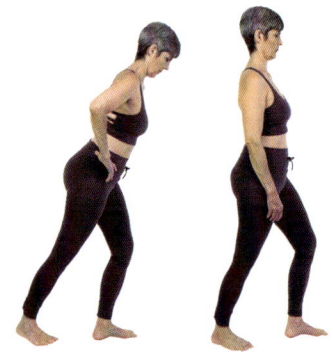

Another common mistake is to change the angle of the torso rather than keeping the incline constant during the entire stride.

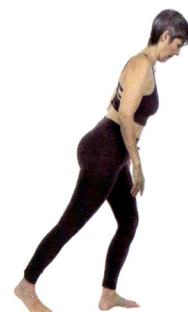

Once you have memorized the 4-point Checklist stance going backwards, look for the same stance walking forwards.

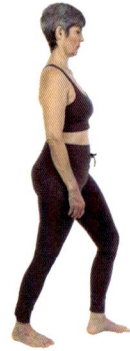

Avoid reaching the ball of the back foot, rather than the heel, to the ground.

PART C: BREAKING DOWN A STRIDE

This section examines the 4-point Checklist in the context of a stride. Here we will talk about the leg-coming-forward and the leg-going-back, rather than the "front leg" and the "back leg."

LEG-GOING-BACK GLUTES ENGAGED

1 ADOPT THE 4-POINT CHECKLIST STANCE, WITH YOUR LEFT FOOT FORWARD

Make sure you are leaning forward from the hips so your behind is behind you; this places the glutes in a position of biomechanical advantage.

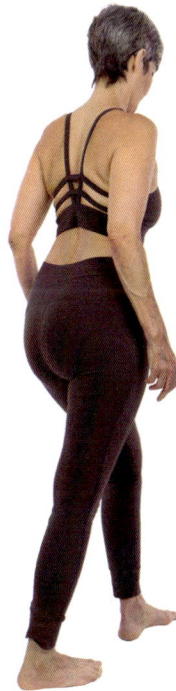

2 AS YOU BEGIN TO TRANSFER YOUR WEIGHT TO YOUR FRONT (LEFT) FOOT, INCREASINGLY CONTRACT YOUR LEFT BUTTOCK

The left leg begins to straighten.

You would like all the left buttock muscles to engage, including *gluteus medius* (in the upper outer quadrant of your buttock). Having your feet slightly pointed outwards (5–10°) and maintaining weight on your left foot enables and encourages this action.

USING THE BUTTOCKS FOR PROPULSION

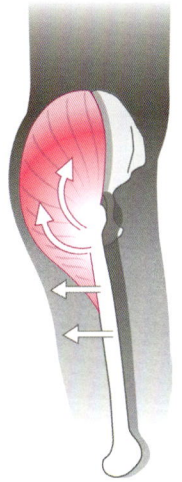

Contracting the buttock muscles pulls the upper part of the femur back within the flesh of the thigh.

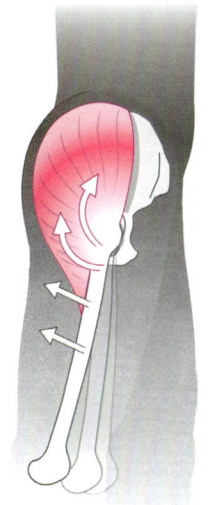

Further contacting the buttock muscles pivots the leg back relative to the torso. Because the foot is firmly positioned on the floor, this action propels the body forward.

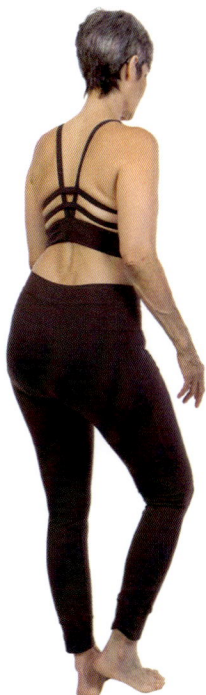

EXAMPLES OF
LEG-GOING-BACK
GLUTES ENGAGED

EXAMPLES OF LEG-GOING-BACK GLUTES ENGAGED

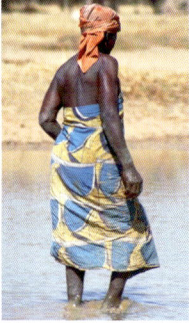

(Burkina Faso)

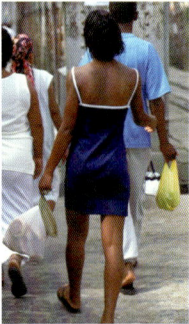

(Brazil)

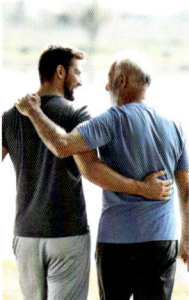

(Serbia)

Strong gluteal activation in gait facilitates pelvic anteversion, better balance, and powerful forward propulsion of the body.

3 CONTINUE STRONGLY SQUEEZING YOUR LEFT BUTTOCK AS YOU TAKE A STEP FORWARD

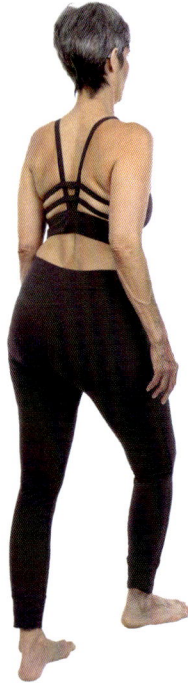

Do not allow the contraction of your gluteal muscles to be abrupt, causing a jerky, upward, prancing motion. Rather, make the contraction crescendo, compelling a smooth forward propulsion.

At the end of Step 3 you should be in the 4-point Checklist stance with your right foot forward.

4 IN EACH SUCCESSIVE STRIDE, FOCUS ON CONTRACTING THE BUTTOCK OF THE LEG-GOING-BACK

If you find it challenging to quickly switch your focus from one side of the body to the other, try focusing on a single side at a time (i.e., every other stride).

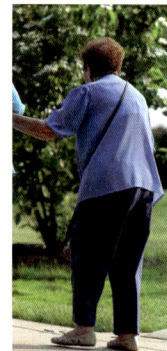

A common mistake is to not keep the gluteal muscles engaged until the heel of the leg-coming-forward touches the ground. This will result in a heavy landing.

In case your gluteus medius needs strengthening, the exercise on page 213 will assist you in locating and toning this muscle.

The Backwards Walking Drill on page 178 is also an effective way to practice engaging the gluteal muscles.

LEG-GOING-BACK STRAIGHTENS

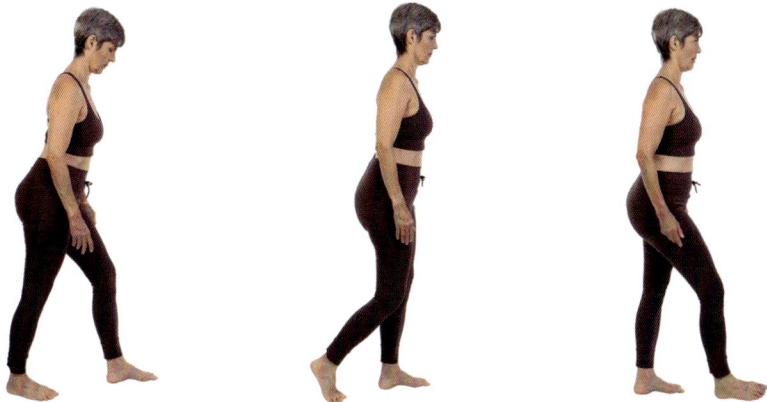

Each step starts with a bent front knee…

…which becomes straight by mid-stride…

…and remains straight to become the straight back leg of the 4-point Checklist.

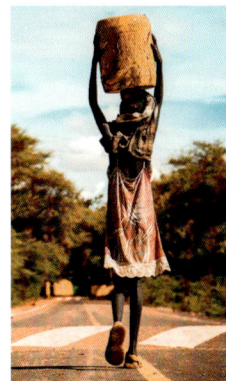

(Kenya)

1 ADOPT THE 4-POINT CHECKLIST STANCE, WITH YOUR LEFT FOOT FORWARD

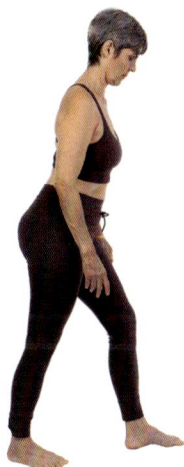

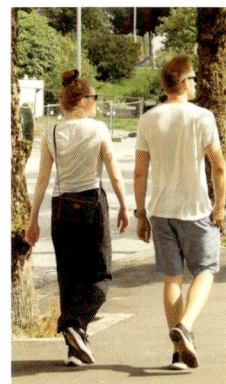

(Norway)

2 DO THE FOLLOWING ACTIONS SIMULTANEOUSLY TO ARRIVE AT MID-STRIDE:

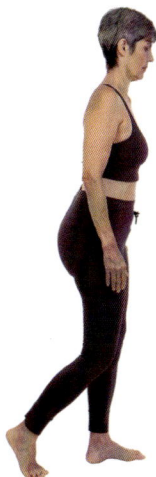

- Straighten out your front (left) knee
- Transfer your weight to your front (left) foot
- Relax all the muscles in your back (right) leg while rolling onto the point of the big toe of your back foot

Notice your knees are now next to each other and your hips are stacked above them. Your leg-going-back (left leg) should be straight (but not locked).

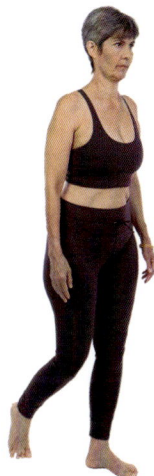

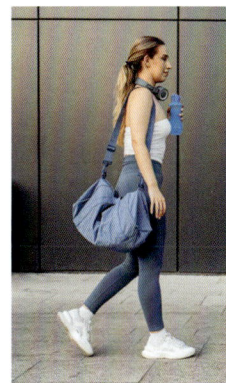

(Serbia)

EXAMPLES OF THE LEG-GOING-BACK REMAINING STRAIGHT UNTIL THE COMPLETION OF THE STRIDE

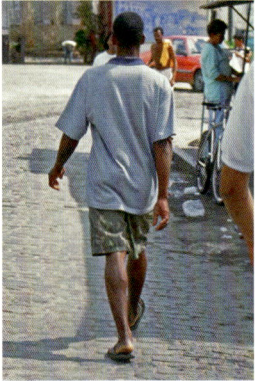

(Brazil)

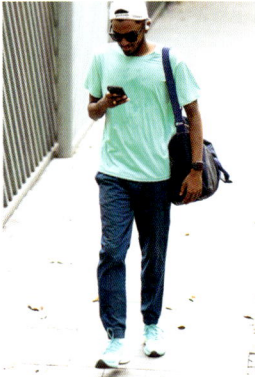

(India)

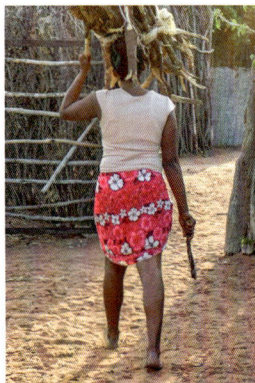

(Botswana)

Keeping the back leg straight facilitates stretch in the psoas and calf.

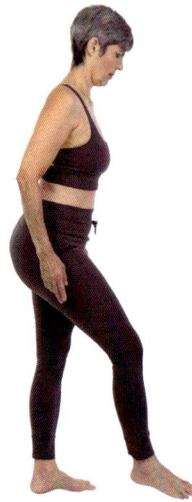

3 **KEEP THE LEG-GOING-BACK (LEFT LEG) STRAIGHT, AS THE LEG COMING FORWARD SWINGS OUT AHEAD**

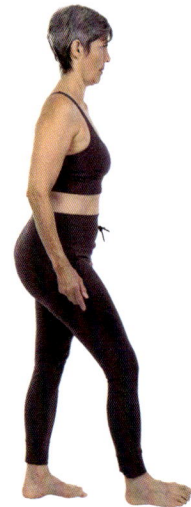

4 **LAND YOUR RIGHT FOOT, HEEL SLIGHTLY BEFORE THE REST OF THE FOOT**

At this point, your back (left) leg should still be straight, but the heel may begin to lift if you took a large step.

5 **REPEAT STEPS 2–4 SLOWLY, ALTERNATING LEGS**

Gradually build up speed until you are confidently able to maintain straightness in the leg-going-back at a brisk pace.

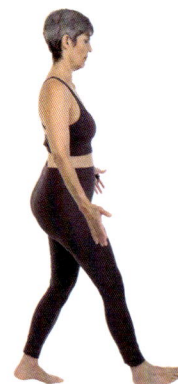

A common mistake is to straighten the leg too late or not keep the leg straight through the completion of the stride.

Another common mistake is to take strides that are too long for the current state of weakness/tightness in your muscles.

LEG-GOING-BACK HEEL DOWN

EXAMPLES OF LEG-GOING-BACK HEEL DOWN

1 ADOPT THE 4-POINT CHECKLIST STANCE

Make sure you are leaning forward from the hips, so your behind is behind you.

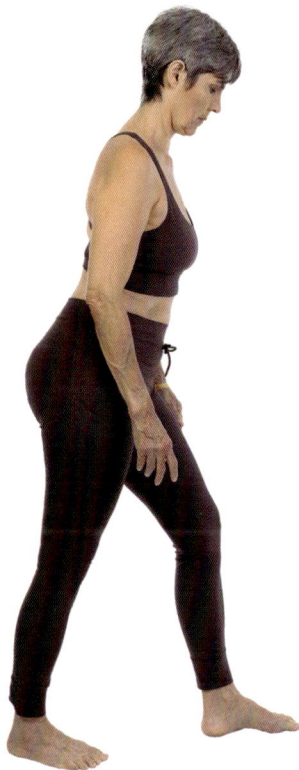

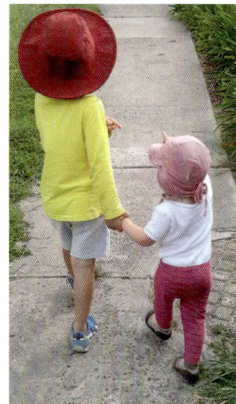

(Australia)

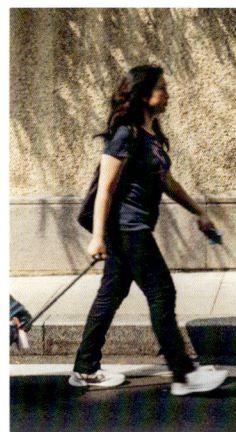

(China)

2 PROCEED TO THE 4-POINT CHECKLIST STANCE ON THE OTHER SIDE

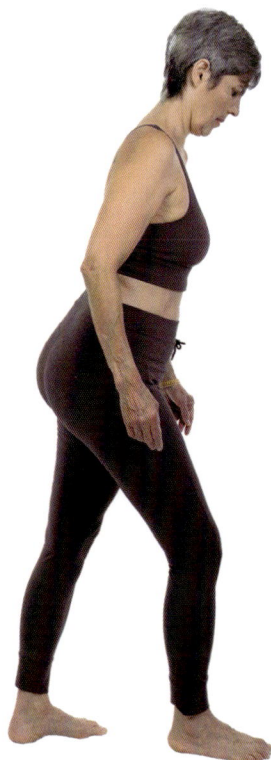

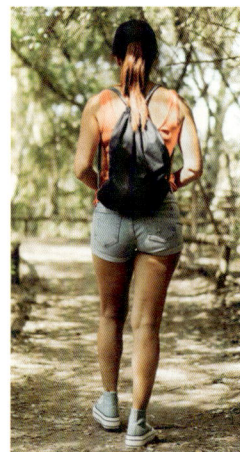

(Spain)

Keeping the weight in the back heel protects the front of the foot from unhealthy pressure.

EXAMPLES OF LEG-GOING-BACK HEEL DOWN

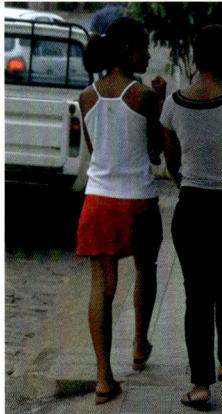

(Brazil)

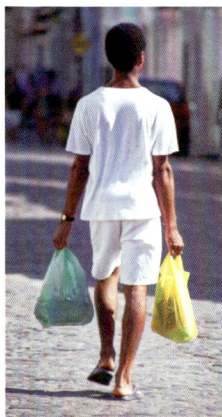

(Brazil)

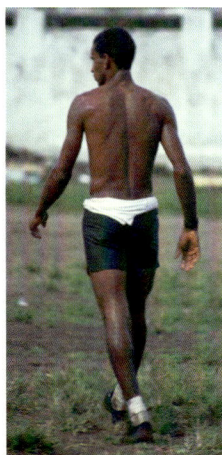

(Brazil)

3 WALK SLOWLY WITH SMALL STEPS, CHECKING THAT YOUR BACK HEEL STAYS DOWN—WITH MUCH OF YOUR BODY'S WEIGHT ON IT—FOR THE DURATION OF THE STRIDE

Use a visualization to help you keep your back heel down:

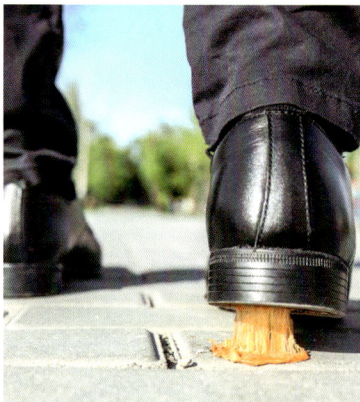

Gum stuck to the bottom of the heel

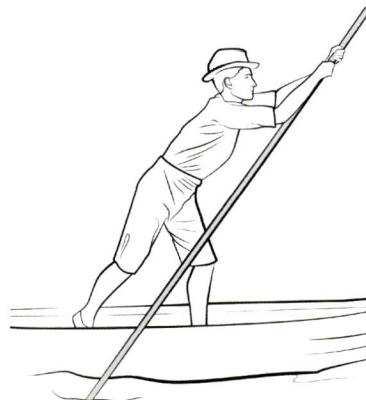

The heel as the point of a ski pole, walking pole, or punting pole, driving into the ground

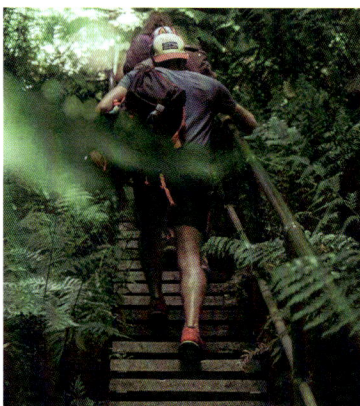

Walking uphill

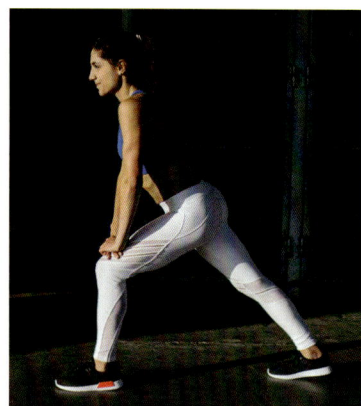

Doing a calf stretch

4 GRADUALLY INCREASE YOUR WALKING SPEED AND STRIDE LENGTH TO NORMAL

You may notice that with the increased stride length, your back heel begins to lift off the ground before your front foot lands. This effect should be quite small, and is a part of natural walking. On page 188, you'll learn to grip the ground with your feet; this action keeps your foot shape intact, protecting you from damage even when the heel is raised.

LEG-COMING-FORWARD KNEE BENT

1 ADOPT THE 4-POINT CHECKLIST STANCE

Make sure you are leaning forward from the hips, so your behind is behind you. This makes meeting the ground with a bent front knee easier.

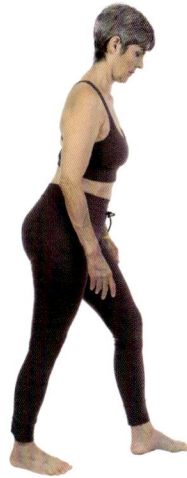

2 TAKE A STEP, FOCUSING ON LANDING WITH A BENT FRONT KNEE

3 TAKE SEVERAL SLOW STEPS, FOCUSING ON LANDING WITH A BENT KNEE

It can help to imagine you are climbing a hill. Your knee will be slightly bent, and your lower leg will align vertically. Note that the bend does not need to be exaggerated; a small bend is sufficient to cushion your joints.

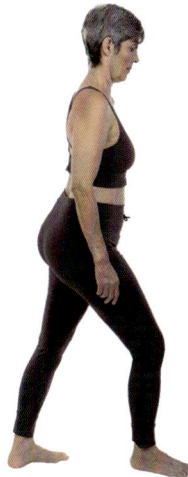

4 GRADUALLY INCREASE YOUR SPEED

⊗

Try to avoid these common mistakes:

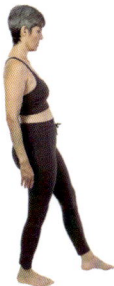 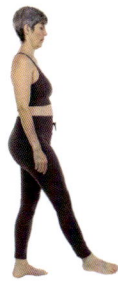 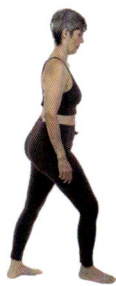 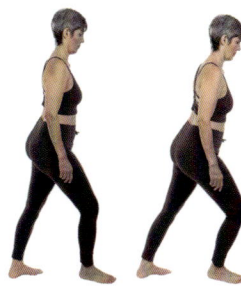

Not leaning forward enough.

Landing on a straight leg and then bending the knee, rather than landing with the knee already bent.

Landing on a bent knee, but then sinking into a deeper bend.

EXAMPLES OF LEG-GOING-FORWARD KNEE BENT

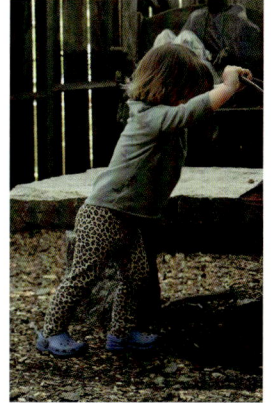

(USA)

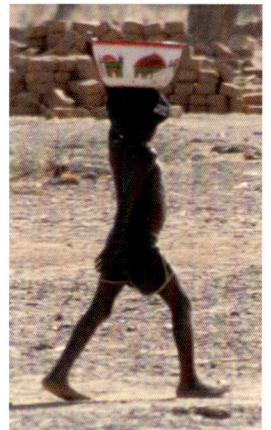

(Burkina Faso)

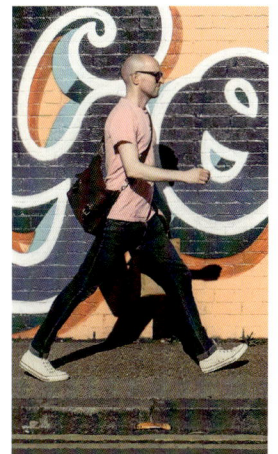

(UK)

Landing with a bend in the front knee protects the knee joint from damage.

EXAMPLES OF FEET GRABBING THE GROUND

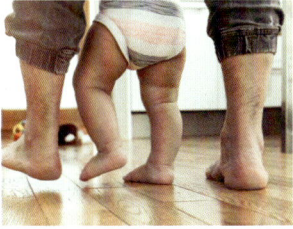

(Slovenia)

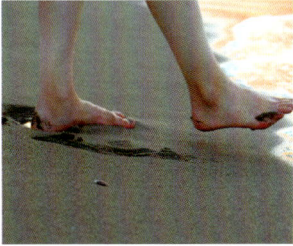

(Turkey)

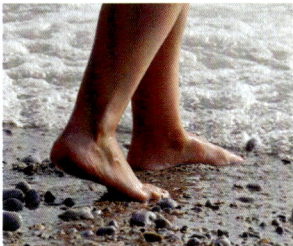

(Turkey)

PART D: ACTIVE FOOTWORK

In this section, you will relearn to grip and push the ground with your feet as you walk. This is a part of normal walking, is protective for the feet, and creates power and speed.

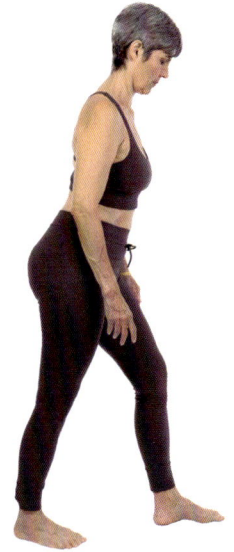

1 ADOPT THE 4-POINT CHECKLIST STANCE, WITH YOUR LEFT FOOT FORWARD

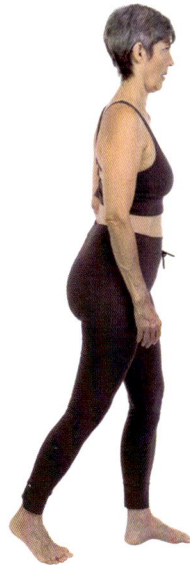

2 TRANSFER WEIGHT TO YOUR FRONT (LEFT) FOOT WHILE BEGINNING TO CONTRACT THE ARCH MUSCLES OF THE LEFT FOOT

The aim is to contract the muscles forming all three arches of the foot (the *inner*, *outer*, and *transverse arches*).

3 INCREASINGLY CONTRACT YOUR LEFT FOOT ARCH MUSCLES AS YOU COMPLETE THE STRIDE

Your foot will first pull and then push the ground backwards.

Your foot grabs the ground in sync with the glute action (see page 181) on the same side. Both foot and glute engagement crescendo to reach maximum squeeze at the end of each stride.

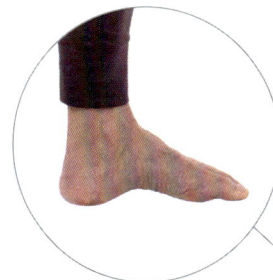

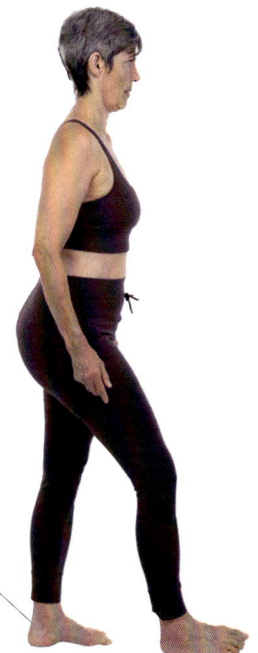

4 REPEAT ON THE OTHER SIDE, FOCUSING ON CONTRACTING THE "FOOT-GOING-BACK"

It may help to imagine the following:

- Jumpstarting a broken treadmill using your feet
- Grabbing clumps of dirt or grass in the savanna
- A monkey's feet grabbing branch after branch, swinging through the forest.

5 WHEN YOU CAN RELIABLY GRIP THE GROUND WITH EACH STEP, PRACTICE PUSHING OFF OF THE BIG TOE AT THE END OF EVERY STRIDE

Keeping the arch muscles contracted during push off mostly preserves the convex shape of your foot. This prevents strain in the forefoot and plantar fascia.

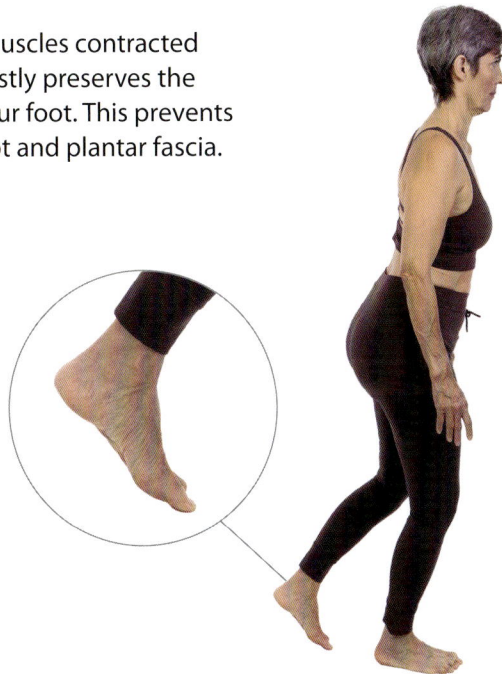

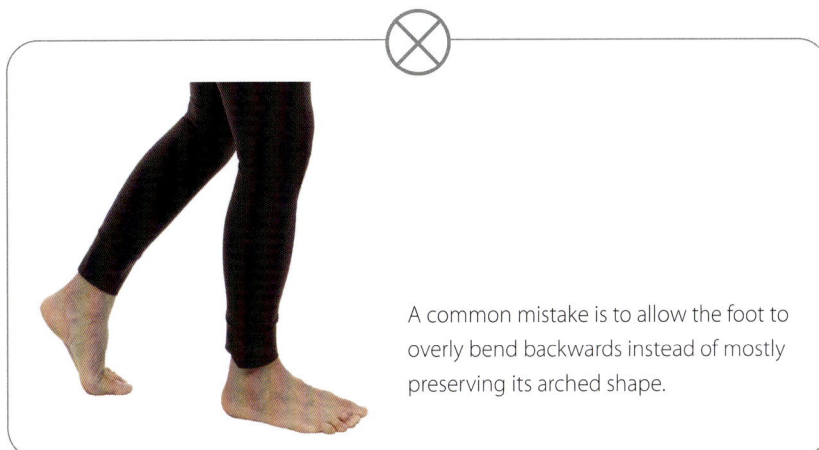

A common mistake is to allow the foot to overly bend backwards instead of mostly preserving its arched shape.

EXAMPLES OF FOOT ARCH MUSCLE ENGAGEMENT AT PUSH OFF

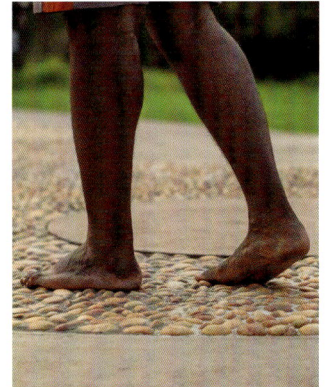

(India)

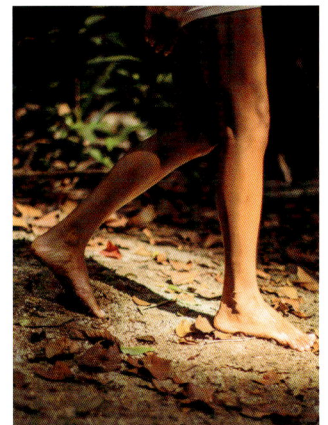

(Thailand)

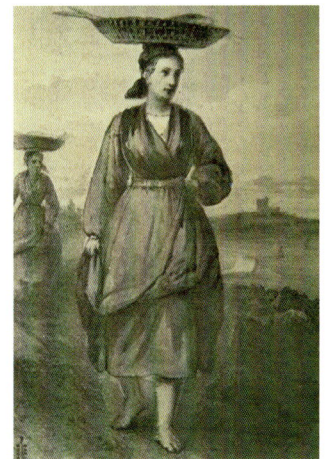

(France)

EXAMPLES OF HEALTHY
RELAXATION IN THE
LEG-COMING-FORWARD

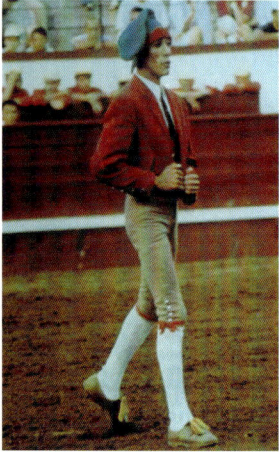

(Portugal)

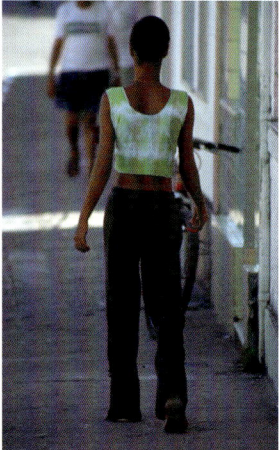

(Brazil)

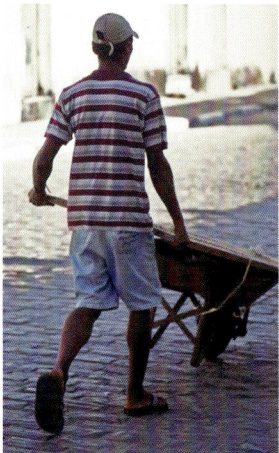

(Brazil)

PART E: THE PASSIVE PHASE OF WALKING

So far, the focus has been on the action in the leg-going-back:
the muscles of that leg, foot, and buttock contract strongly to propel
you forward in each stride. In a healthy gait, the passive phase is as
important as the active phase. As the front foot and leg increasingly
take your weight, the muscles in the back leg that have just worked
hard can profoundly relax as the leg swings forward.

1 ADOPT THE 4-POINT
CHECKLIST STANCE, WITH
YOUR LEFT FOOT FORWARD

Your right leg is straightened behind
you, your right buttock is contracted,
and your right heel is pressed into
the ground.

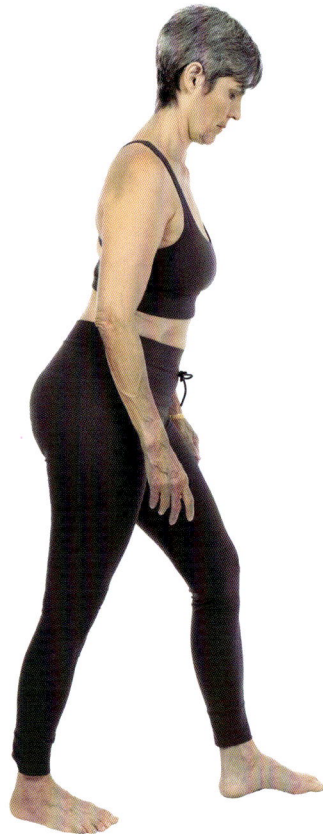

2 SHIFT YOUR WEIGHT ONTO YOUR
LEFT LEG BY STRAIGHTENING
IT UNDERNEATH YOU

Maintain your forward lean and
check that your hips haven't tucked
or migrated ahead of your left heel.

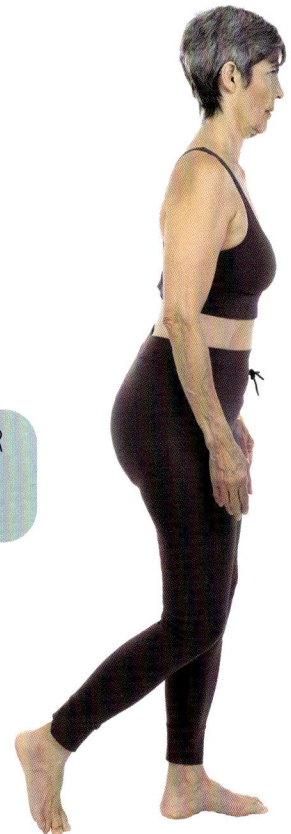

3 COMPLETELY RELAX ALL THE MUSCLES IN THE RIGHT LEG

Allow the right foot to pivot onto the tip of the big toe, the knee to bend, and the thigh to hang vertically and freely from its socket. (This is only an approximation of what happens in actual walking, where the right foot becomes airborne.)

Note: you may need to shorten your stride to allow the thighs to line up vertically when you pivot on the point of the big toe.

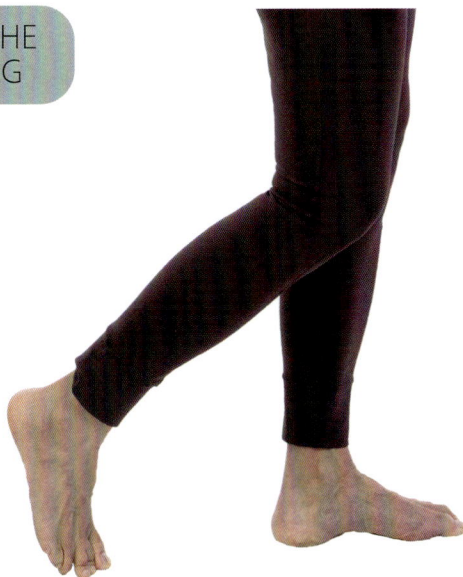

4 CHECK THAT YOUR RIGHT LEG IS RELAXED: PLACE YOUR RIGHT HAND ON YOUR RIGHT THIGH AND GIVE A GENTLE PUSH

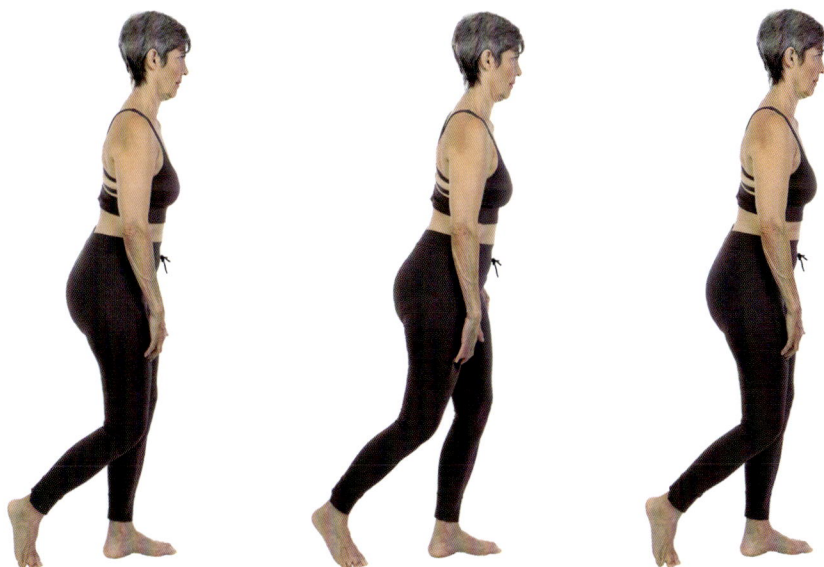

Your right leg should swing freely like a pendulum, with the big toe resting on the same spot on the ground. It will likely take some practice to relax all the muscles in the entire leg so that it truly dangles. It may help to think of your leg going limp or your knee hanging heavily towards the ground.

5 PRACTICE THIS TRANSITION FROM ENGAGEMENT TO RELAXATION IN THE LEG-COMING-FORWARD ON BOTH SIDES

THE LEG AS A PENDULUM

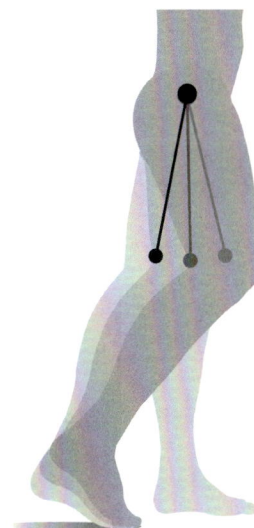

When the muscles around the hip joint relax during the passive phase of the stride, the leg-coming-forward will dangle and swing like a pendulum.

191

EXAMPLES OF THE PASSIVE PHASE OF WALKING

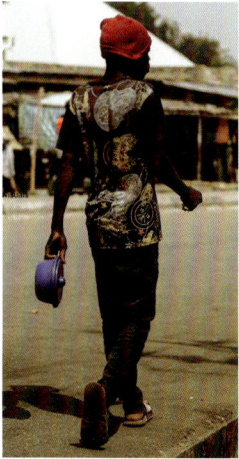

(Nigeria)

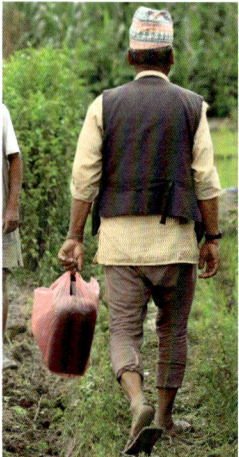

(Nepal)

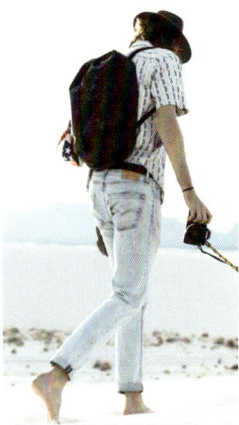

(USA)

PART F: PUTTING IT ALL TOGETHER: REFINING YOUR GAIT

As you walk, each leg alternates between an active, weight-bearing phase and a passive, swing phase. The active phase contributes power and speed to your gait; the passive phase contributes relaxation and grace. In this section, you will combine the phases to walk with strength *and* grace.

Because this is the most complex technique in the book, it is easy to feel overwhelmed. Only add the following refinements after you have digested the basics of glidewalking.

TRANSITION FROM ACTIVE PHASE TO PASSIVE PHASE

Take several steps. Focus on the transition between the active phase and the passive phase in only one of your legs. After a while, switch your focus to that transition in your other leg.

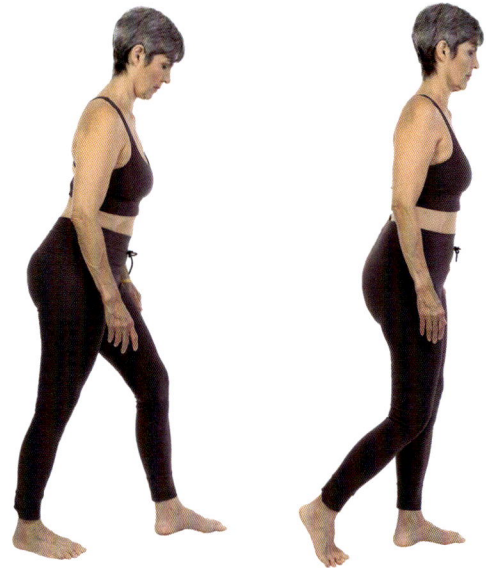

You want to feel the following changes:

	LEG-GOING-BACK	LEG-COMING-FORWARD
WEIGHT POSITIONING	Non-weight-bearing → Weight-bearing	Weight-bearing → Non-weight-bearing
LEG ACTION	Relaxed → Contracting; Bent → Straight	Contracting → Relaxed; Straight → Bent
FOOT ACTION	Relaxed → Contracting	Contracting → Relaxed

As you practice, focus on one cell of the table above at a time. (Note: this table presents a partial description of walking transitions; nuances such as "relatively relaxed" and "relatively non-weight-bearing" have been glossed over for the purpose of simplicity.)

You want these transitions of weight and work from one leg to the other to become ingrained in your muscle memory and not need your attention.

If you find it difficult, as most students do, to alternate between extreme contraction and extreme relaxation in your muscles, slow your pace to give yourself more time to track the transitions.

KNEE AND HIP POSITIONING AT MID-STRIDE

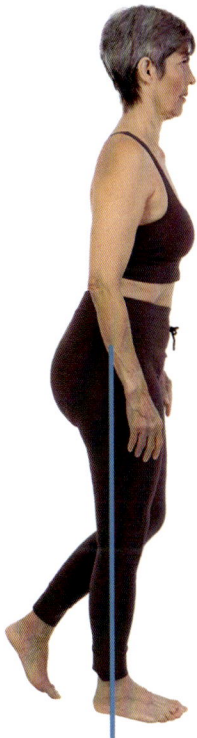

Pause in your gait just as your back knee settles alongside your front knee. Check your hip position in a mirror. At this point in the step, your pelvis should be anteverted and stacked over the straightened, vertical, weight-bearing leg.

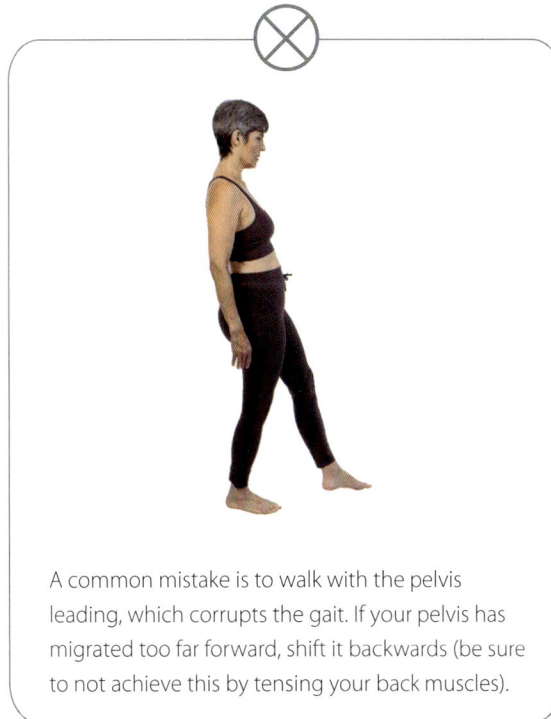

A common mistake is to walk with the pelvis leading, which corrupts the gait. If your pelvis has migrated too far forward, shift it backwards (be sure to not achieve this by tensing your back muscles).

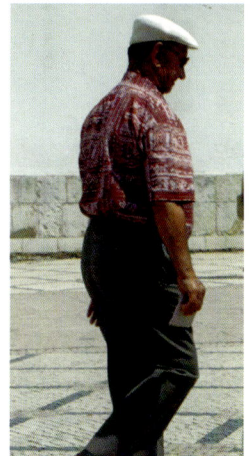

(Portugal)

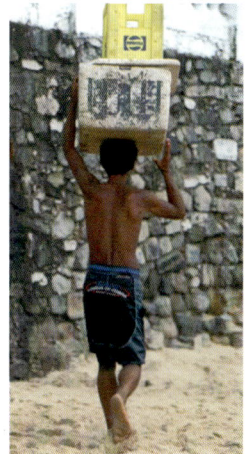

(Brazil)

FOOT POSITIONING

WALK ON A LINE, WITH THE INNER EDGE OF EACH HEEL TOUCHING THE LINE, AND THE FRONT OF THE FOOT ANGLED 5–10° OUTWARDS

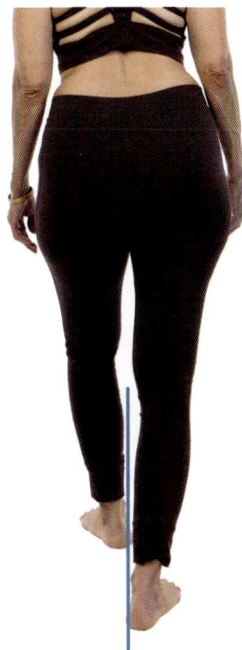

Find a surface with lines, such as a hardwood floor or striped carpet, and straddle one line. Walk in the direction of the line, noticing the orientation of your feet as they contact the floor.

You may feel your inner thigh muscles (*adductors*) working to bring your inner heels to this line.

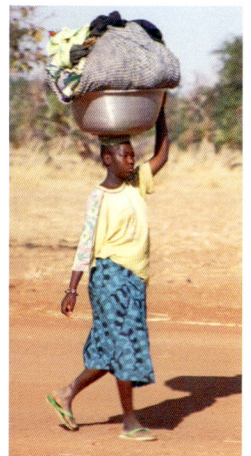

(Burkina Faso)

EXAMPLES OF WALKING ON A LINE WITH FEET ANGLED OUTWARDS

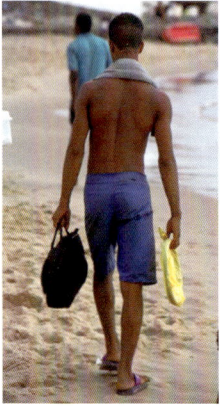

(Brazil)

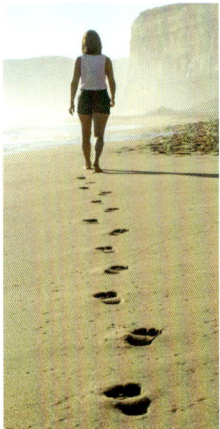

(Australia)

EXAMPLE OF HEALTHY SHOULDER POSITION WHILE WALKING

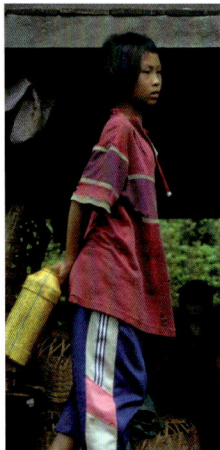

(Thailand)

Common mistakes include:

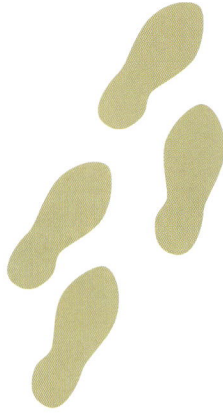

Pointing the toes in

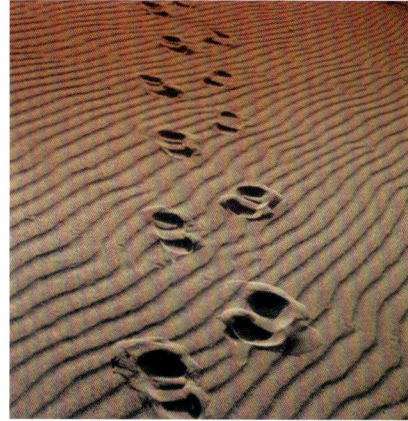

Pointing the feet out excessively

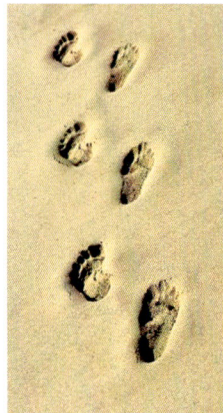

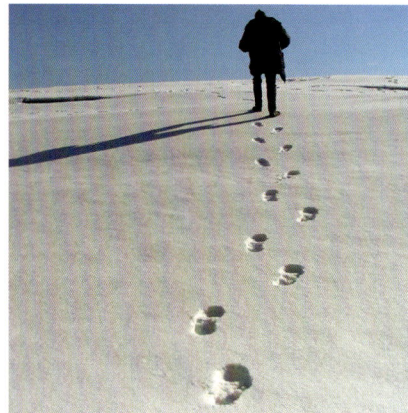

Walking on two lines

UPPER BODY POSITIONING

Anchor your ribs, lengthen the back of your neck, and do a shoulder roll with each shoulder. Then place your arms behind your back with one hand clasping the other hand or wrist. This will help you position your shoulders in a healthy way without having to pay attention to them. Try to position the backs of your wrists on your buttocks. This will help you monitor the action of your gluteal muscles. Most students feel they are leaning exaggeratedly forward when they walk correctly; resist the urge to "straighten up."

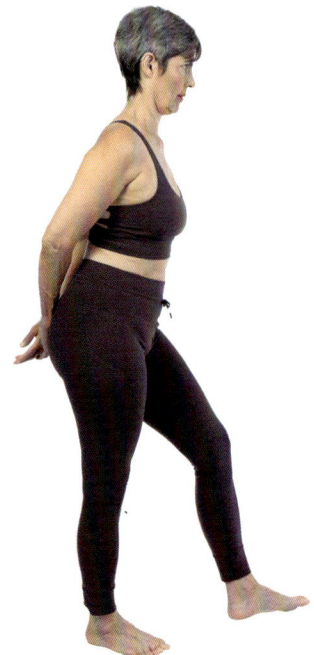

EXAMPLES OF GLIDEWALKING

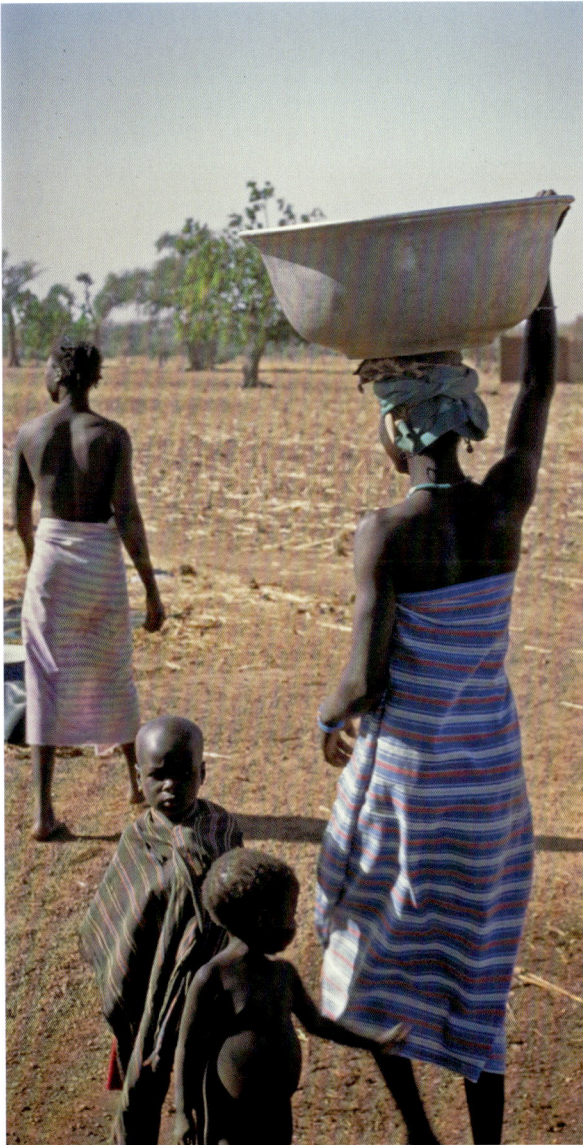

(Burkina Faso)

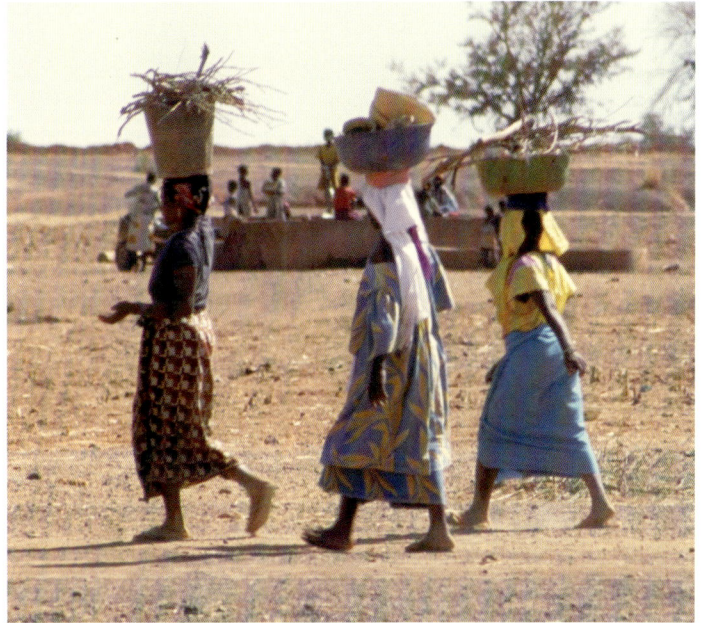

(Burkina Faso)

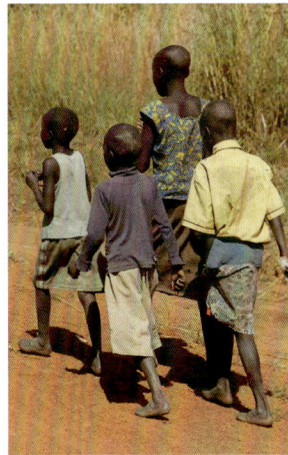

(Uganda)

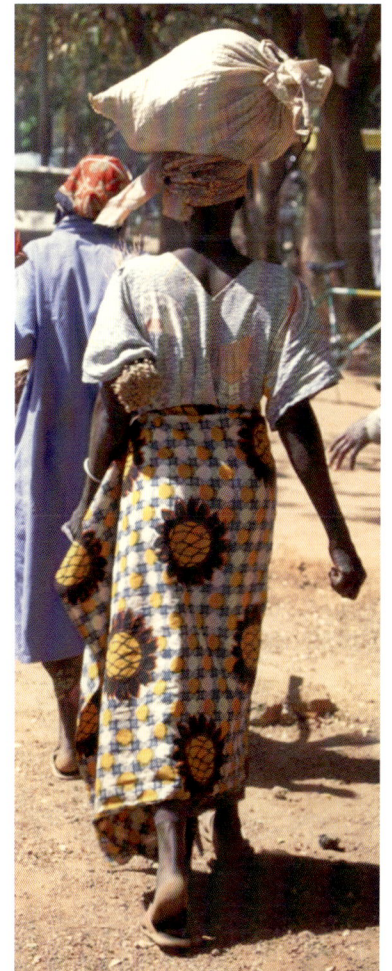

(Burkina Faso)

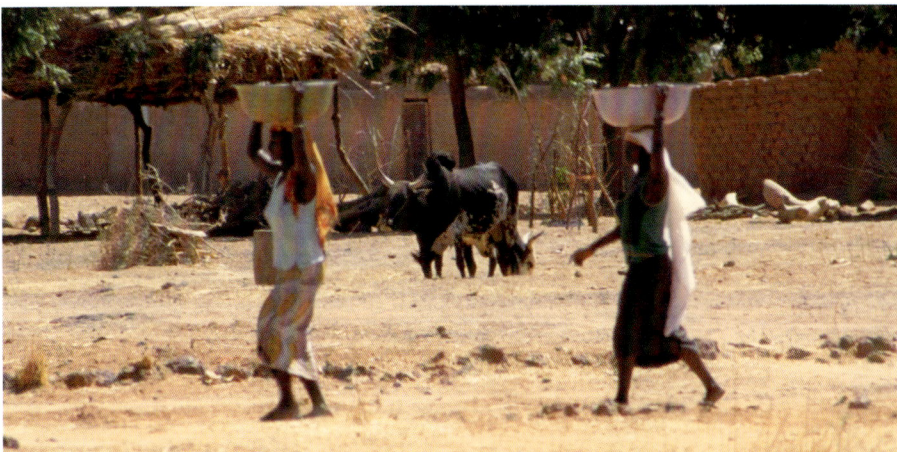

(Burkina Faso)

INDICATIONS OF IMPROVEMENT

Your musculature may change profoundly in the first weeks of learning to glidewalk. Students often report that their glutes are sore the day after their first walking session. Over time, they develop stronger, firmer glutes. Every step done well is similar to the "donkey kick" exercise on page 213, adding up to a lot of repetitions.

When your walking becomes a series of controlled forward propulsions, your tread is lighter, your movement is more graceful, and your walking experience becomes smoother and calmer. Over time you will strengthen the gluteal, leg, and foot muscles, and, from walking briskly, the inner corset. You may notice additional length in your psoas muscles, where previously they were tight.

This book is, of course, a static medium. Just as it is difficult to learn to play tennis or golf from a book, expect glidewalking to also be difficult to learn from a book. At some point you will benefit from working with a coach. Our community of Gokhale Method teachers around the world offer coaching, in-person and online, to help you learn and master glidewalking. See gokhalemethod.com for more information.

TROUBLESHOOTING

FEELING THAT YOU ARE LEANING FORWARD
If you felt as though you were leaning forward in tallstanding, glidewalking is likely to feel very peculiar. We teach a natural, slight forward lean as part of glidewalking technique. If you are used to arching back in your stance and gait, this slight forward lean is going to feel like an extreme forward lean. A glance in the mirror will reassure you that you do not look as strange as you feel, and that, in fact, your stance looks rather athletic. The forward lean puts the glutes in a position of mechanical advantage so they can work optimally; it also facilitates the other elements of the 4-point Checklist.

TENDENCY TO TUCK OR LEAD WITH THE PELVIS
Even if you understand the concept of leaving your pelvis anteverted throughout your gait, you may find that you have a strong tendency to tuck or lead with the pelvis. Understanding why this is so can help reduce the tendency.

You have probably been using your thigh *(quadriceps)* muscles to advance your front leg and pelvis in your gait. Now you need to use your psoas muscle to advance your front leg and your buttock (gluteal) muscles in the rear leg to advance your pelvis. Whereas your quads can work more efficiently when your pelvis is tucked, your psoas and gluteal muscles work more efficiently when your pelvis is anteverted. Changing your pelvic position changes much of the muscle action underlying your gait. This may not be an easy transition, but sticking with it will yield many benefits.

UNSURE OF GLUTEAL ACTION
You can check for gluteus medius action in the back leg with your fingertips in the upper outer quadrant of the buttock. Press firmly to feel the contraction; it is somewhat like a bicep bulging. Over time, as your glutes strengthen and the sensation of contracting these muscles becomes more familiar, the coordination with the forward propulsion will become clearer. You will no longer need to use your quadriceps inappropriately to move forward.

SORENESS IN THE HIPS, GROIN, OR LOWER BACK
If you have a tight psoas muscle, too long a stride will pull your lower back into a sway and/or inflame the attachment on the *lesser trochanter* of the femur (inner thigh). Try taking smaller strides. This will have the added advantage of allowing your back heel to remain in contact with the ground for longer, improving your balance. As glidewalking becomes your habit, you will find your psoas muscles gradually lengthen and you will no longer need to restrict your stride length.

LOSING TRACK OF YOUR POSTURE
When learning this new gait, students often regress in their overall posture, returning to old habits. Pause for a moment to reset your shoulders, your neck and head, and your lower back. Be careful not to tuck or lead with the pelvis, or sway the lower back in an effort to "straighten up." Look at Troubleshooting in

Chapter 6 for reminders on how to align the shoulders and achieve optimal stacking. Tying your arms behind your body (see fig.6-13 on page 143) will help you align your shoulders without having to pay attention to them.

CANNOT COORDINATE ALL THE ELEMENTS OF GLIDEWALKING

For some people it is very difficult to edit their deeply ingrained walking pattern. If you find the material in this chapter too challenging, try an alternative approach: learn and practice the basic Samba step! Chances are, you do not know how to dance the Samba, so you will start with a clean slate, with nothing to unlearn. You can learn the glidewalking motion without the difficulty of unlearning your old gait. This approach works very well.

Learning the Samba

The step taught here is slightly different from the classic three-beat, hip-swinging Samba. This version emphasizes the movements needed for glidewalking (fig.8-10).

1. Take a small step back with the right leg and press the heel into the ground, straightening the right leg and tightening the right buttock muscles. You will need to bend the left (front) knee a little to enable the back heel to reach the floor. This constitutes the first beat.
2. Hold that position for a second beat.
3. Move the right leg forward to return to the starting position.
4. Perform the same motions with the left leg: step back, press the heel into the ground, straighten the leg, and contract the buttock muscles; hold for a beat; return to the starting position.
5. Repeat the movements, alternating the left and right legs, until the movements become familiar.

When you have mastered this movement on both sides and have "memorized" the stance of the first beat (i.e. the 4-point Checklist stance), step *forward* into the same stance. Practice this with each leg, going forward and holding each pose for one beat. Next, practice moving forward, alternating steps and smoothing out the action until it feels like walking. You have just learned the glidewalking motion without the difficulty of unlearning your old gait.

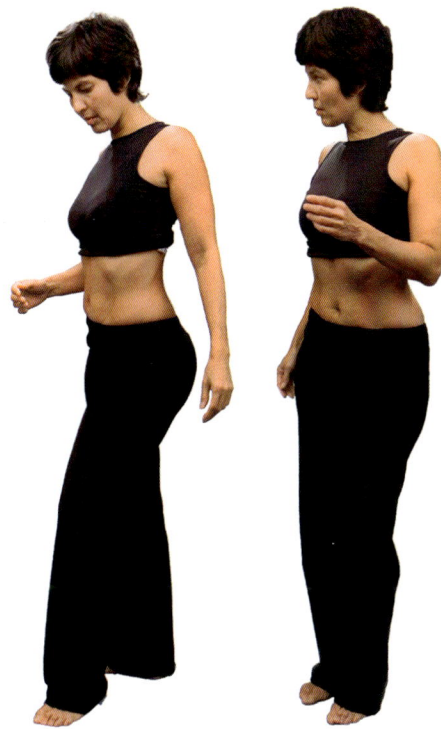

fig.8-10

Learning walking through a modified Samba step provides a "clean slate" that can be very effective.

FURTHER INFORMATION

Glidewalking is complex. We have curated some videos of people glidewalking at gokhalemethod.com to help educate and inspire you.

GLIDEWALKING VIDEOS

WALKING ON ONE LINE

The feature of "walking on one line" that you learned in "Leg-Going-Back Heel Down" on page 193 has an interesting anthropological history. The oldest known human footprints were found at the Laetoli site in the Olduvai Gorge in northern Tanzania (fig.8-11). They consist of two parallel tracks, thought to belong to an adult and a child. Both individuals walked "on a line;" that is to say, the inner heels of each individual touched a single line. This finding has been used as evidence of evolutionary distance between the ancient pair and modern man. The argument, which is correct, is that modern man walks on two lines. But walking on two lines is a very recent cultural distortion in modern industrialized societies. Modern man in more traditional societies elsewhere in the world (as well as in our society until a century ago) walks on one line. The finding that the Laetoli duo walked on a line then becomes an argument not for evolutionary distance, but rather for evolutionary proximity to modern man.

fig.8-11

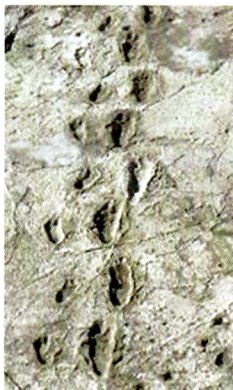

The Laetoli footprints, estimated to date from ~3.7 million years ago, show that the bipedal individuals walked "on a line," much as people do today in traditional cultures.

GETTING EXTRA POWER AND SPEED IN YOUR STRIDE

Many activities, such as running, hiking uphill, and skating, require extra power in each stride. In these activities we naturally lean forward to put our glutes in a position of maximum mechanical advantage (fig.8-12). The goal is to use the glutes in the same way when walking, which is typical in kinesthetically intact cultures. Using strong foot muscle activation to push ourselves forward will also contribute power and speed.

fig.8-12

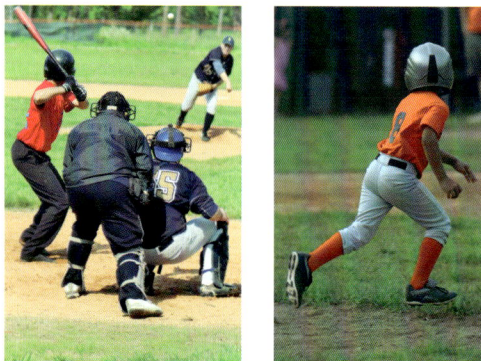

We naturally lean forward when doing demanding activities, as this puts the gluteal muscles in a position of mechanical advantage.

RUNNING

Although many of the principles of glidewalking transfer over to running, there are important additional principles that apply. For further information about "gliderunning" see our series of blog posts. The most important difference between glidewalking and gliderunning is that there is more impact in gliderunning than in glidewalking. The impact requires more recruitment of the inner corset (see Chapter 5) to prevent degeneration and damage.

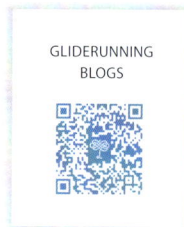

GLIDERUNNING BLOGS

If you have observed Kenyan and some other elite runners, you may notice that they run with upright torsos. Their stance may seem to contradict the theory that leaning forward puts your glutes into a position of mechanical advantage. Most of these elite runners have a marked angle at L5-S1, allowing for both an anteverted pelvis (providing the necessary mechanical advantage to the gluteal muscles) and an upright torso. The important factor is the anteverted pelvis, which these runners achieve without leaning forward (fig.8-13).

fig.8-13

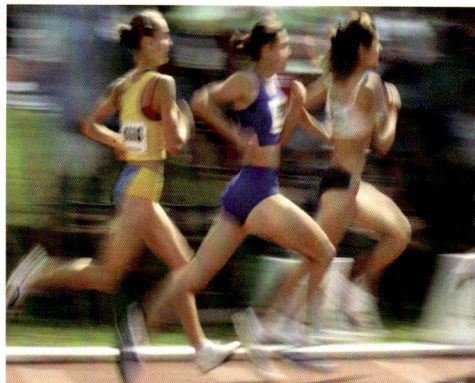

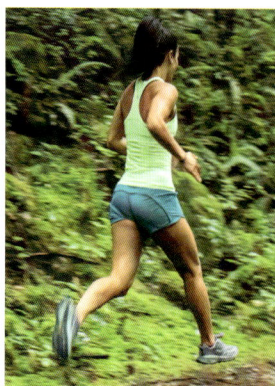

These elite runners show both an anteverted pelvis and an upright torso.

RECAP

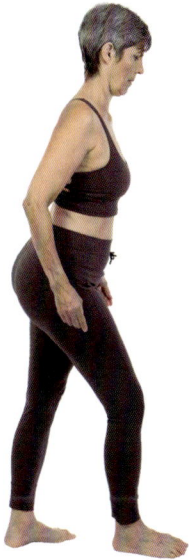

a. **Adopt 4-point Checklist stance, right foot forward; lean forward from hips**

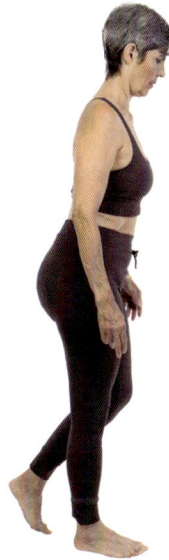

b. **Straighten right leg; tighten right buttock; press right heel into ground; relax and bend left leg**

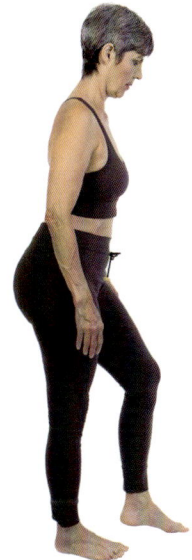

c. **Extend left leg forward; keep right leg straight, and right buttock and foot contracted**

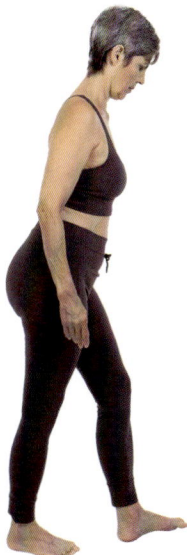

d. **Push off strongly through right heel; gently land left foot, heel first**

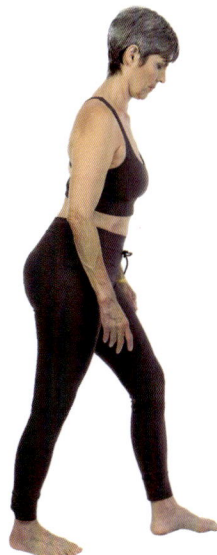

e. **Check left knee is bent and left foot points 5–10° outwards**

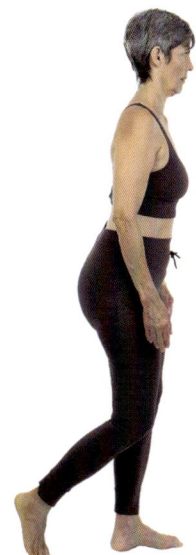

f. **Transfer weight to left foot; relax and bend right leg**

APPENDIX 1
OPTIONAL
EXERCISES

Strengthening and lengthening key muscles to accelerate your progress

One of the special benefits of the Gokhale Method is that it does not require setting aside time for special exercise regimens. However, you may want to perform a few optional exercises early in your training to help you reach a threshold level of strength or flexibility in key muscles. The exercises in this appendix are safe, efficient, and relevant to good posture. Eventually, you will not need them, because as you perform your daily activities with good form, and include appropriate physical exertion in your life, you will meet most of your muscle lengthening and strengthening needs in your everyday life. You will then be in a self-sustaining cycle of healthy posture supporting healthy musculature supporting healthy posture.

When you perform these exercises, especially if your muscles are not warm, be sure to tune in to your body. Do not push yourself to the point of injury or pain.

HOW MUCH AND HOW LONG?

In general, do as much as is comfortable. The exercises should leave you feeling pleasantly fatigued. Many people find it feels right to hold each stretch or pose 30 seconds to a minute. If repetitions are involved, try starting with eight to ten, in two sets.

The exercises are organized into the following categories:

- Strengthening torso muscles

- Strengthening key muscles used in walking

- Strengthening and stretching shoulder muscles

- Strengthening and stretching neck muscles

- Stretching key muscles connecting the torso and legs

EQUIPMENT

You will need the following:
- *A TheraBand™ or strap*
- *One or two pillows*
- *Rolls made of towels or cotton batting*
- *Hard synthetic balls of various diameters, from 1/2" (1cm) to 1" (2.5cm)*
- *A piece of sturdy fabric about 6' (2m) long*
- *A small hand towel or flannel square*
- *A steady object to lean on, such as a desk or counter*
- *A carpeted surface or mat*

STRENGTHENING THE TORSO MUSCLES

Three sets of muscles in your torso warrant your attention. The first, the "rib anchor," holds the front lower edge of the rib cage flush with the abdomen. This maintains the shape of the torso and helps eliminate a sway. The second and third sets of muscles comprise the "inner corset." They lengthen the torso and protect the spine from compression and possible injury. The front part of the inner corset includes the *obliques* and the *transversus*. The back part of the inner corset is composed of the deepest layer of back muscles, the *rotatores* and *multifidus*.

STRENGTHENING THE ABDOMINAL MUSCLES

The most important exercise for your abdominal muscles should occur throughout the day as they work to maintain the shape and length of your torso against gravity and stress. It is *for* performing this function that we want the abdominal muscles to be strong; it is *in* performing this function that the abdominals can become and remain strong. In our society, where many of us engage in sedentary activities for long hours, our abdominal muscles may not be adequately challenged throughout the day. Because they are not kept at a baseline level of strength, the muscles are not up to their task of protecting the spine.

The standard approach for strengthening the abdominals involves exercises such as sit-ups and crunches that distort the spine. Such exercises do strengthen the abdominals, but at the expense of discs and ligaments in the spine.

In the Gokhale Method, you use your abdominal muscles to prevent this distortion and maintain the shape of your spine. In this way you strengthen your abdominals in their natural function of preserving the shape of the spine.

Many exercises for the abdominal muscles are done lying on your back. You will begin by engaging the rib anchor to attain a safe and healthy baseline position.

ENGAGING THE RIB ANCHOR

1. LENGTHEN YOUR BACK AS YOU LIE DOWN, AS YOU LEARNED TO DO IN CHAPTER 2

You will work to preserve the shape of your spine as you do these exercises, but some distortion may occur. Lengthening your back at the start will prevent the distortion from causing problems to your discs. If you do not lengthen your back first and you have some compressed discs, any distortion from the exercises may cause damage.

2. USE ONE OR MORE PILLOWS UNDER YOUR HEAD AND SHOULDERS. PLACE YOUR ARMS COMFORTABLY AT YOUR SIDES

When you lie completely flat, the abdominal muscles are close to the end of their range of motion where they are at their weakest. The pillows help to rotate the rib cage forward, putting the abdominal muscles in a position of mechanical advantage. This way you will not strain your neck to achieve a favorable body configuration for working your abdominal muscles.

3. PRESS THE BACK OF YOUR RIB CAGE AGAINST THE FLOOR WITHOUT LIFTING YOUR "TAIL" OFF THE FLOOR. IT IS EASIEST TO FIND THIS ACTION ON THE EXHALATION. MAINTAIN THE POSITION WHILE CONTINUING TO BREATHE IN AND OUT

This is a difficult action for many people, but it is important to work toward achieving it. The idea is to isolate the action of the rib cage without tucking the pelvis. Slowing the action down will help you find this isolation. Consider placing your hand under your mid-back, and feel your rib cage pressing against your hand.

Now you are ready to proceed with the first set of exercises.

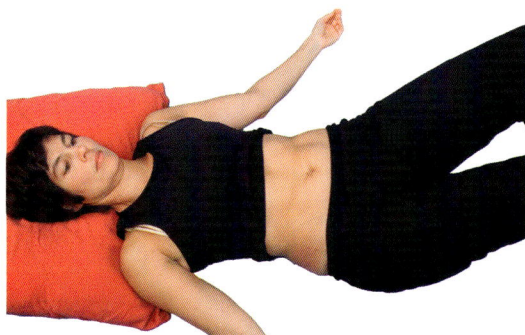

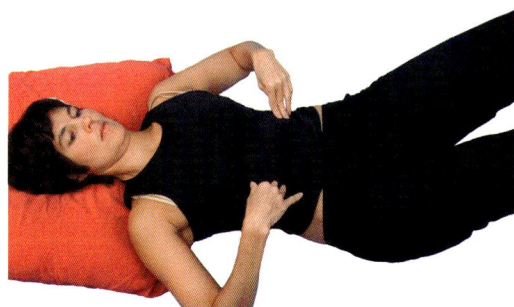

The following is a series of related, increasingly difficult exercises. It's important to master each exercise before progressing to the next.

CYCLING

1. FROM THE RIB ANCHOR POSITION, BEND YOUR KNEES AND BRING THEM TO YOUR CHEST

2. STRAIGHTEN YOUR LEGS SO THEY FORM A 90° ANGLE WITH YOUR TORSO

   Be sure to maintain even pressure against the floor with the back of your rib cage. You will find this especially difficult when moving your legs into and out of the starting position above your body. You must use your upper abdominal muscles to anchor your ribcage and prevent your back from swaying.

3. WHILE KEEPING THE BACK OF THE RIB CAGE PUSHING INTO THE FLOOR, ADD THE ACTION OF CYCLING WITH YOUR FEET

4. USE YOUR ABDOMINAL MUSCLES TO STEADY YOUR TORSO

   If your abdominal muscles are lax, your rib cage will lift from the floor, and your torso will tend to squirm from side to side.

5. WHEN THIS CYCLING EXERCISE FEELS VERY EASY AND YOUR ABDOMINAL MUSCLES ARE READY FOR A GREATER CHALLENGE, MOVE YOUR IMAGINARY BICYCLE PEDALS CLOSER TO THE FLOOR

   With your legs in this position, your abdominal muscles have to work harder to keep the back of your rib cage pressed against the floor. Make sure you do not over challenge your abdominals. Preserve the shape of the spine throughout the exercise. In this way, your abdominals get a good workout without damaging the discs and ligaments of the spine.

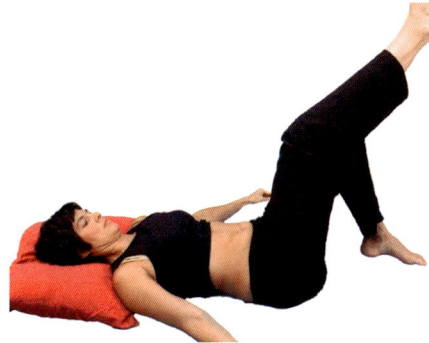

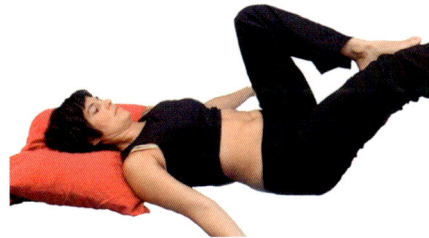

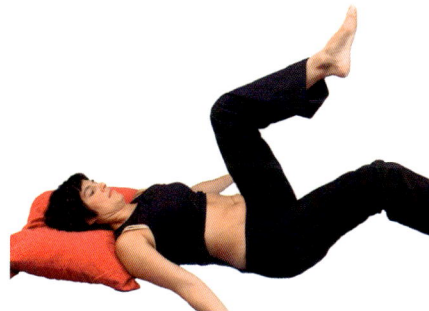

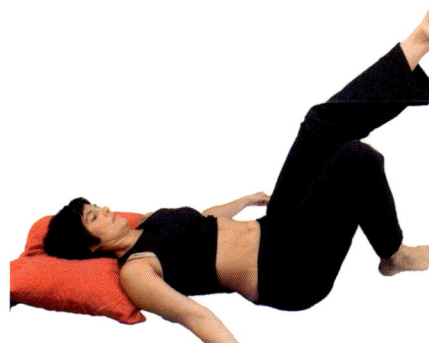

205

LEG SLIDE

1. FROM THE RIB ANCHOR POSITION, BEND YOUR KNEES AND PLACE YOUR FEET ON THE FLOOR

2. SLOWLY STRAIGHTEN ONE LEG, SLIDING THE FOOT ALONG THE FLOOR
Keep the weight of the foot light on the floor.

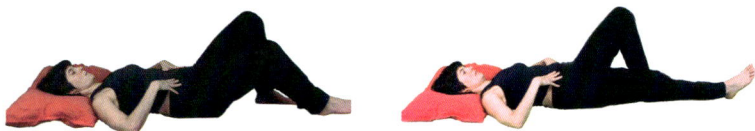

3. WHEN YOUR LEG IS NEARLY STRAIGHT, SLIDE THE FOOT BACK TO ITS STARTING POSITION
Throughout the range of motion, maintain the pressure of the back of your rib cage against the floor.

4. REPEAT THIS MOTION SEVERAL TIMES AND THEN SWITCH LEGS

5. AS YOUR ABDOMINAL MUSCLES STRENGTHEN, LIGHTEN THE WEIGHT OF YOUR FOOT ON THE FLOOR UNTIL YOUR FOOT IS OFF THE FLOOR

6. WHEN YOUR ABDOMINAL MUSCLES ARE READY FOR EVEN MORE CHALLENGE, DO THE SAME EXERCISE WITH BOTH LEGS AT ONCE

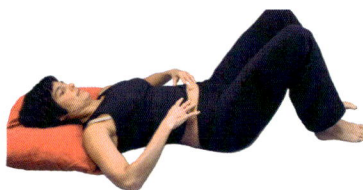

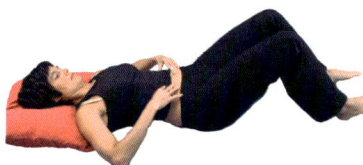

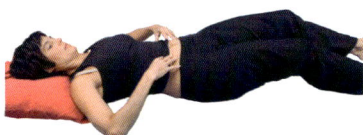

ARM RAISE

1. FROM THE RIB ANCHOR POSITION, RAISE YOUR ARMS TOWARD THE CEILING AND THEN OVER YOUR HEAD
Be sure to keep pressing the back of your rib cage against the floor. The most challenging position is when your arms approach the floor over your head. Raising the arms tends to rotate the rib cage backwards and sway your lower back. Your abdominal muscles are challenged to counteract this effect.

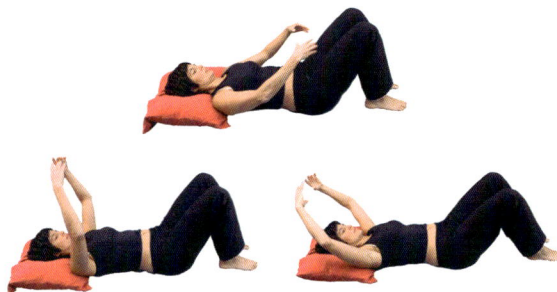

2. LOWER YOUR ARMS BACK TO YOUR SIDES

3. REPEAT THIS MOVEMENT A FEW TIMES
This exercise also patterns you to reach for things above your head without swaying your back.

4. WHEN YOU ARE FAMILIAR WITH THIS EXERCISE, COMBINE THE LEG SLIDE AND ARM RAISE EXERCISES
Remember to maintain the "J" shape of your spine while you are moving and stretching all four limbs. This is an excellent exercise for strengthening your core and patterning your muscles.

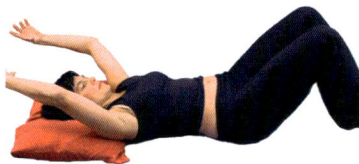

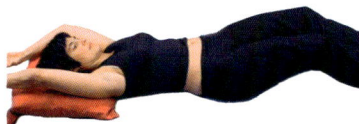

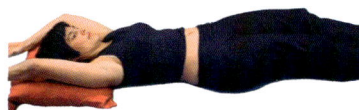

LEG LIFTS

1. FROM THE RIB ANCHOR POSITION, BEND YOUR KNEES AND BRING THEM TO YOUR CHEST

2. STRAIGHTEN YOUR LEGS SO THEY FORM A 90º ANGLE WITH YOUR TORSO

3. LOWER YOUR LEGS TOWARD THE FLOOR WITHOUT MOVING YOUR SPINE
   The challenge here is to keep your spine immobile as your legs travel through their range of motion. If you feel your rib cage begin to lift from the floor, you have gone too far.

4. RETURN YOUR LEGS TO THEIR STARTING POSITION

5. REPEAT THIS MOVEMENT SEVERAL TIMES

LEG SCISSORS

1. FROM THE RIB ANCHOR POSITION, BEND YOUR KNEES AND BRING THEM TO YOUR CHEST

2. STRAIGHTEN YOUR LEGS SO THEY FORM A 90º ANGLE WITH YOUR TORSO

3. SLICE YOUR LEGS THROUGH THE AIR IN A SIDEWAYS SCISSOR MOVEMENT
   a) Widen your legs.
   b) Bring them together.
   c) Cross one over the other, alternating which leg is on top.

4. FOR A GREATER CHALLENGE, MOVE YOUR LEGS CLOSER TO THE FLOOR
   Again, go only to the point where your abdominals are still able to press your rib cage firmly to the floor.

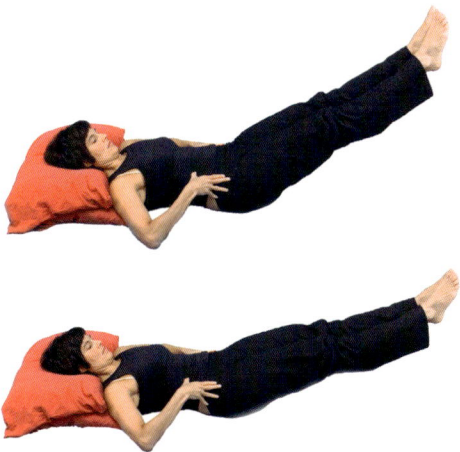

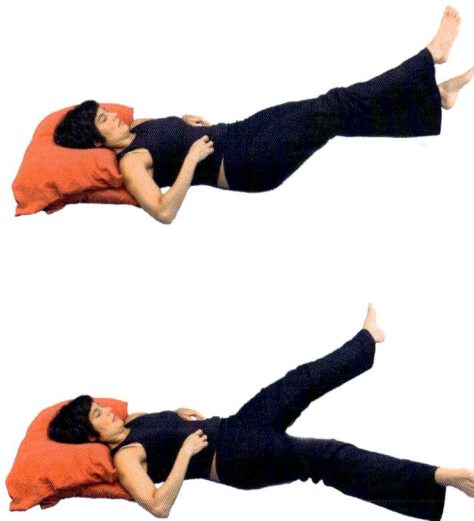

ALPHABET

1. FROM THE RIB ANCHOR POSITION, BEND YOUR KNEES AND BRING THEM TO YOUR CHEST

2. STRAIGHTEN YOUR LEGS SO THEY FORM A 90º ANGLE WITH YOUR TORSO

3. KEEPING YOUR LEGS TOGETHER AND STRAIGHT, USE THEM TO WRITE THE LETTERS OF THE ALPHABET IN THE AIR
   Be sure to keep your rib cage firmly pressed to the floor.

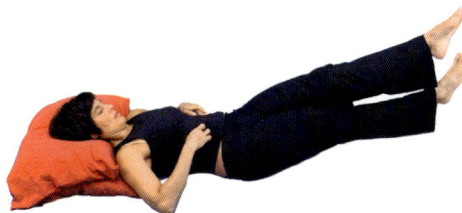

Three yoga poses are particularly effective for strengthening the abdominals: the plank, the side plank, and the boat. Engage your inner corset (Chapter 5) for extra safety and exercise while doing these poses.

PLANK

1. **GET INTO A POSITION ON ALL FOURS, WITH YOUR SHOULDERS DIRECTLY ABOVE YOUR HANDS AND YOUR HIPS DIRECTLY ABOVE YOUR KNEES**
   In yoga, this is known as Table Pose.

2. **ROLL OPEN YOUR SHOULDERS**

3. **EXTEND ONE LEG BACK WITH THE TOES CURLED UNDER, THEN EXTEND YOUR OTHER LEG**
   You are now in push-up position with your arms straight.

4. **CHECK YOUR POSITION AND MAKE THE FOLLOWING ADJUSTMENTS AS NECESSARY:**
   a. Aim for a J-spine and a straight line from your legs through your torso to your neck.
   b. Resist the tendency to sag or elevate the buttocks out of this line.
   c. Keep the shoulders rolled back and down. Use your muscles to maintain the original relationship between the shoulder blades and the spine.

5. **HOLD THIS POSITION UNTIL YOUR MUSCLES FATIGUE**
   As you gain strength, you will find you can hold the position longer and longer.

6. **REPEAT TWO OR THREE TIMES**

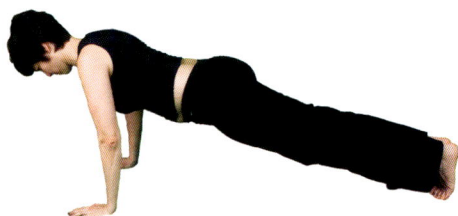

If you find this is too difficult for you, modify your position: Rest your upper body on your forearms rather than your hands, and/or rest your lower body on your knees rather than your feet.

SIDE PLANK

1. **LIE ON YOUR SIDE**

2. **ROLL YOUR SHOULDERS OPEN AND RAISE YOUR UPPER BODY ONTO YOUR LOWER ARM**

3. **RAISE YOUR HIPS OFF THE FLOOR SO YOU ARE BALANCING ON YOUR LOWER ARM AND FOOT**
   Your body should form a straight line. Don't let the hips sag toward the floor.

4. **HOLD THIS POSITION FOR A FEW SECONDS**

5. **REPEAT ON THE OPPOSITE SIDE**

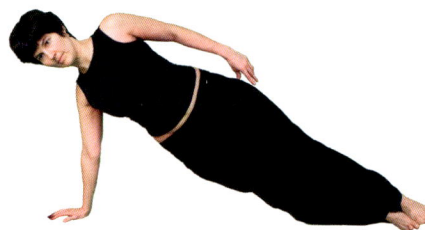

If you find this is too difficult for you, modify your position: Rest your upper body on your forearm rather than your hand, or rest your lower body on your knee rather than your foot.

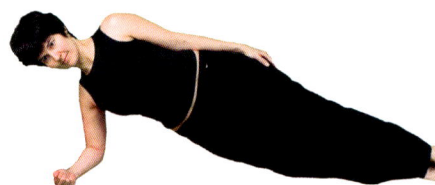

BOAT

1. **SIT ON THE FLOOR, WITH YOUR ARMS BEHIND YOU FOR SUPPORT AND WITH YOUR KNEES BENT**

   Be sure your shoulders are rolled back and down, your rib cage is strongly anchored, your inner corset is engaged (see Chapter 5), and your neck is well aligned with the spine.

   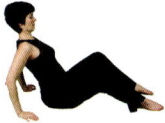

2. **GRADUALLY LESSEN THE WEIGHT ON YOUR HANDS UNTIL YOU CAN BRING THEM TO YOUR SIDES AND YOUR INNER CORSET FULLY SUPPORTS YOUR BACK**

   Be sure to maintain the alignment in the neck and shoulders.

   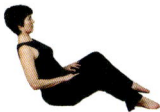

3. **LEAN BACK SLIGHTLY, REDUCING THE WEIGHT ON YOUR FEET, TO FIND A NATURAL BALANCE POINT**

   As you do this, work to maintain the original alignment throughout your torso.

   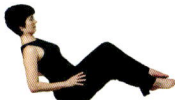

4. **LIFT YOUR FEET FROM THE FLOOR WITH BENT KNEES**

   Be sure you don't tuck your pelvis as you lift your feet.

   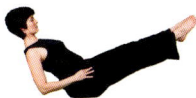

5. **IF POSSIBLE, STRAIGHTEN YOUR LEGS**

   Again, be sure to hold your torso steady.

6. **HOLD THIS POSITION UNTIL MUSCLE FATIGUE**

7. **REPEAT TWO OR THREE TIMES**

SAMBA

Another very effective—and fun—way to strengthen your abdominal muscles is to practice the Samba. Refer to page 197 in Chapter 8 to learn the basic dance steps. Then consider taking a class or finding an instructional video. You will learn to move your hips a great deal, motored by action in the legs, while your upper torso remains still or moves with a separate action. Isolating the actions of the upper and lower body challenges the abdominal muscles in complex and constantly changing ways. If you engage your inner corset to lengthen your torso as you twist and undulate, your abdominal muscles will get an even more intense workout and your back will be safeguarded.

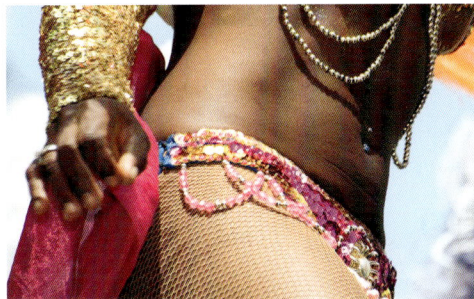

(Brazil)

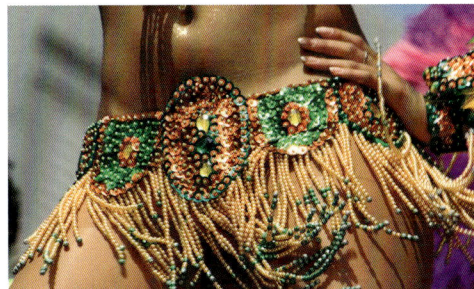

(Brazil)

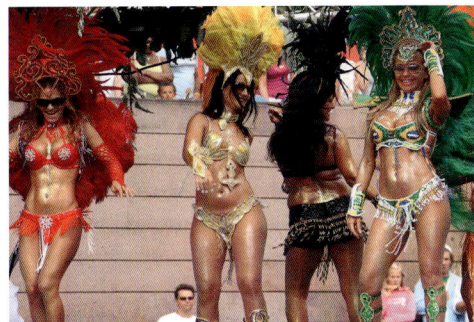

(Norway)

STRENGTHENING THE DEEP MUSCLES OF THE BACK

When you engage your inner corset, you contract the deep muscles of the back bilaterally (both sides at once). The exercises in this section are particularly effective at isolating these muscles, one side at a time, to strengthen them.

OPPOSITE ARM/LEG STRETCH

1. **BEGIN ON ALL FOURS, WITH YOUR HANDS BENEATH YOUR SHOULDERS AND YOUR KNEES BENEATH YOUR HIPS**
   Engage your abdominal muscles so that your back does not sway. Allow your pelvis to tip forward comfortably. Be sure that your shoulders remain rolled back.

2. **STRAIGHTEN YOUR RIGHT ARM OUT IN FRONT OF YOU AS YOU LIFT AND STRAIGHTEN YOUR LEFT LEG BEHIND YOU. HOLD FOR A FEW SECONDS**
   Maintain your torso position (that is, a J-spine) throughout this movement.

3. **REPEAT WITH THE OPPOSITE ARM AND LEG**

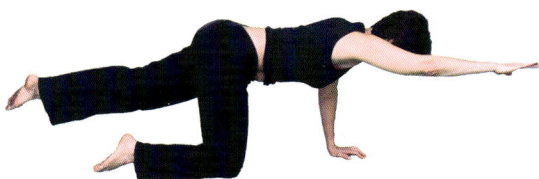

WARRIOR III

1. **BEGIN IN A COMFORTABLE STANDING POSITION**
   Be sure your feet are in kidney bean shape and your legs are externally rotated. This will enable your pelvis to settle well in Step 2.

2. **KEEPING THE HIPS SQUARE, HINGE FORWARD AT THE HIPS AS YOU LIFT YOUR LEFT LEG STRAIGHT BEHIND YOU**
   Do not sway your back. Use your *gluteus medius* muscles, not your back, to raise the leg. Use the abdominals to prevent any distortion in the torso.

3. **WHEN YOU ARE BALANCED IN THIS POSITION, RAISE YOUR ARMS OVER YOUR HEAD SO THEY FORM A STRAIGHT LINE WITH YOUR TORSO AND RAISED LEG**
   Your body forms an extended "T" shape, balanced on the left leg. Bend the left leg to help maintain balance. If necessary, perform this exercise beside a wall or chair that you can use for balance.

4. **HOLD THIS POSITION FOR A FEW SECONDS**

5. **REPEAT WITH THE RIGHT LEG ON THE OTHER SIDE**

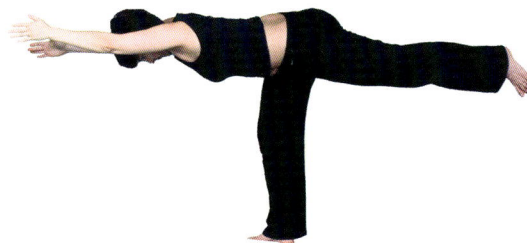

STRENGTHENING KEY MUSCLES USED IN WALKING

Strong arch muscles are essential to the health of the foot and protect foot ligaments from being overstretched. These muscles contribute to a strong push off when walking. The gluteus medius muscles of the buttocks help give you a healthy gait with a soft landing, contribute to pelvic anteversion, and help externally rotate your legs. The tibialis anterior muscles help you create and support a kidney bean shape in your feet and help externally rotate your knees.

STRENGTHENING THE ARCH MUSCLES

Achieving a kidney bean shape in your foot substantially restores the inner arch, the most important of the three arches of the foot. The following exercises further strengthen it, as well as the outer and transverse arches.

BALLET SNATCH

1. SIT OR STAND WELL

2. BALANCE ONE FOOT ON THE TIP OF ITS LONGEST TOE. BEGINNERS OFTEN NEED TO SUPPORT THE WEIGHT OF THEIR LEG USING THEIR HANDS

3. CONTRACT YOUR ARCH MUSCLES SO YOUR FOOT BECOMES SHORTER AND CURVED, LIKE A BALLET DANCER STANDING *EN POINTE*

4. RELAX, THEN REPEAT SEVERAL TIMES WITH EACH FOOT

INCHWORM

1. WHILE STANDING OR SITTING WELL, PLACE YOUR FEET INTO KIDNEY BEAN SHAPE

2. RELEASE MOST OF THE WEIGHT FROM ONE FOOT (a)

3. FIX THE TOES OF THAT FOOT TO THE FLOOR AND CONTRACT ALL THE ARCH MUSCLES IN THE BOTTOM OF THE FOOT (b)

Your objective is to shorten the foot into an arched shape, drawing the heel closer to the toes.

4. NOW FIX THE HEEL TO THE FLOOR, RELEASE THE TOES AND RELAX ALL THE ARCH MUSCLES (c)
Allow your foot to return to its longer length. Your foot should be slightly ahead of its starting position; it has "inched" forward.

5. REPEAT STEPS 1–4 SEVERAL TIMES UNTIL YOUR FOOT HAS CREPT ABOUT 6 INCHES (15CM) FORWARD

You will now reverse the action to move your foot backwards instead of forwards:

6. FIX THE HEEL TO THE FLOOR (d)

7. CONTRACT THE ARCH MUSCLES TO DRAW THE TOES BACK TOWARD THE HEEL (e)
The foot shortens.

8. NOW FIX THE TOES TO THE FLOOR AND RELEASE THE CONTRACTION OF THE ARCH MUSCLES (f)
This allows the heel to move backwards.

9. REPEAT STEPS 7–9 SEVERAL TIMES UNTIL YOUR FOOT HAS RETURNED TO ITS STARTING POSITION
It is common for beginners to contract their toes more than their arches. Try to maximize the contraction of your arches while minimizing the contraction of your toes. Over time you will improve your ability to isolate these muscles.

10. REPEAT STEPS 2–9 WITH THE OTHER FOOT

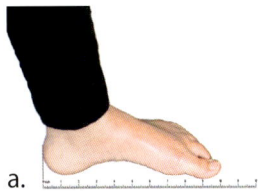
a.

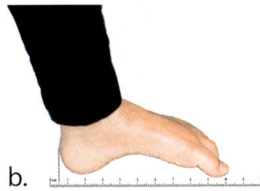
b.

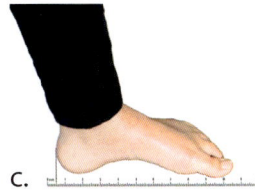
c.

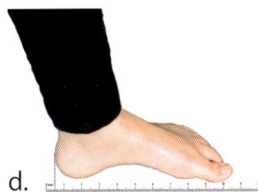
d.

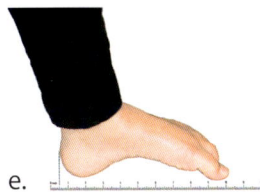
e.

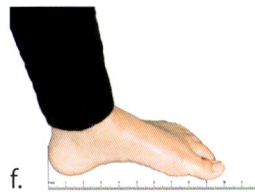
f.

INCHWORM VIDEO

EAT THE CLOTH

1. **SPREAD A HAND TOWEL OR SMALL CLOTH ON THE FLOOR**
Use a cloth with some texture, such as terry cloth. Avoid slippery fabrics like silk.

2. **WHILE STANDING OR SITTING WELL, PLACE ONE FOOT ON THE EDGE OF THE CLOTH CLOSEST TO YOU (a)**

3. **USING JUST YOUR FOOT, TRY TO GATHER THE CLOTH UNDER THE FOOT (b)**
This exercise strengthens the muscles that control the underside of your foot.

4. **REPEAT WITH THE OTHER FOOT**

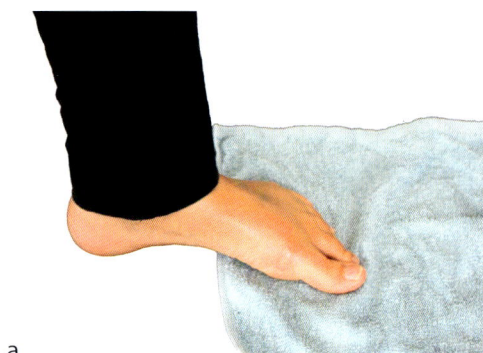

a.

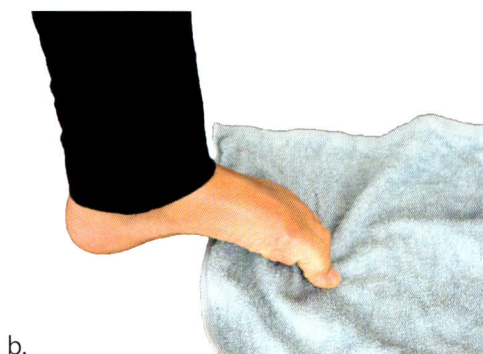

b.

GRAB THE BALL

1. **PLACE A SMALL BALL ON THE FLOOR**
It is useful to have various-sized balls for this exercise. Most students begin with a ball of half-an-inch (1cm) to one inch (2.5cm) in diameter.

2. **WHILE STANDING OR SITTING WELL, TRY TO GRAB THE BALL WITH ONE FOOT**
Initially, you may only be able to grab the ball with your toes. Work to grab increasingly larger balls. As your arches grow stronger, you may be able to grab a ball under your transverse arch.

3. **REPEAT THESE STEPS WITH THE OTHER FOOT**

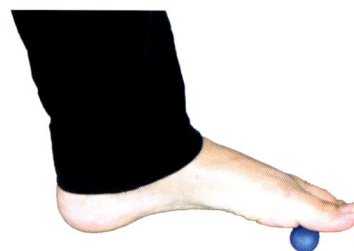

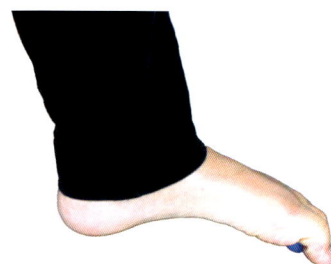

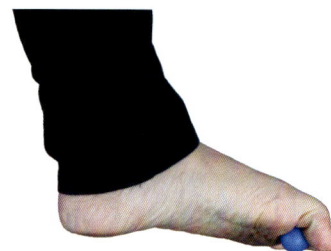

STRENGTHENING THE GLUTEUS MEDIUS MUSCLES

In this exercise, as you lift your leg, you will feel the gluteus medius muscle on that side contract. However, you will also be exercising the same muscle on the other side as it works to maintain a level pelvis.

1. STAND WITH SOFT KNEES AND KIDNEY BEAN-SHAPED FEET

2. SHIFT YOUR WEIGHT TO YOUR LEFT FOOT
   Try to minimize any disturbance to the rest of your body.

3. BEND YOUR BODY FORWARD, HINGING AT THE GROIN (a)
   If necessary, steady yourself by holding onto a chair or wall. With practice you may no longer need to use a support.

4. ROTATE THE RIGHT LEG OUTWARD AT THE HIP, PIVOTING YOUR HEEL (b)
   The toes of your right foot are now pointing to the side. This outward rotation isolates the gluteus medius muscle of your right leg.

5. BEND YOUR RIGHT KNEE AND RAISE THE LEG BACKWARDS (c)
   Become aware that you are engaging your gluteal muscles. Leave the pelvis in its original position as you raise your leg. Do not sway or tuck.

6. PLACE YOUR LEFT HAND ON YOUR LOWER BACK TO ENSURE YOU KEEP THIS AREA STRAIGHT (d)
   Use your abdominal muscles to keep your back steady.

7. LOWER YOUR LEG A LITTLE AND RAISE IT AGAIN (e,f)

8. REPEAT THESE STEPS ON THE OPPOSITE SIDE
   Repeat this motion in sets of 20 (or a number of your choice). It is helpful to do this to the beat of music you enjoy.

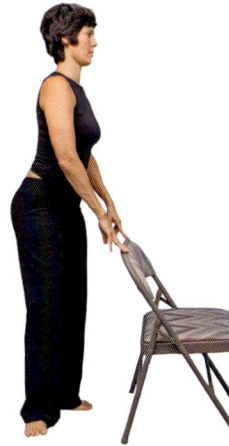
a.
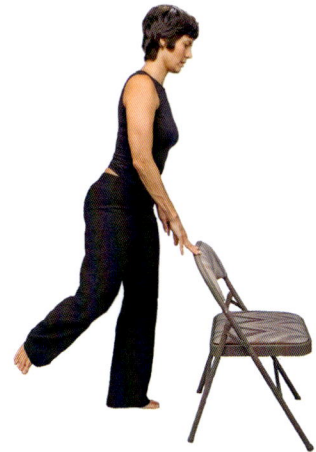
b.
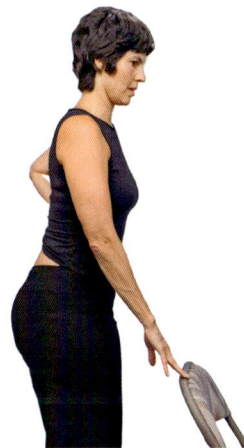
c.
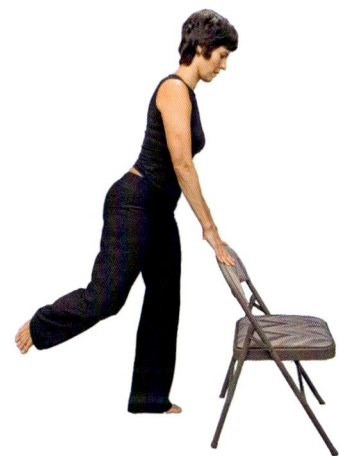
d.
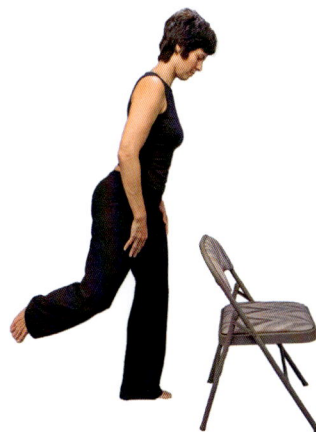
e.
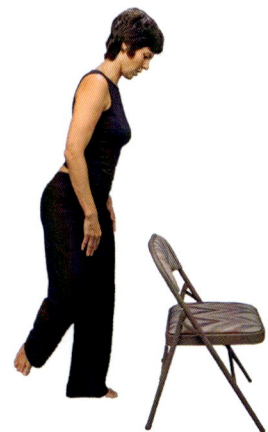
f.

213

STRENGTHENING THE TIBIALIS ANTERIOR

This muscle enables you to create and maintain a kidney bean shape in your foot. It is also the muscle associated with shin splints and fallen arches. When the muscle is weak and you place demands on it, as in running and long-distance walking, it can cause significant pain. The following "toe tap" exercise, which you might want to do to music with a driving beat, strengthens the muscle very efficiently.

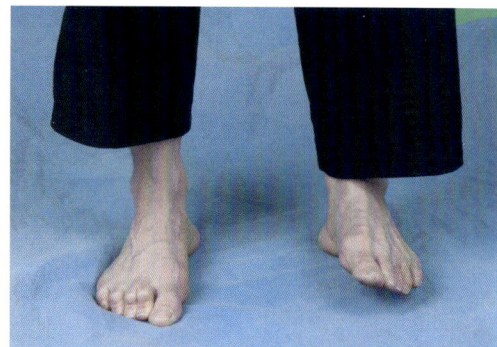

a.

1. STAND WITH SOFT KNEES AND KIDNEY BEAN-SHAPED FEET

Engage all the arch muscles of the foot to emphasize its convex shape.

2. SHIFT ALL YOUR WEIGHT ONTO YOUR HEELS

Allow your body to hinge forward slightly at the hip joint to maintain your balance.

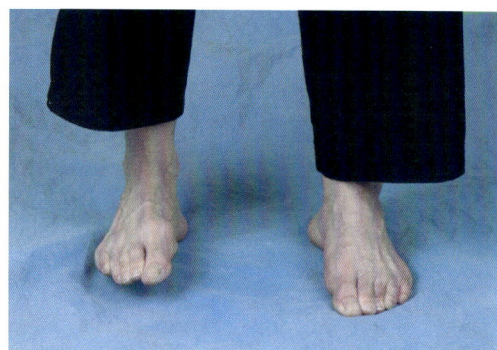

b.

3. WHILE MAINTAINING YOUR CONVEX FOOT SHAPE, LIFT THE FRONT OF ONE FOOT OFF THE FLOOR (a)

Do not to curl your toes upward as you do this.

4. REPLACE THAT FOOT TO THE FLOOR AS YOU LIFT THE OTHER FOOT (b)

Notice that your entire weight remains on your heels.

TOE TAP
VIDEO

5. REPEAT THE MOVEMENT, INCREASING THE SPEED UNTIL YOU FEEL MUSCLE FATIGUE

6. ALLOW YOUR MUSCLES TO RECOVER. THEN REPEAT THE EXERCISE

STRENGTHENING AND STRETCHING THE MUSCLES IN THE SHOULDER AREA

To settle the shoulders in a healthy position requires relaxed *pectoral* and *trapezius* muscles, and toned *rhomboid* muscles. All these muscles affect shoulder and arm posture, which influences how the spine stacks. Relaxed pectoral muscles allow the chest cavity to expand freely, facilitating inhalation. Relaxed trapezius muscles allow a healthy spacing in the upper thoracic and cervical spine. Relaxed pectoral and trapezius muscles permit the arms to move independently of the torso. Strong rhomboid muscles help peg the shoulders down and back along the torso.

For some people, shoulder rolls (see page 42) performed several times a day may be enough to return the shoulders to a good baseline position. For others, one or more of the following exercises may be helpful.

PECTORAL STRETCH

Begin by positioning yourself well, tallstanding or stacksitting. For all of these exercises, maintaining a good baseline position is important to protect your muscles and joints.

VARIATION 1

1. BEGIN BY PERFORMING A SHOULDER ROLL
If you start with your shoulders in a healthy position, that position becomes locked into place during this exercise.

2. INTERLACE THE FINGERS BEHIND THE BACK WITH PALMS FACING EACH OTHER

3. ANCHOR THE RIBCAGE
Contract the *internal oblique* abdominal muscles to prevent a sway in your back.

4. MOVE THE SHOULDERS FURTHER BACK AND DOWN. ACTIVELY LENGTHEN THE BACK OF YOUR NECK WITH YOUR CHIN ANGLED DOWN WHILE DOING THIS

5. STRAIGHTEN AND RAISE THE ARMS
Be sure to stop short of distorting your torso or straining your neck or upper shoulders.

6. HOLD FOR A FEW SECONDS

VARIATION 2

In Step 2 above, with fingers interlaced, try rotating palms inward and downward. Continue with the remaining steps.

VARIATION 3

In Step 2 above, with fingers interlaced, try rotating palms outward and downward. Continue with the remaining steps.

VARIATION 4

1. BEGIN BY PERFORMING A SHOULDER ROLL

2. WRAP A STRAP OR THERABAND™ BEHIND THE BACK AND HOLD ONE END IN EACH HAND
Hold each end so that the band lies along the inner forearms and your palms face up.

3. ATTEMPT TO LIFT THE BAND BACK AWAY FROM YOUR SPINE BY MOVING YOUR ARMS OUT AND BACK
Be sure to anchor the rib cage, avoiding a sway, and maintain length in the back of the neck.

4. HOLD THE POSITION FOR 30 SECONDS

5. REPEAT SEVERAL TIMES

RHOMBOID TONER

1. BEGIN BY PERFORMING A SHOULDER ROLL

    It's important to begin with a healthy shoulder position to place the rhomboids in a position of mechanical advantage.

2. PIN YOUR ELBOWS TO YOUR SIDES AND BEND YOUR ELBOWS TO A 90º ANGLE IN THE FRONT

    The position is similar to when you're carrying a tray.

3. GRAB A THERABAND™ OR STRAP

    Be sure not to distort the wrists; keep them firm to avoid unnecessary strain.

4. PRESSING YOUR ELBOWS AGAINST YOUR SIDES, DRAW YOUR SHOULDER BLADES AS CLOSE TOGETHER AS YOU CAN

    Naturally your hands will move away from each other. The band or strap provides resistance to this motion, challenging the rhomboids.

    Be sure not to tense the shoulders or neck.

5. HOLD FOR A FEW SECONDS

TRAP STRETCH

Caution: **If you have neck problems (herniated discs or bone spurs), skip this exercise.**

1. BEGIN BY PERFORMING A SHOULDER ROLL

    Be sure to begin with a healthy shoulder position so that the exercise targets the most relevant part of the trapezius muscle.

2. PLACE THE PALM OF YOUR RIGHT HAND OVER YOUR HEAD NEAR YOUR LEFT EAR

3. USE YOUR HAND TO LENGTHEN YOUR NECK AS YOU GENTLY ALLOW THE WEIGHT OF YOUR RIGHT ARM TO PULL YOUR HEAD CLOSER TO YOUR RIGHT SHOULDER

    Do not force this movement.

4. GENTLY PRESS THE HEEL OF YOUR LEFT HAND DOWN TO AUGMENT THE STRETCH

5. HOLD THIS POSITION FOR A FEW SECONDS

6. REPEAT ON THE OTHER SIDE

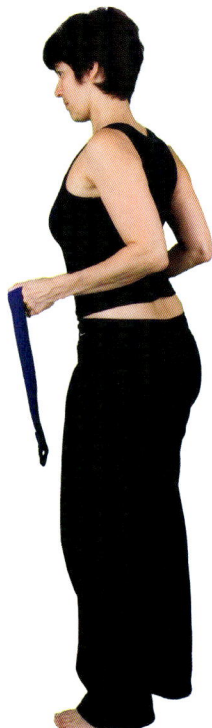

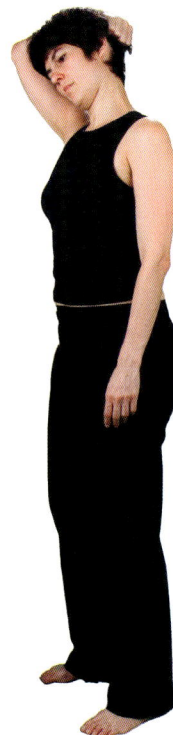
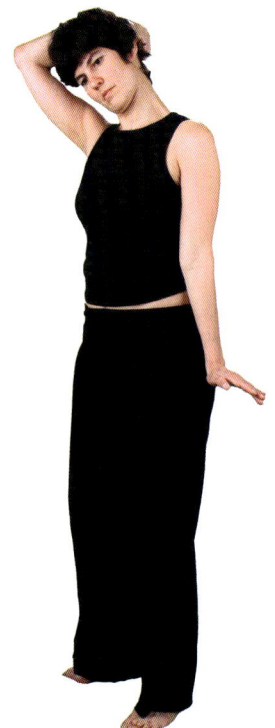

STRENGTHENING THE NECK MUSCLES

1. FOLD A 6-FOOT (2M) LENGTH OF FABRIC INTO A 6-INCH (15CM) WIDE BAND

2. WRAP THE BAND BEHIND THE NECK AND HOLD ONE END IN EACH HAND

3. GET INTO A POSITION ON ALL FOURS, WITH YOUR SHOULDERS DIRECTLY ABOVE YOUR HANDS AND YOUR HIPS DIRECTLY ABOVE YOUR KNEES

4. ANCHOR THE BAND SECURELY UNDER YOUR HANDS
Be sure the band is snug against the back of the neck.

5. USE YOUR NECK MUSCLES TO PULL BACK (UP) AGAINST THE BAND

6. HOLD FOR 10 SECONDS

7. REPEAT SEVERAL TIMES

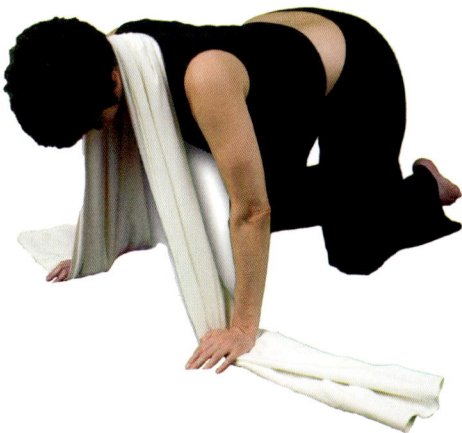

STRETCHING THE NECK MUSCLES

1. BEGIN BY POSITIONING YOURSELF WELL, TALLSTANDING OR STACKSITTING (a)

2. TRANSLATE YOUR FACE FORWARD TILL YOU FEEL A SIGNIFICANT STRETCH IN YOUR NECK MUSCLES (b,c)
Your face remains in the same orientation to the ground throughout the stretch.

3. HOLD THE STRETCH FOR A FEW SECONDS

4. SHIFT YOUR FACE BACKWARDS BEYOND WHERE YOU WERE AT THE START OF THE EXERCISE (d)
You will feel a stretch as you lengthen the back of your neck.

5. AUGMENT THE STRETCH BY PULLING BACKWARDS AND UPWARDS ON THE HAIR AT THE BASE OF YOUR SKULL

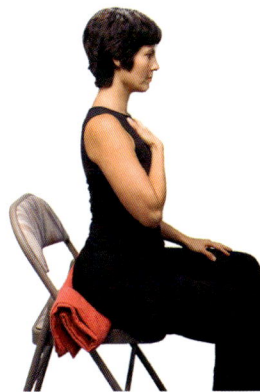

a.

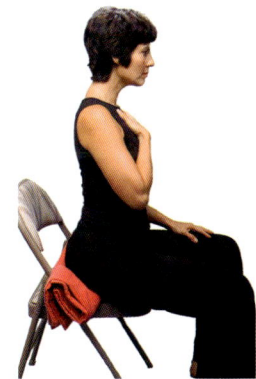

b.

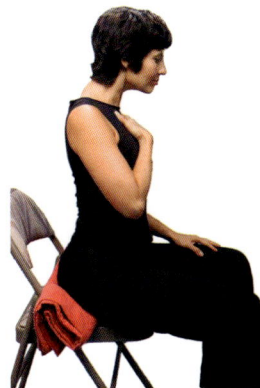

c.

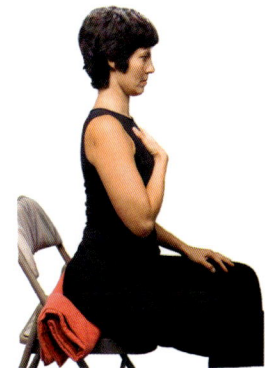

d.

STRETCHING THE KEY MUSCLES THAT CONNECT THE TORSO AND LEGS

Ideally, your legs are able to move independently of your torso. This requires flexibility in several muscles, such as the *hamstrings*, *psoas*, and *external hip rotators*. Length in the hamstring muscles is essential to a healthy pelvic position and healthy bending. A lengthened psoas, one of the key muscles in the groin, facilitates good alignment in the lumbar spine and a healthy stride. Flexible external hip rotator muscles permit the pelvis to form an acute angle with the leg bones for deep hip-hinging.

STRETCHING THE HAMSTRINGS

These two stretches are safe and effective for lengthening the hamstring muscles. The hamstrings attach to the sitz bones, and tight hamstrings force the pelvis into a tuck (*retroversion*). If you have short hamstrings, lengthening them is vital to the success of your posture work.

WALL STRETCH

1. **STAND WELL, ABOUT TWO TO THREE FEET (30CM) FROM AND FACING A WALL**
   The distance depends on your hamstring flexibility and the length of your upper body. You may need to adjust your position.

2. **HINGE AT YOUR HIPS AS YOU PLACE YOUR HANDS ON THE WALL**
   Do not allow your pelvis to tuck.

3. **LEAVE YOUR HANDS ON THE WALL ABOVE YOUR HEAD**
   This lets your shoulders stretch backwards.

4. **IF YOU CAN BEND FURTHER, LET YOUR TORSO MOVE TOWARD THE FLOOR AS FAR AS THE HAMSTRINGS WILL TOLERATE**
   This will increase your shoulder stretch. If it is too intense, let your hands slide down the wall as you move your torso.

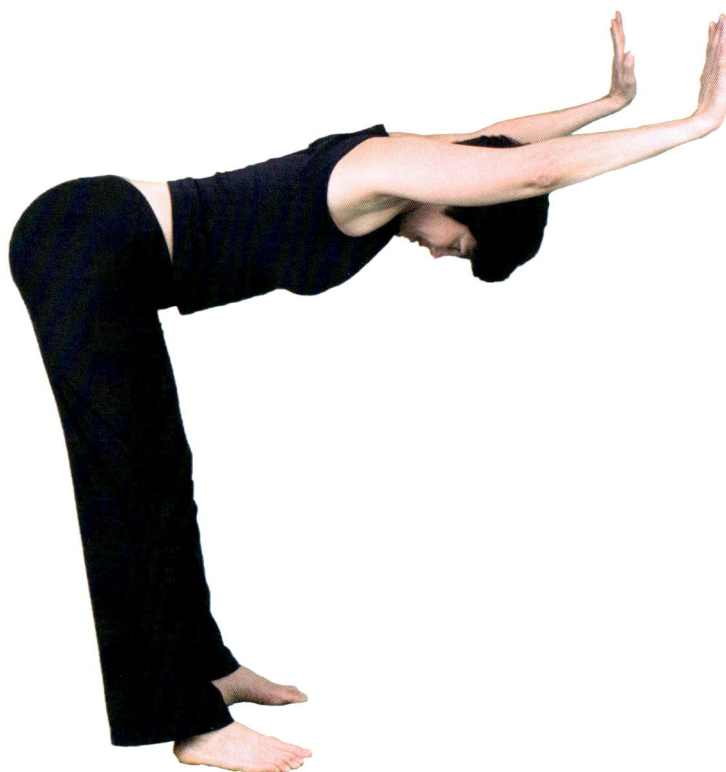

LYING HAMSTRING STRETCH

1. LENGTHEN YOUR BACK AS YOU LIE DOWN, AS YOU LEARNED TO DO IN CHAPTER 2

2. PLACE A PILLOW UNDER YOUR HEAD AND SHOULDERS

3. HOLDING ONE END OF A STRAP IN EACH HAND, LOOP THE STRAP AROUND THE BALL OF YOUR RIGHT FOOT, AND THEN MOSTLY STRAIGHTEN YOUR LEG (a)
Keep your arms outstretched and your shoulder blades fixed in position. Don't allow your shoulders to pull forward.

4. LIFT YOUR RIGHT LEG UPWARD TOWARD YOUR HEAD UNTIL YOU FEEL A SIGNIFICANT HAMSTRING STRETCH
Do not overstretch.

5. HOLD BOTH STRAP ENDS WITH THE RIGHT HAND

6. GENTLY ALLOW THE LEG TO MOVE TO THE RIGHT, TOWARD THE FLOOR, WITHOUT RAISING YOUR LEFT HIP FROM THE FLOOR (b)
If it helps, use your left hand to hold your left hip to the floor.

7. MOVE YOUR RIGHT LEG BACK UPWARD

8. SWITCH THE STRAP ENDS TO THE LEFT HAND

9. ALLOW YOUR LEG TO FALL GENTLY TO THE LEFT, ACROSS YOUR BODY, TOWARD THE FLOOR (c)
Do not let your right hip lift from the floor. Your leg will probably not travel very far from vertical.

10. REPEAT THESE STEPS WITH THE LEFT LEG (d,e,f)

a.

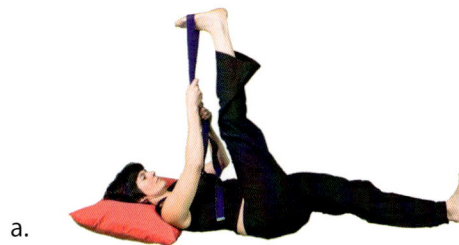

b.

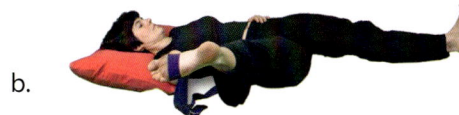

c.

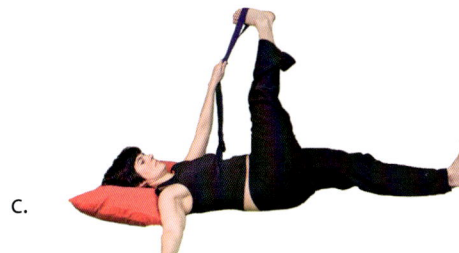

d.

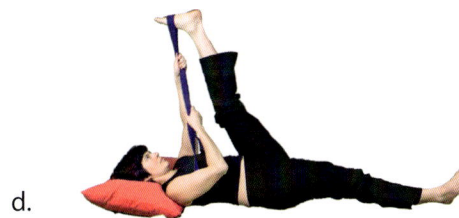

e.

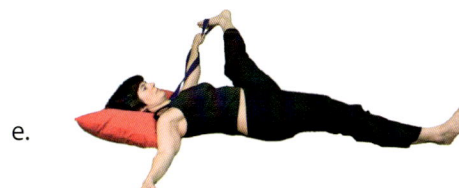

f.

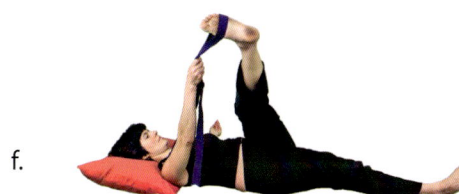

STRETCHING THE EXTERNAL HIP ROTATOR MUSCLES

PAPER CLIP

1. LENGTHEN YOUR BACK AS YOU LIE DOWN, AS YOU LEARNED TO DO IN CHAPTER 2

2. PLACE A PILLOW UNDER YOUR HEAD AND SHOULDERS

3. BEND BOTH KNEES AND PLACE YOUR FEET ON THE FLOOR

4. PLACE THE RIGHT ANKLE ACROSS THE LEFT KNEE

5. INTERLACE YOUR FINGERS EITHER BEHIND YOUR LEFT THIGH OR AROUND YOUR LEFT SHIN, LIFTING YOUR LEFT FOOT OFF THE FLOOR (a)
You can use a strap to prevent any distortion in your shoulders or torso (b).

6. DRAW BOTH LEGS TOWARD YOUR CHEST UNTIL YOU SENSE A SIGNIFICANT STRETCH
Again, do not stretch to the point of discomfort.

7. LOWER THE LEGS UNTIL YOUR LEFT FOOT IS ON THE FLOOR; THEN RELEASE

8. REPEAT ON THE OTHER SIDE (c,d)

LENGTHENING THE PSOAS MUSCLES

LUNGE

1. STAND WELL WITH YOUR FEET ABOUT HIP-WIDTH APART

2. BEND FORWARD WITH A STRAIGHT BACK, PLACING YOUR HANDS TO THE FLOOR OUTSIDE YOUR FEET OR RESTING ON YOUR KNEES
Bend your knees as necessary.

3. EXTEND ONE LEG FAR BACK, OPTIONALLY RESTING THE KNEE ON THE GROUND
Keep the hips square to the ground. Be sure the forward knee does not bend more than 90° or extend in front of the ankle.

4. LET THE PELVIS SINK TOWARD THE FLOOR
This results in a strong stretch in the groin.

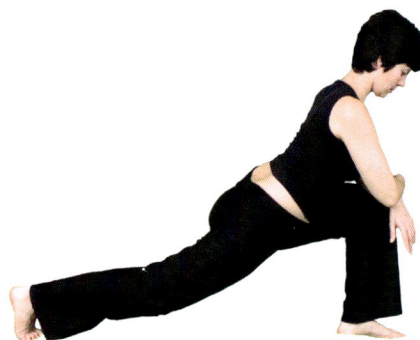

5. REPEAT ON THE OTHER SIDE

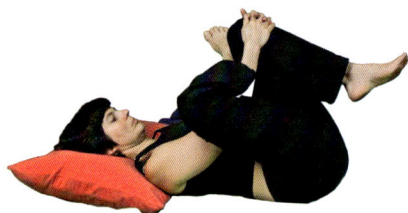 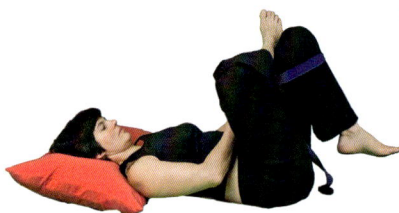

a.   b.

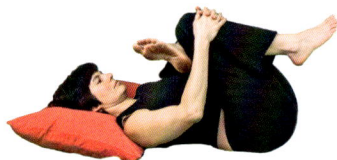 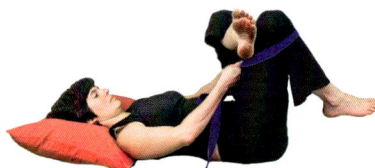

c.   d.

TROUBLESHOOTING

STIFFNESS OR PAIN

You may experience some soreness or stiffness in the days following these exercises. This is completely normal when you exercise muscles that are out of shape. However, if you experience significant pain during or after performing any of these exercises, you may be stretching or strengthening too vigorously. Let your body recover for a day or two. Then proceed, building up more slowly in intensity and repetitions.

LACK OF IMPROVEMENT

Many of these exercises help you create additional length in your muscles. However, maintaining the new length requires that you use the lengthened muscles in your everyday stance and activities. Brief minutes spent performing targeted exercises may not be sufficient to overcome hours of poor posture. The combination of working on your posture and performing relevant exercises is the fastest way of making change.

FAILURE TO EXERCISE

Some of you will have trouble finding time to perform even a few targeted exercises. If you simply cannot work them into your routine, don't worry about it! If you perform your everyday activities with increased awareness and improved form, you will still make good progress.

FURTHER INFORMATION

Of the countless exercises and regimens available today, many have relatively little value, and some can even cause damage. For example, traditional back extension exercises strengthen the *erector spinae* muscles. However, often the problem with these muscles is that they are too tight, not too weak. In this case, performing back extensions may exacerbate the real problem.

Similarly, traditional crunches target the *rectus abdominus* muscle, can put strain on the lumbar and cervical discs and ligaments, potentially causing serious damage.

People often ask me about the value of the exercise circuits at gyms and fitness centers. In a society where some people interface with little more than their computer all day long, a gym can provide valuable human interaction. Weight machines target specific muscles and track specific actions, thus, adequately challenging major muscle groups safely. In addition, users benefit from feedback on their strength and progress. However, because circuit machines control your actions, they do not provide the opportunity for the mixed movements of everyday activities. It is best to mix any exercise regimen with a variety of physical activities.

APPENDIX 2
ANATOMY

Pectorals (pecs)

Deltoid

Trapezius (traps)

Latissimus dorsi (lats)

External Oblique

Gluteus medius

Gluteus maximus

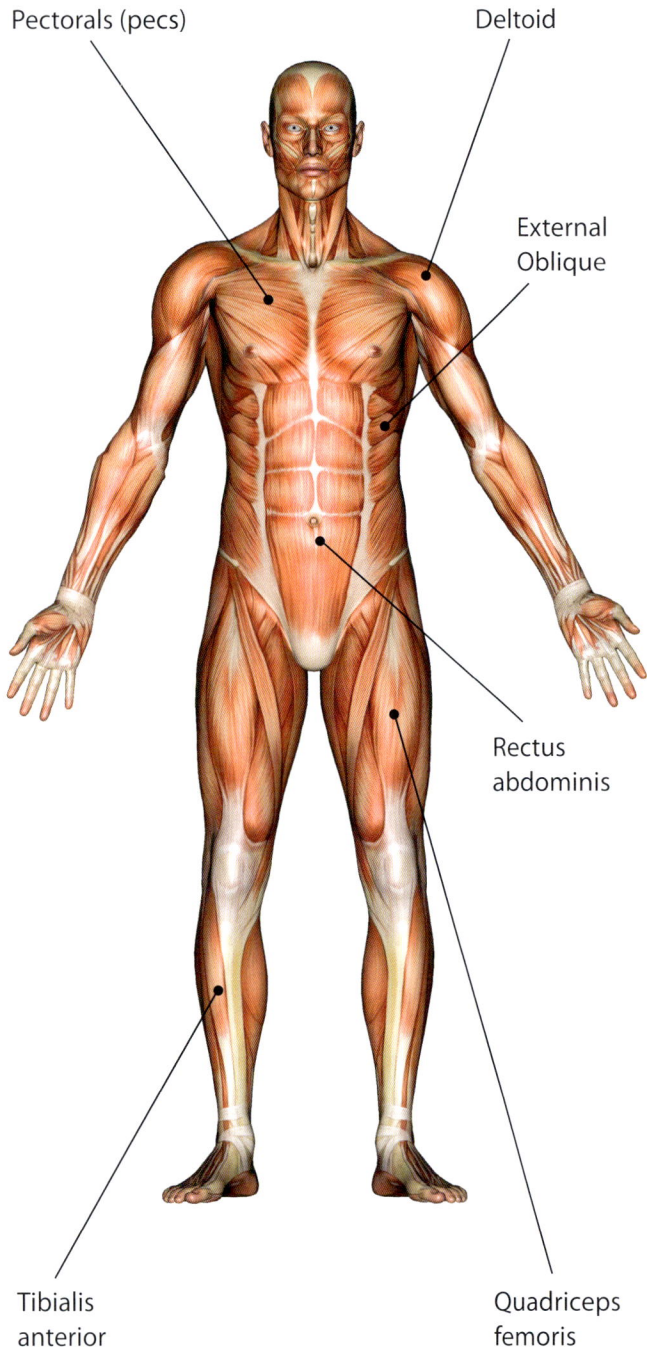
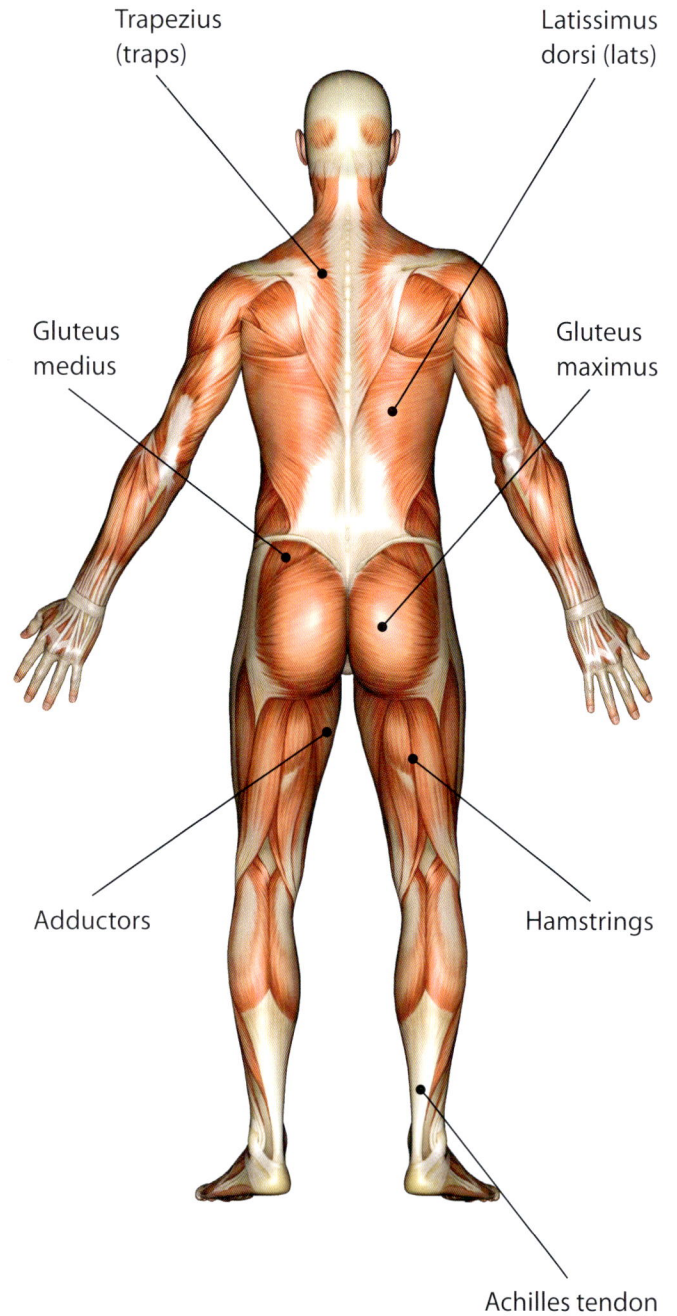

Rectus abdominis

Adductors

Hamstrings

Tibialis anterior

Quadriceps femoris

Achilles tendon

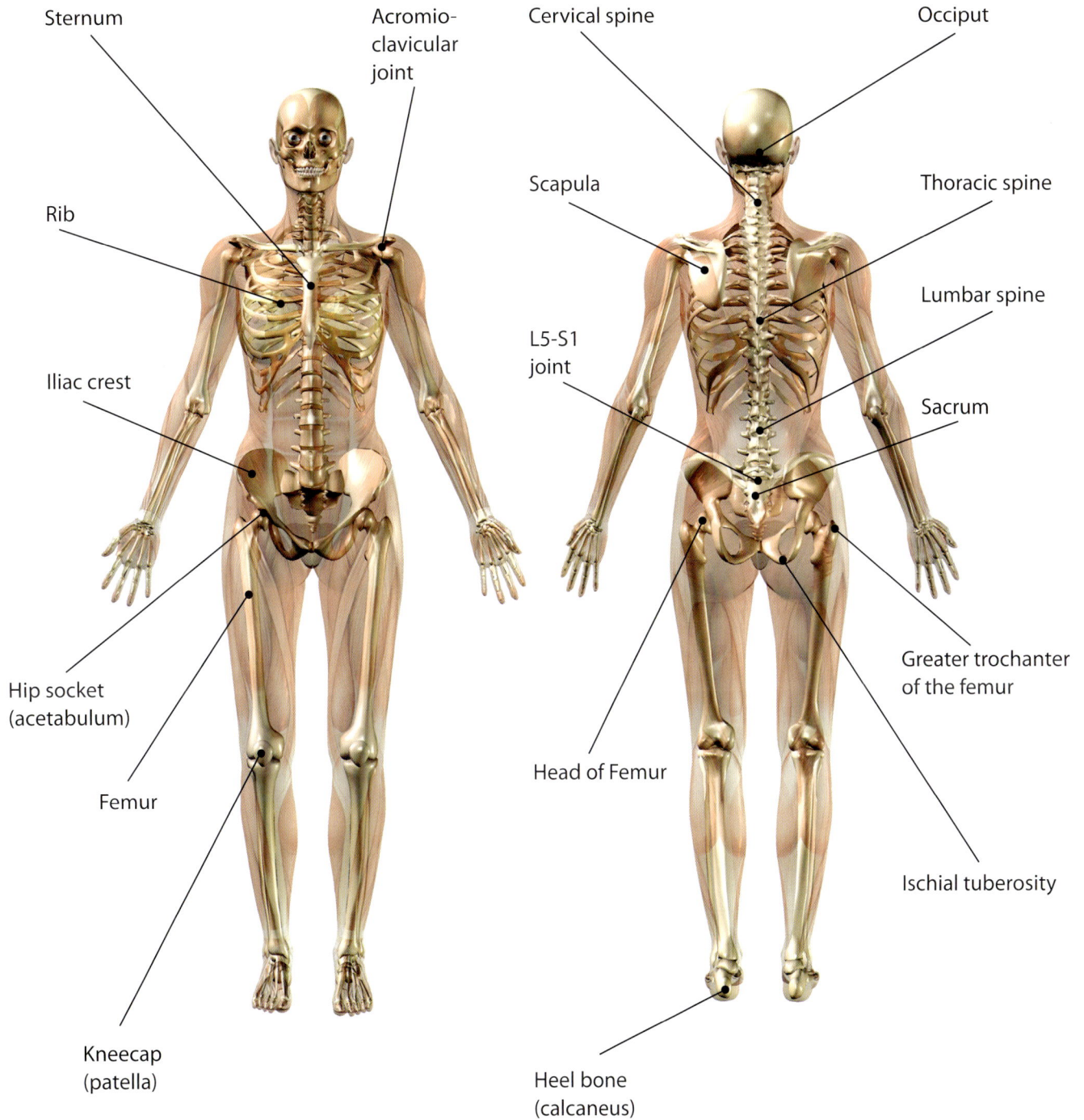

Sternum

Acromio-
clavicular
joint

Rib

Iliac crest

Hip socket
(acetabulum)

Femur

Kneecap
(patella)

Cervical spine

Occiput

Scapula

Thoracic spine

L5-S1
joint

Lumbar spine

Sacrum

Head of Femur

Greater trochanter
of the femur

Ischial tuberosity

Heel bone
(calcaneus)

GLOSSARY

ABDOMINAL OBLIQUE MUSCLES
See Oblique muscles.

ACETABULUM
The socket of the hip bone (Os Coxae) into which the head of the femur fits.

ACHILLES TENDON
The tendon of the gastrocnemius (large muscle on the posterior of the leg) and soleus (broad, flat calf muscle).

ARCHES OF THE FOOT: INNER, OUTER, AND TRANSVERSE
The inner or medial longitudinal arch runs on the inside of the foot. The outer or lateral longitudinal arch runs along the outside of the foot. The transverse or metatarsal arch runs across the ball of the foot.

ACROMIOCLAVICULAR JOINT
The joint between the clavicle (the long bone of the shoulder girdle running between the sternum and the shoulder blade) and the scapula (the shoulder blade).

ANTEVERSION
Inclining forward without bending (cf. retroversion).

ANTEVERTED PELVIS
The natural human pelvic position, defined by a significant lumbosacral angle at L5-S1 (cf. pelvic tilt).

BACKBONE
The set of vertebrae that extends from the cranium to the coccyx, and provides support and a flexible bony case for the spinal cord. The backbone is composed of 33 vertebrae (7 cervical, 12 thoracic, 5 lumbar, 5 fused sacral—forming the sacrum, 4 fused coccygeal—forming the coccyx).

BODY SCAN
A conscious and systematic focusing of one's attention on each part of the body. One method is to begin with the toes

and feet, move upward through the legs and torso to the shoulders, then down the arms to the hands and fingers. Last, scan the neck and head.

BRACHIAL PLEXUS
A complex network of nerves originating from the spinal cord (C5–T1) that supplies the shoulder, arm, and hand.

CERVICAL SPINE
The neck portion of the spine, composed of the first seven vertebrae (C1–C7) (cf. thoracic spine, lumbar spine).

CLAVICLE, OR COLLAR BONE
A doubly curved long bone that connects the arm to the body. It is located directly above the first rib.

DOWAGER'S HUMP
An extreme forward bending or curving of the spine.

ELECTROMYOGRAPHY (EMG)
A method of recording the electrical currents generated in an active muscle.

ERECTOR SPINAE MUSCLE (SACROSPINALIS)
A large muscle of the back that supports the spinal column and head.

EXTERNAL OBLIQUE MUSCLES
Paired muscles originating from the lower eight ribs and inserting into the iliac crest and linea alba, with the fibers running downward and medially (perpendicular to the internal oblique fibers). They lie beneath the rectus abdominis muscle and above the internal oblique muscles.

EXTERNAL HIP ROTATOR MUSCLES
A group of deep muscles responsible for rotating the hip outward and stabilizing the hip joint, including piriformis and gluteus medius.

EXTERNAL ROTATION (OF THE HIP)
The process of turning the leg outward at the hip joint, so the legs and feet are not parallel, but angled outward with the heels closer together than the toes.

FEMUR
The large bone of the thigh extending from the hip to the knee; the longest and strongest bone of the skeleton.

GLUTEAL MUSCLES
The gluteus maximus, gluteus medius, and gluteus minimus muscles that form the buttocks.

GLUTEUS MEDIUS MUSCLE
One of three major muscles of the buttocks. Located in the upper, outer quadrant of the buttock, the gluteus medius moves the leg to the side and rotates the thigh.

HAMSTRING MUSCLES
The group of three muscles at the back of the thigh.

ILIAC CREST
The upper, outer free edge of the ilium (part of the pelvis)

INNER ARCH
See arches of the foot.

INNER CORSET
The collection of muscles between the ribs and hips that help lengthen and support the spine.

INTERNAL OBLIQUE MUSCLES
Paired abdominal muscles that originate from the iliac crest and insert onto the lower ribs and linea alba. They lie beneath the external oblique and above the transversus abdominis muscles, running upward and medially (perpendicular to the external oblique fibers).

ISCHIAL TUBEROSITIES
The rounded portion of the lower hip bones (ischia); also called sitz bones.

KIDNEY BEAN-SHAPED FEET
The healthy shape of the feet with the heels pivoted inward and strong inner arches.

KYPHOSIS
Forward bending or curving of the spine, particularly in the thoracic spine. Extreme forms are known as Dowager's hump and humpback. Even minor forms contribute to back pain (cf. lordosis).

KYPHOTIC
Characterized by extreme forward curvature (cf. lordotic).

INTERCOSTAL MUSCLES
Muscles that run between the ribs, helping to form and move the chest wall.

L5-S1
The portion of the lower back where the lumbar and sacral spines meet, specifically the junction between the fifth lumbar vertebra and the first sacral vertebra.

LESSER TROCHANTER
See Trochanter, lesser.

LONGUS COLLI MUSCLE
A long muscle that twists and bends the neck forward.

LORDOSIS
Backward bending or arching of the spine, particularly in the lumbar area (cf. kyphosis).

LORDOTIC
Characterized by extreme backward curvature (cf. kyphotic).

LOWER BACK
The lower portion of the spine, composed of five vertebrae (L1–L5). Same as lumbar spine.

LUMBAR SPINE
The lower portion of the spine, composed of five vertebrae (L1–L5) (cf. cervical spine, thoracic spine).

LUMBOSACRAL ARCH/ ANGLE/CURVE
The natural arch of the lower back, between the last lumbar vertebra and the sacrum (L5-S1).

LYMPHATIC VESSELS
A network of channels that collect and transport lymph—a clear fluid containing immune cells, waste products, and excess interstitial fluid—from tissues back into the circulatory system.

MIDLINE GROOVE
A long, narrow furrow running vertically along the spine.

MULTIFIDUS MUSCLES
Deep muscles located on either side of the vertebral column spanning from the sacrum to the cervical spine, providing stability and support.

NEUTRAL SPINE
The state of the spine when it is neither overly flat nor overly curved, but held in a normal state of balanced tension.

OBLIQUE MUSCLES
Muscles at the side of the abdomen about at the level of the waist that compress the viscera and flex the thorax forward (cf. internal oblique, external oblique).

OUTER ARCH
See arches of the foot.

PECTORAL MUSCLES
The muscles of the chest: pectoralis major (which flexes, rotates, and adducts the arm), pectoralis minor (which raises the ribs and draws down the shoulder blades), and subclavius (which elevates first rib and draws clavicle down).

PELVIC RIM
See iliac crest.

PELVIC TILT, PELVIC TUCK
Two positions of the pelvis. A pelvic tilt moves the upper portion of the pelvis anterior to the lower portion. A slight pelvic tilt is desirable; an exaggerated pelvic tilt can lead to lordosis. A pelvic tuck moves the lower portion of the pelvis in line with, or even anterior to, the upper portion. An exaggerated pelvic tuck can lead to kyphosis.

PIRIFORMIS MUSCLE
A deep muscle located in the buttock, involved in hip rotation and stabilization of the pelvis. In close proximity with the sciatic nerve.

PRONATION OF FEET (FLAT FEET, FALLEN ARCHES)
A condition where the arch or instep of the foot collapses and approaches or comes in contact with the ground.

PSOAS MUSCLES
Two deep muscles of the lower spine: psoas major (which rotates the thighs and bends the spine) and psoas minor (which flexes the spine).

PUBOCOCCYGEUS MUSCLE (PC, KEGEL MUSCLE)
A hammock-like muscle, found in both sexes, that stretches from the pubic bone to the tail bone forming the floor of the pelvic cavity.

QUADRICEPS MUSCLE
A large muscle on the anterior surface of the thigh that extends the leg, and is composed of four smaller muscles: the rectus femoris, the vastus lateralis, the vastus medialis, and the vastus intermedius.

RECTUS ABDOMINUS MUSCLE
A paired muscle that runs vertically on each side of the abdomen from the pubis to the lower costal cartilages.

RETROVERSION
Inclining backward without bending (cf. anteversion).

RHOMBOID MUSCLES
Muscles that connect the inner borders of the scapula (shoulder blades) to the thoracic spine.

ROTATORES
Muscles of the back that rotate and extend the vertebral column.

SACRUM
The triangular bone that is located at the top of the pelvis and the base of the spine.

SITZ BONES
See ischial tuberosities.

SPINAL COMPRESSION
The act of applying an unusual amount of pressure on the spinal column, often resulting in pain due to damage to a spinal disc, fracture of a vertebra, or pressure on a nerve.

STERNUM
The long, flat bone in the middle of the rib cage. Also called the breastbone.

SWAY BACK
See lordosis.

THORACIC SPINE
The middle portion of the spine, composed of 12 vertebrae (T1–T12) (cf. cervical spine, lumbar spine).

TIBIALIS ANTERIOR
A muscle that runs from the outer lower leg to the inner foot. It acts to dorsiflex and invert the foot.

TRACTION
The process of pulling a limb, bone, or muscle group to align it or relieve pressure on it.

TRANSVERSE ARCH
See arches of the foot.

TRANSVERSUS MUSCLE
A flat muscle that forms the lateral and anterior walls of the abdominal cavity.

TRAPEZIUS MUSCLE
Muscle in the upper back that rotates the shoulder blades (scapula), and draws the head back and to the side.

TROCHANTER, LESSER
A small, bony prominence on the medial and posterior aspect of the femur, located just below the femoral neck. The site of attachment of the iliopsoas muscle.

VERTEBRAL LEVEL
Any reference point along the vertebral column.

BIBLIOGRAPHY

(1) Volinn, E. (1997). The epidemiology of low back pain in the rest of the world: A review of surveys in low- and middle-income countries. Spine, 22(15), 1747-1754.

(2) Fahrni, W.H. (1975). Conservative treatment of lumbar disc degeneration: Our primary responsibility. Orthop Clin North Am, 6, 93-101.

(3) Darmawan, J., et al. (1992). Epidemiology of rheumatic diseases in rural and urban populations in Indonesia: World Health Organisation International League Against Rheumatism COPCORD study, stage 1, phase 2. Annals of Rheumatic Diseases, 51, 525-528.

(4) Darmawan, J., Valkenburg, H.A., & Muirden, K.D. (1995). The prevalence of soft tissue rheumatism. A WHO-ILAR COPCORD study. Rheumatology International, 15, 121-124.

(5) Wigley, R.D., et al. (1994). Rheumatic diseases in China: ILAR-China study comparing the prevalence of rheumatic symptoms in northern and southern rural populations. J Rheumatol, 21(8), 1480-1490.

(6) Dixon, R.A., & Thompson, J.S. (1993). Base-line village health profiles in the E.Y.N rural health programme area of north-east Nigeria. African Journal of Medical Science, 22, 75-80.

(7) Anderson, R.T. (1984). An orthopedic ethnography in rural Nepal. Med Anthropol, 8(1), 46-59.

(8) Farooqi, A., & Gibson, T. (1998). Prevalence of the major rheumatic discords in the adult population of North Pakistan. British Journal of Rheumatology, 37, 491-495.

(9) Chaiamnuay, P., et al. (1998). Epidemiology of rheumatic disease in rural Thailand: A WHO-ILAR COPCORD study. Journal of Rheumatology, 25, 7.

(10) Andersson, G.B.J. (1998). Epidemiology of low back pain. Acta Orthopaedica Scandinavica, 69(sup281), 28-31.

(11) Freburger, J.K., Holmes, G.M., Agans, R.P., et al. (2009). The rising prevalence of chronic low back pain. Arch Intern Med, 169(3), 251-258.

(12) Rubin, D.I. (2007). Epidemiology and risk factors for spine pain. Neurologic Clinics, 25(2), 353-371.

(13) de Souza, I.M.B., et al. (2019). Prevalence of low back pain in the elderly population: A systematic review. Clinics, 28, 74.

(14) Atlas, S., et al. (2001). Evaluating and managing acute low back pain in the primary care setting. J Gen Intern Med, 16, 120-131.

(15) Global Burden of Disease Study. (2017). Global Burden of Disease Study 2017 data. Institute for Health Metrics and Evaluation.

(16) Hoy, D., et al. (2014). The global burden of low back pain: A systematic analysis. The Lancet, 384(9946), 971–981.

(17) Waddell, G., & Burton, A.K. (2006). Is work good for your health and well-being? The Stationery Office.

(18) Bigos, S.J., et al. (2009). Acute low back problems in adults: A clinical practice guideline from the American College of Physicians. Annals of Internal Medicine, 150(6), 447-458.

(19) World Health Organization & The Bone and Joint Decade. (2001).

(20) Deyo, R.A., & Phillips, W.R. (1996). Low back pain: A primary care challenge. Spine, 21(24), 2826-2832.

(21) Siambanes, D., Martinez, J.W., Butler, E.W., et al. (2004). Influence of school backpacks on adolescent back pain. J Pediatr Orthop, 24(2), 211-217.

(22) Luo, X., et al. (2004). Estimates and patterns of direct health care expenditures among individuals with back pain in the United States. Spine, 29(1), 79-86.

(23) Global, regional, and national burden of low back pain, 1990-2020, its attributable risk factors, and projections to 2050: A systematic analysis of the Global Burden of Disease Study 2021. (2023). Lancet Rheumatol, 5, e316-329.

(24) Global, regional, and national burden of low back pain, 1990-2020, its attributable risk factors, and projections to 2050: A systematic analysis of the Global Burden of Disease Study 2021. (2023). Lancet Rheumatol, 5, e316-329.

(25) Mattiuzzi, C., Lippi, G., & Bovo, C. (2020). Current epidemiology of low back pain. Journal of Hospital Management and Health Policy, 4.

(26) Lucas, J.W., Connor, E.M., & Bose, J. (2021). Back, lower limb, and upper limb pain among U.S. adults, 2019. NCHS Data Brief, no. 415. Hyattsville, MD: National Center for Health Statistics.

(27) Feldman, D.E., & Nahin, R.L. (2022). Disability among persons with chronic severe back pain: Results from a nationally representative population-based sample. The Journal of Pain, 23(12), 2144-2154.

(28) Siambanes, D., Martinez, J.W., Butler, E.W., et al. (2004). Influence of school backpacks on adolescent back pain. J Pediatr Orthop, 24(2), 211-217.

(29) Dagenais, S., Caro, J., & Haldeman, S. (2008). A systematic review of low back pain cost of illness studies in the United States and internationally. The Spine Journal: Official Journal of the North American Spine Society, 8, 8-20. https://doi.org/10.1016/j.spinee.2007.10.005.

(30) Shelerud, R.A. (2006). Epidemiology of occupational low back pain. Clin Occup Environ Med, 5(3), 501-528.

(31) Punnet, L., Pruss-Ustun, A., Nelson, D.I., et al. (2005). Estimating the global burden of low back pain attributable to combined occupational exposures. American Journal of Industrial Medicine.

(32) Hartvigsen, J., Leboeuf-Yde, C., Lings, S., et al. (2000). Is sitting-while-at-work associated with low back pain? A systematic, critical literature review. Scand J Public Health, 28(3), 230-239.

(33) Leboeuf-Yde, D.C. (2000). Body weight and low back pain: A systematic literature review of 56 journal articles reporting on 65 epidemiologic studies. Spine, 25(2), 226.

(34) Heliovaara, M. (1989). Risk factors for low back pain and sciatica. Annals of Medicine, 21(4), 257-264.

(35) Swiss Masai. (n.d.). www.swissmasai.com.

(36) MacGregor, A.J., Andrew, T., Sambrook, P.N., et al. (2004). Structural, psychological, and genetic influences on low back and neck pain: A study of adult female twins. Arthritis Care and Research, 51(2), 160-167.

(37) Battie, M.C., & Videman, T. (2006). Lumbar disc degeneration: Epidemiology and genetics. J Bone Joint Surg Am, 88 Suppl 2, 3-9.

(38) Leboeuf-Yde, C. (1999). Smoking and low back pain: A systematic literature review of 41 journal articles reporting 47 epidemiologic studies. Spine, 24(14), 1463-1470.

(39) Katz, J.N. (Ed.). (2006). A special health report from Harvard Medical School: Low back pain: Healing your aching back. Boston: Harvard Health Publications.

(40) Harkness, E.F., Macfarlane, G.J., Silman, A.J., et al. (2005). Is musculoskeletal pain more common now than 40 years ago?: Two population-based cross-sectional studies. Rheumatology, 44, 890-895.

(41) Gerrish, F.H. (Ed.). (1911). A textbook of anatomy. W.B. Saunders Company.

(42) Rouvière, H. (1990). Anatomie humaine. Éditions Masson.

(43) White, A.H. (2001). The Posture Prescription: A Doctor's Rx for Eliminating Back, Muscle, and Joint Pain, Achieving Optimum Strength and Mobility, Living a Life of Fitness and Well-Being. Three Rivers Press.

(44) Weiniger, S. (2009). The posture prescription. Hachette Books.

(45) Harvard Women's Health Watch. (2005, August). Posture and back health: Paying attention to posture can help you look and feel better. Harvard Women's Health Watch, 6-7.

(46) Consumer Reports on Health. (2006, February). Position yourself to stay well: The right body alignment can help you avoid falls and prevent muscle and joint pain. Consumer Reports on Health, 8-9.

(47) Jackson, R.P., & McManus, A.C. (1994). Radiographic analysis of sagittal plane alignment and balance in standing volunteers and patients with low back pain matched for age, sex, and size: A prospective controlled clinical study. Spine, 19(14), 1611-1618.

(48) Fahrni, W.H., & Trueman, G.E. (1965). Comparative radiological study of the spines of a primitive population with North Americans and Northern Europeans. The Journal of Bone and Joint Surgery, 47-B(3), 552.

(49) Fullenlove, T.M., & Williams, A.J. (1957). Comparative roentgen findings in symptomatic and asymptomatic back. Radiology, 68, 572.

(50) Hult, L. (1954). The Munkfors investigation. A study of the frequency and causes of the stiff neck-brachialgia and lumbago-sciatica syndromes. Acta Orthopaedica Scandinavica, Supplementum No. 16.

INDEX

SUMMARY GUIDE

1. STRETCHSITTING

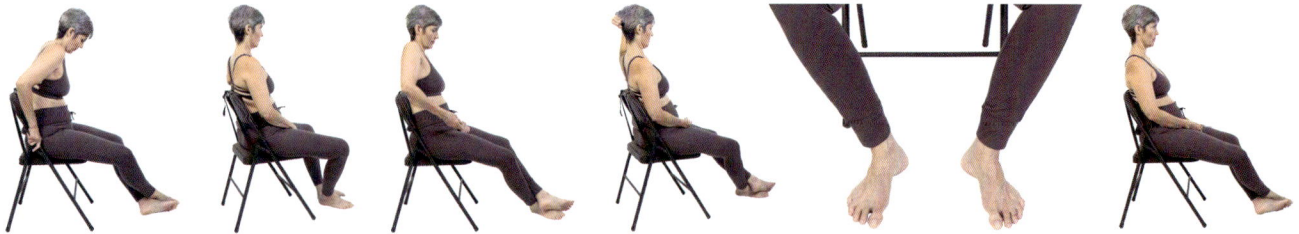

2. STRETCHLYING ON YOUR BACK

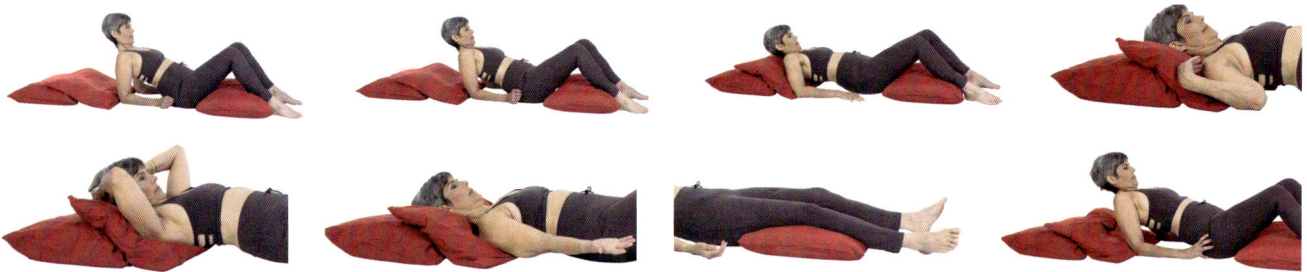

3. STACKSITTING

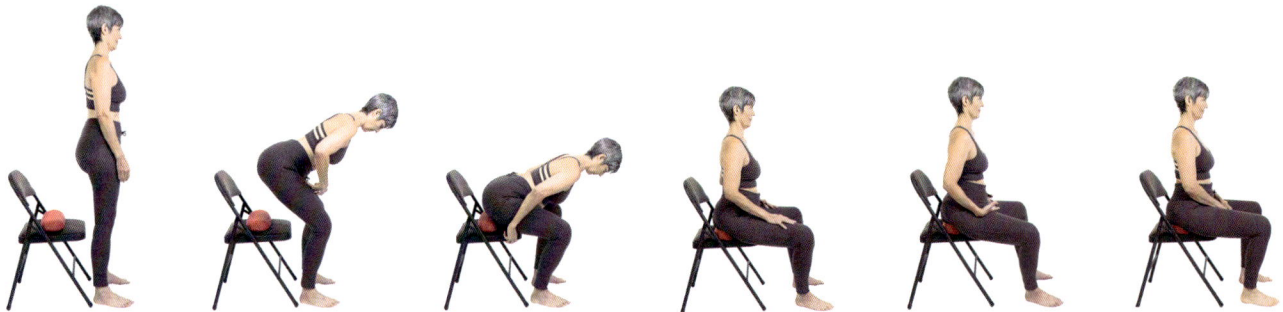

4. STRETCHLYING ON YOUR SIDE

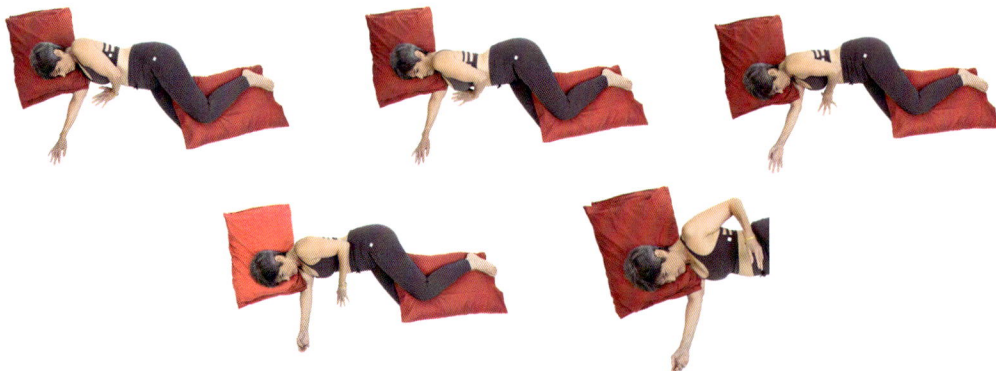

5. USING YOUR INNER CORSET

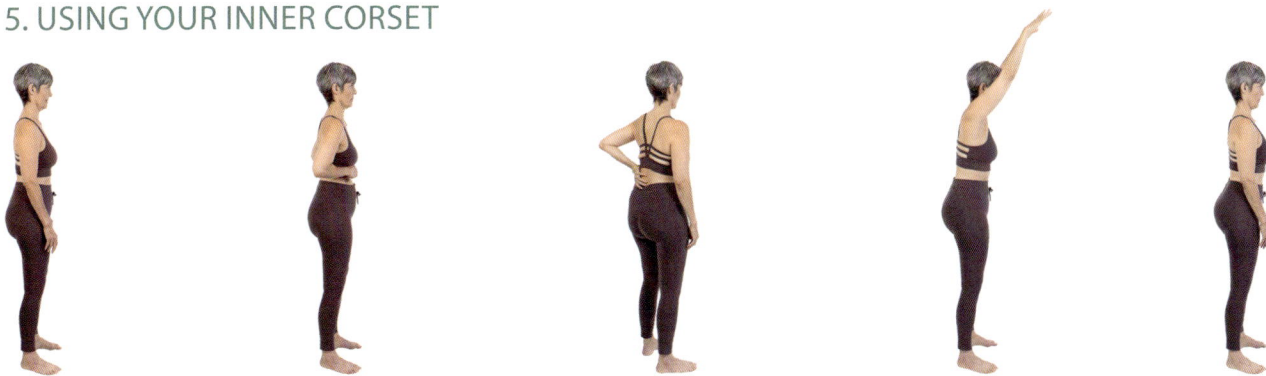

6. TALLSTANDING

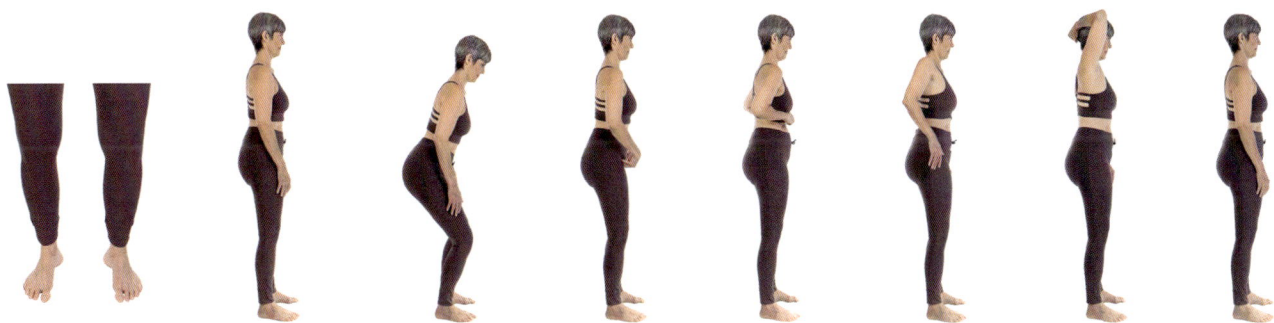

7. HIP-HINGING

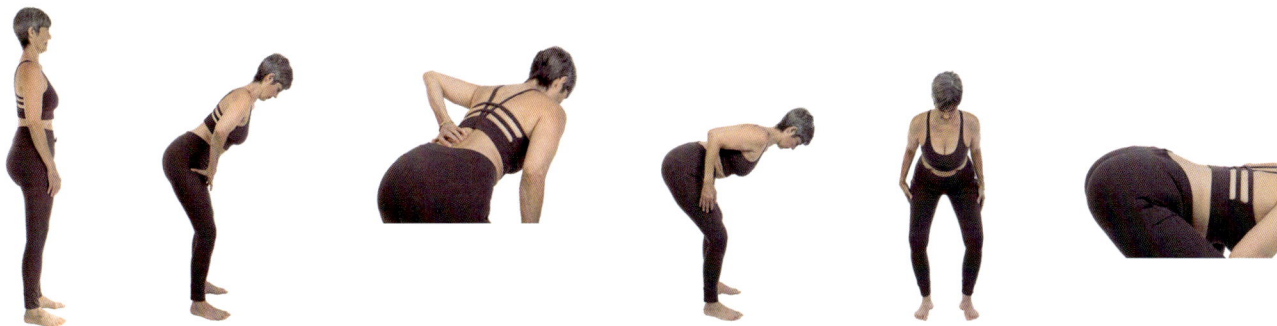

8. GLIDEWALKING

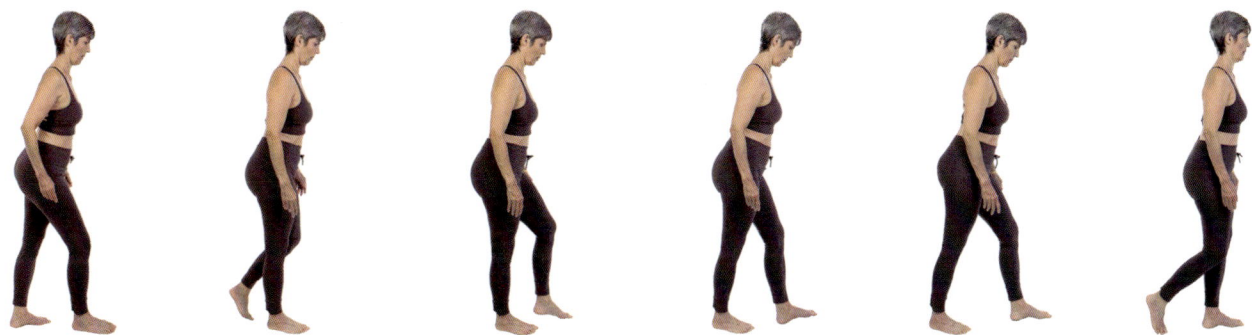

Work With A Qualified Gokhale Method Teacher

It's a rare person who integrates a J-spine into their everyday posture from reading this book alone. Just as learning an instrument or playing a sport greatly benefits from coaching, so does learning posture.

Available **Online** or **In-Person**

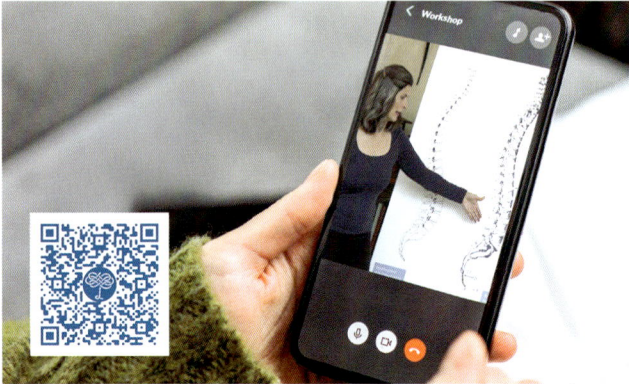

Free Workshops

We offer free workshops online and in-person in various locations worldwide. These sessions are live, interactive, and practical. We will coach you through one of our techniques and take time to answer individual questions.

Learn more at gokhalemethod.com/free_workshops

Gokhale Consultation

It's one thing to understand the logic and concepts in this book; it's another to figure out which ones apply to you and how to implement them. Are your feet pointing outward enough? Is your pelvis tucked? During this 40-minute consultation, a qualified Gokhale Method teacher will guide you through a personalized posture and movement analysis. Learn how the way you're positioning your body is contributing to any pain and dysfunction you may have, discover the optimal sequence in which to integrate the techniques, and take the first step toward moving like you are meant to.

By the end of the session you'll have a clear idea of the path forward, and newfound hope for a healthier, more active future.

Learn more at gokhalemethod.com/consultation

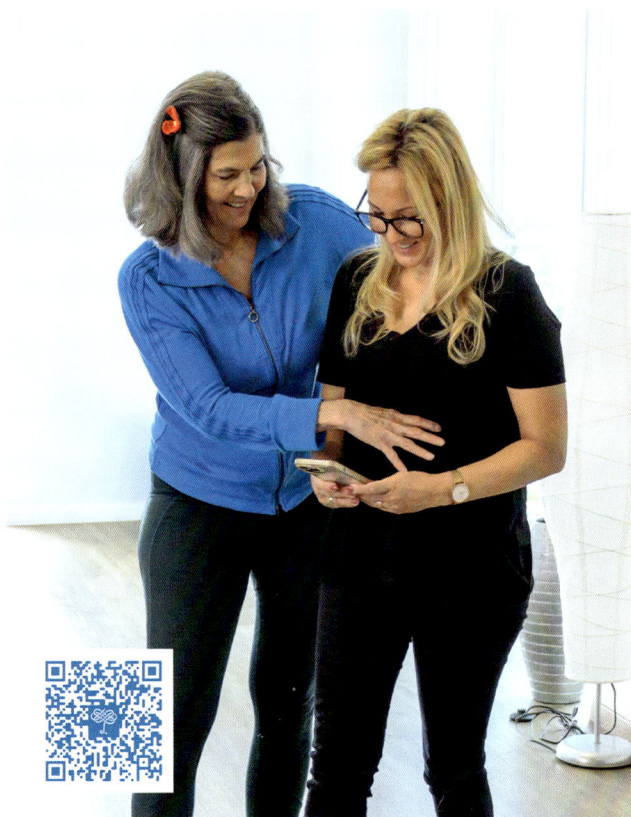

Our mission at the Gokhale Method is to make back pain rare. I am delighted that you have read this book and want you to know that my team of wonderful teachers and I are here for you, to support you through every step of your posture journey.

📞 +1 844 777 0440   ✉️ info@gokhalemethod.com   f in 📷 ▶️ @GokhaleMethod